POLYSOMNOGRAPHY
for the SLEEP TECHNOLOGIST

Instrumentation, Monitoring, and Related Procedures

POLYSOMNOGRAPHY
for the SLEEP
TECHNOLOGIST

Instrumentation, Monitoring, and Related Procedures

Bonnie Robertson, AAHA, CRT, RPSGT
Patient Care Manager
Clinical Sleep Educator
Indianapolis, Indiana
Franciscan St. Francis Health
Franciscan Sleep DME
Indianapolis, Indiana

Buddy Marshall, MEd, CRT-SDS, RST, RPSGT
Sleep Technology Program Director
Baptist Health Schools Little Rock
Little Rock, Arkansas

Margaret-Ann Carno, PhD, MBA, RN, CPNP, D,ABSM, FAAN
Associate Professor of Clinical Nursing and Pediatrics
School of Nursing
University of Rochester
Pediatric Nurse Practitioner
Pediatric Sleep Medicine Service
University of Rochester Medical Center
Rochester, New York

ELSEVIER
MOSBY

3251 Riverport Lane
St. Louis, Missouri 63043

ISBN: 978-0-323-10019-9

Library of Congress Cataloging-in-Publication Data

Robertson, Bonnie, author.
  Polysomnography for the sleep technologist : instrumentation, monitoring, and related
procedures / Bonnie Robertson, Buddy Marshall, Margaret-Ann Carno. -- First edition.
    p. ; cm.
  Includes bibliographical references and index.
  ISBN 978-0-323-10019-9 (pbk. : alk. paper)
  I. Marshall, Buddy, author. II. Carno, Margaret-Ann, author. III. Title.
  [DNLM: 1. Polysomnography--instrumentation.   2. Polysomnography--methods.
3. Sleep Disorders. WL 108]
  RC547
  616.8'498075--dc23
                                                              2013037158

Content Manager: Billie Sharp
Freelance Content Development Specialist: Betsy McCormac
Publishing Services Manager: Julie Eddy
Senior Project Manager: Celeste Clingan
Design Direction: Ashley Miner

Contributors

Carolyn C. Campo, MA, RRT, RPSGT
Director, Sleep Operations
Charlotte, North Carolina

Jacqueline Compton, BA, MAEd, RPSGT, RST
Instructor/Consultant
Highline Community College
Polysomnographic Technology Program
Des Moines, Washington

Mike Longman, RPSGT, RRT
Coordinator, Sleep Disorders Center
Morton Plant Mease Hospitals
Clearwater, Florida

James T. Mitchum, BS, RPSGT
Polysomnographic Technologist
Olathe Medical Center
Olathe, Kansas

K. Wayne Peacock, BS, RST, RPSGT
Manager, Sleep and Neurodiagnostics
Baptist Hospital
Pensacola, Florida

Michael J. Salemi, RPSGT, MBA
Co-Founder and CEO
Actus MSO
Oakland, California

Kristine Bresnehan Servidio, BBA, CRT, RCP, RPSGT
CAAHEP Commissioner
Chair Outcomes Committee
San Marco, California

Kimberly A Trotter, MA, RPSGT
Administrative Director
University of California-San Francisco
San Francisco, California

Robyn Woidtke, RN, RPSGT
Principal Clinical Consultant
RVW Clinical Consulting
Castro Valley, California

Reviewers

S. Gregory Marshall, PhD, RRT, RPSGT, RST
Chair/Associate Professor
Texas State University
College of Health Professions
Department of Respiratory Care & Texas State
Sleep Center
San Marcos, Texas

Susan L. Townsley, RRT, RPSGT, RPFT
Sleep Coordinator
SSM St. Joseph Health Center
Sleep Disorders Center
St. Charles, Missouri

S. R. Pandi-Perumal, MSc
President and Chief Executive Officer
Somnogen Canada Inc.
Toronto, Ontario, Canada

*In memory of my loved ones: Daddy
and my brothers Bob and Jerry.*

Bonnie Robertson

*To my Mom, without her love, support,
and encouragement, I would not be where I am today.*

Margaret-Ann Carno

Foreword

A woman attending her son's graduation, at her own alma mater, ran into her old science teacher. She couldn't help but ask him, "I've noticed that you haven't changed any of the questions in your exams. The ones you gave my son were the same questions you asked me 25 years ago." "Ah yes," he replied, " . . . but the answers are all different."

Sleep technology is still sleep technology; yet, it is, undoubtedly, not the same sleep technology of 25 years ago. The tools have changed since that time as has its techniques and rules. The main dilemma with change is that it, too, is eternally changing. Once a new tool has been mastered, a new technique learned, or a new rule adopted, the field of sleep technology lurches forward with even better tools. The continuation of improved techniques or newer rules will once again leave uncertainty and confusion in its wake and have loftier goals and greater expectations in its sight. The only way to keep up with change is to somehow stay ahead of it. One needs to know where the future of sleep technology is headed! But how does one do so?

To predict the future of sleep technology, one can start by recalling its past, analyzing patterns of change, and learning from them. Better still, one can look at the present changes in the field. It has been suggested that the "future" has already arrived – it is just not evenly distributed; i.e., some technologists or sleep centers are relatively more advanced than others; and certain regions are more affected by specific market forces than others. Discerning what works and what does not work, one can copy or correct, respectively, these specific changes; however, the best way to predict the future of sleep technology, I propose, is to create its future yourself.

Many a naysayer has predicted the demise of sleep technology with the advent of home sleep apnea testing, automation of positive airway pressure titration, and outsourcing of sleep scoring. I disagree. I see these developments as opportunities to reinvent the field and redefine a larger role for sleep technologists in sleep testing, clinical care, management, research, education, outreach, community service, audit and review, legislation, and entrepreneurship. Sleep technologists should help direct market reforms in the health industry by serving as key opinion leaders to hospitals, health plans, and state/regional regulators that are embarking upon policy changes affecting sleep medicine. They should champion the creation of disease management programs and disease registries to measure treatment outcomes in their laboratories and clinics and to decrease inefficiencies in service utilization. They should develop new care delivery models for sleep medicine that use their expertise more fully. These new responsibilities require educated, trained sleep technologists.

The driving force for this new sleep technology must, at its core, be the provision of cost-effective, comprehensive, multidisciplinary, accountable, socially responsible, long-term care in partnership with persons who have sleep-related complaints.

Cost-effectiveness might include better assessment and monitoring tools and measures to improve clinical efficiency. *Comprehensiveness* requires the full integration of psychological, medical, dental, and surgical sciences into sleep technology; creation of "full-service" sleep centers with assistance from durable medical equipment suppliers; and, an expanded role for the sleep technologist in the management of persons with sleep disorders. *Accountability* refers to quality control and performance measures as well as continued professional career development. *Partnership* demands the creation of systems that foster patient empowerment and self-management. *Social responsibility* ensures availability of, and access to, sleep services for the medically indigent; and the education of students, trainees, and the lay public.

The "storm of change" is upon us. Only through greater advocacy, leadership, and mentoring by the entire community of sleep technologists, united in commitment to their craft, peers, and patients, can we create *our* future of sleep technology.

Teofilo Lee-Chiong MD
Professor of Medicine
National Jewish Health
Denver, Colorado

Professor of Medicine
University of Colorado, Denver School of Medicine
Aurora, Colorado

Chief Medical Liaison
Philips Respironics
Murrysville, Pennsylvania

Preface

The field of sleep medicine has grown exponentially in recent years and, with this growth, the role of the sleep technologist has expanded. In the multi-faceted field of polysomnography, the sleep technologist is on the front line, responsible for performing diagnostic tests and therapeutic interventions for patients with sleep disorders. Providing excellent care to patients at clinics and sleep-testing centers is the number-one goal of all sleep technologists.

Our goal in writing this textbook was twofold: first, to produce a "student-friendly," sleep-technology–specific textbook for students entering the field; and second, to provide a valuable reference for the experienced sleep technologist or other healthcare clinician. The sequential learning approach used in writing this text addresses both entry-level foundational material and subsequent advanced-level material.

We feel that no one textbook can cover every facet of this field in a comprehensive way within a single volume of text. For that reason, this text focuses on the knowledge base required of a competent sleep technologist to have a thorough familiarity with, and proficiency in, the areas of electronics, instrumentation, recording parameters, data acquisition, ancillary equipment, troubleshooting, recording quality, infection control, basic positive pressure therapy, and cardiopulmonary monitoring and intervention.

Producing high-quality data clearly relies on the technologist's vigilance; more importantly, to ensure the patient's safety during testing and to ensure delivery of the best possible treatment for the patient's sleep disorder, a thorough understanding of the recording instrumentation, the clinical evaluation, and the physiological monitoring and diagnostic testing are essential competencies for the sleep technologist.

The spectrum of sleep-related disorders and daytime alertness in which polysomnography plays an integral diagnostic and therapeutic role is broad. We have addressed the most commonly encountered of these disorders, along with the diagnostics, prevention, and therapeutic interventions.

With this text, we hope that students will become proficient in evaluating patient sleep concerns and determining the best practices for recording, monitoring, staging, and scoring sleep studies. For students and professionals alike, we hope you find this textbook a constant source of knowledge in delivering the highest level of care to maximize overall quality of life for all sleep patients.

FEATURES

Designed with the student in mind, this book contains the following learning features that will help guide the student to mastery of the content:
- Chapter outlines
- Learning objectives
- Key terms (bolded and defined in context)
- Bulleted chapter summary
- Review questions appear at the end of each chapter and provide a review so the student can assess what they have retained from reading each chapter. An answer key to the questions appears at the end of the book.
- List of references
- The field of sleep technology is rich in terminology that is unique and specific to this area of healthcare. A comprehensive **glossary** at the end of the text provides students with a quick alpha reference to access terms and definitions identified as key terms throughout the text.

FOR EDUCATORS

Evolve is an interactive teaching and learning environment designed to work in coordination with *Polysomnography for the Sleep Technologist: Instrumentation, Monitoring, and Related Procedures*. Educators may use Evolve to provide an internet-based course component that reinforces and expands the concepts presented in class. Evolve may be used to publish the class syllabus, outlines, and lecture notes; set up "virtual office hours" and e-mail communication; share important dates and information through the online class calendar; and encourage student participation through chat rooms and discussion boards. Evolve also allows educators to post exams and manage their grade books online.

EVOLVE RESOURCES

- PowerPoint slide presentations for each chapter, which can be edited as desired.
- An image collection for each chapter, which can be used to create new PowerPoint slides.
- A question test bank for each chapter containing multiple choice questions.

For more information, visit http://evolve.elsevier.com/Robertson/polysom/ or contact an Elsevier sales representative.

Acknowledgements

We are profoundly grateful to all the contributors to this first edition of the textbook. We also wish to thank all of our students over the years who have inspired us to write this textbook. Finally, we wish to thank the Elsevier publishing team, especially Betsy McCormac, Content Development Specialist, and Billie Sharp, Content Manager, for guiding us through this process. We know that working with three different editors with different styles was not easy, but Betsy and Billie managed to keep us on track.

Bonnie Robertson
Buddy Marshall
Margaret-Ann Carno

Contents

Chapter 1

Overview of Sleep Medicine Physiology and Technology

Jackie Compton • Bonnie Robertson

CHAPTER OUTLINE

LEARNING OBJECTIVES

After reading this chapter, you will be able to:
  1. Identify the medical discoveries that led to the development of sleep medicine and technology.
  2. List the key people involved in the development of sleep medicine and their contributions.
  3. List hallmark publications related to sleep medicine and technology.
  4. Provide an overview of technological advances in sleep medicine and technology.
  5. Describe the circadian variations related to wake and sleep.
  6. Explain the opponent process model of sleep.
  7. Describe how the body changes between sleep and wake.
  8. Identify the structures and neurotransmitters that are involved in the sleep and wake process.
  9. Explain the normal stages of sleep and the histogram.
  10. Define the different breathing patterns.
  11. Describe the different sensors used during a polysomnogram.
  12. Differentiate between analog and digital polysomnography.
  13. List the basic waveforms of sleep and the cycles of sleep.
  14. Explain how the sleep technologist position was created.
  15. Detail the scope of practice of a sleep technologist.
  16. List the duties of a sleep technologist.
  17. List the training and education required for credentialing.

KEY TERMS

ascending reticular activating
   system (ARAS)
capnography
cerebral cortex
circadian rhythm
electrocardiogram (ECG)
electroencephalogram (EEG)
electromyogram (EMG)
electrooculogram (EOG)
epoch
histogram
hypnogram
hypopnea
K complex
melatonin

multiple sleep latency test (MSLT)
narcolepsy
nasal pressure transducer
neurotransmitters
non–rapid eye movement
   (NREM) sleep
obstructive sleep apnea (OSA)
opponent process model of sleep
oronasal sensor
oximeter
paradoxical sleep
parasomnias
Pickwickian syndrome
polysomnogram (PSG)
polysomnography

rapid eye movement (REM)
   sleep
respiratory belt
reticular formation
sawtooth waves
scoring
sleep architecture
sleep spindle
snore sensor
snoring
suprachiasmatic nucleus (SCN)
thalamus
zeitgeber

Sleep medicine is a vibrant and exciting field of study. Sleep technologists are an integral part of the medical team and are on the front lines, providing one-on-one care to patients with sleep disorders. Care comes in the form of sleep education, diagnostic testing, and application of treatment according to established protocols. The provision of quality care by skilled sleep technologists changes people's lives.

Currently, the sleep technologist position is more important than ever. The provision of quality care by skilled sleep medicine and technology practitioners changes the lives of many people seeking treatment for a sleep-related issue. Sleep deprivation is at epidemic proportions, causing traffic accidents and work injuries and increased risk of heart disease, heart attack, high blood pressure, stroke, diabetes, and death. A well-educated and skilled technologist helps patients understand the devastating effects of their sleep disorder. Education and empathy go a long way in assisting patients to comply with treatment. A compliant patient proactively assists in his or her own healthcare pathway.

Conducting an accurate, well-documented, and interpretable sleep study takes skill and practice. Valid and reliable data enables the sleep physician to make a well-informed, accurate diagnosis. This text provides the learner with the information needed to conduct quality sleep studies.

A HISTORY OF SLEEP MEDICINE TECHNOLOGY

SLEEP MEDICINE THROUGHOUT HISTORY

The intrigue of sleep has been one of humanity's most fascinating curiosities since the dawn of time. As far back as ancient times, sleep has mystified us. From Hippocrates and Sigmund Freud to the present, writers and scientists have delved into the unknown depths of sleep and the mystery of dreams. It is important for sleep technologists to have a basic knowledge of the history of sleep medicine. Only then can one appreciate the successions and rapid advancements of the field.

The recognition and attributes given to sleep and sleep disorders and their treatments throughout time coincided with humanity's belief systems and level of technology. The present-day words for hypnosis, insomnia, and somnolence come from the Greek words *hypnos* and *somnus*. Interestingly, Hypnos was the Greek god of sleep, whereas Somnus was the Roman god of sleep.[1,2] Ancient civilizations believed many illnesses, including sleep disturbances, were caused by angry gods or spirits. To appease their deities, chanting, ceremonies, and other activities were offered.

As far back as 3000 BCE, Mesopotamians attempted to treat insomnia by forcing the insomniac to eat plants and animal parts and by administering enemas or bloodletting to appease the angry gods. In Sumaria, opium may have been used for treating insomnia and could have been the earliest medicinal treatment for a sleep disorder.[3]

Thomas Willis authored four chapters on insomnia and insomnolence in his work *Practice of Physick*.[4] He also wrote about restless legs syndrome and nightmares. Hippocrates hypothesized that sleep was due to blood moving from the limbs to the inner regions of the body.[5] As late as the 1800s, it was believed that sleep was a passive process in which the sleeper was in an unconscious state between wake and death.[6]

Research and Theories

Early research on the **circadian rhythm** (a daily cycle of biological activity), electrical brain activity, and nervous system functions paved the way for the emergence of the sleep medicine field in the twentieth century.

During the seventeenth century, Santorio Sanctorius designed the thermometer and collected his own physiologic changes for 30 years.[7] Current medical guidelines note that temperature is associated with the circadian rhythm, and Sanctorious may have been one of the first scientists to accumulate data on biological temperature cycles known to be a part of normal circadian changes.

It was assumed that the circadian rhythm was influenced by environmental cues and in 1729, Jean Jacques d'Ortous de Mairan noticed that the leaves of flowers opened during the day and closed at night.[8] Because he assumed the movement of the flowers was caused by light and dark fluctuations, de Mairan placed plants in total darkness 24 hours a day and observed that the leaves still opened and closed in the same rhythmic cycle as observed in the light of day. This botanic experiment demonstrated how circadian rhythms occur without the influence of environmental factors for all living things.

Along with the development of theories based on chemistry and neurology, after the discovery of oxygen (O_2) a theory that sleep was caused by a lack of O_2 was developed. Some theorists speculated that mysterious poisons accumulated during the day and the elimination of those poisons at night provoked sleep. Others suggested the animal spirits within people rested at night, causing sleep, or that sleep was caused by an overabundance of carbon dioxide (CO_2) in the blood.[9]

Each historical investigation and medical advancement brought humanity closer to the true nature of sleep.

- In 1771, when Italian physician Luigi Galvani caused the leg muscles of a dead frog to twitch when touched with a spark, he demonstrated the electrical activity of the nervous system.[10]
- Camillo Golgi, an Italian physician, was the first to see a nerve cell under a microscope.[11]
- Jean Baptist Edouard Gélineau clearly documented and named **narcolepsy**, a disorder of uncontrolled sleepiness.[12]
- Wilhelm Griesinger reported eye movement changes during the dreaming state.
- In his work with dreams, Sigmund Freud recognized and wrote about skeletal muscle paralysis during sleep.[13]
- Other scholars explored the causes of sleep, the relationship between body temperature and biologic rhythms, pharmacology and medications, insomnia, abnormal breathing during sleep, night terrors, nocturnal epilepsy, and effects of stimulants on insomnia.

With continuing major advancements in medical knowledge and technology, the twentieth century brought sleep research to a new level. In 1907 French scientists Rene Legendre and Henri Pieron removed blood serum from sleep-deprived dogs and injected it into dogs that were not sleep deprived; the serum induced sleep.[14] This experiment demonstrated the presence of a chemical factor associated with sleep induction. Pieron's 1913 book, *Le Probleme Physiologique du Sommeil,* described sleep in physiologic, scientific terms, and this work is regarded as a milestone in sleep medicine.[15]

Sleep and wake continued to be an area of intense interest during the early twentieth century, and in 1929 Constantin von Economo argued that a "center for regulation of sleep" was controlled by substances that circulated in the blood and exerted an inhibitory influence on the **cerebral cortex**, leading to sleep.[16] The cerebral cortex is the part of the brain responsible for the sleep-wake drive and the circadian rhythms.

Walter Rudolf Hess confirmed von Economo's findings by stimulating the **thalamus** and inducing sleep.[17] The thalamus is the area of the brain that relays signals between the cerebral cortex and the reticular formation.

In 1949 Guiseppe Moruzzi and Horace Magoun published groundbreaking work that stated the stimulation of the **ascending reticular activating system (ARAS)**, located in the thalamus and hypothalamus, produced **electroencephalographic (EEG)** patterns of wakefulness; its deactivation caused sleep.[18]

Richard Caton recorded brain rhythms in rabbits and monkeys in 1875.[19] Caton's discovery was further refined in 1929 when Johannes Hans Berger recorded the first electrical activity of the human brain and differentiated activity between wakefulness and sleep.[20]

THE EVOLUTION OF POLYSOMNOGRAPHY

Pioneers in Sleep Medicine

Polysomnography, which is the measurement of multiple physiologic parameters during sleep, began with Hans Berger's measurements of human brain activity. After Berger's discovery, Alfred Loomis described **non–rapid eye movement (NREM)** sleep in 1935.[21] Just 2 years later, Alfred L. Loomis, E. Newton Harvey, and Garret A. Hobart III classified the EEG sleep patterns into five stages, A-E. In 1939, Nathaniel Kleitman (Figure 1-1), known as the "Father of Sleep Research," wrote the first extensive text on sleep titled *Sleep and Wakefulness*.[22,23]

Nathaniel Kleitman

Kleitman and colleagues found that certain waveforms were more prevalent from specific regions of the brain.[24] Eugene Aserinsky, as a medical student under Kleitman, found it "torturous" observing sleeping persons' eye movements all night, so Kleitman invented a sensor to more accurately measure eye movements during sleep. This sensor measured both slow eye movements and **rapid eye movements (REM)**, which

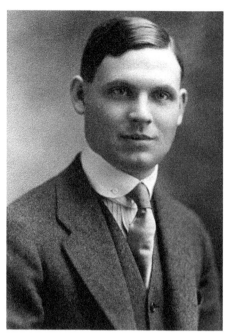

FIGURE 1-1 Nathaniel Kleitman, "father of sleep research." *From Sleep Medicine Clinics, Volume 4, Issue 3, Pages 313-321, September 2009 © Elsevier Inc.*

helped Kleitman determine the relationship between eye movements and sleep cycles.

Kleitman and Aserinsky would wake patients during periods of REM sleep and ask them about their dreams, thus establishing the connection between REM sleep and dreaming.[25]

Until 1957 sleep studies had been conducted only for short periods, rather than through a full night's sleep. When Kleitman and William Dement began performing all-night, uninterrupted sleep studies, they discovered distinct stage patterns in sleep that were consistent among all adults, and thus discovered the cyclical human sleep cycles of NREM and REM sleep.[26]

Sleep Stage Scoring - R&K Manual

Although some researchers began using Kleitman's and Dement's descriptions of sleep stages, others did not. Within a few years, the various methods of measuring and classifying sleep stages made it very difficult to compare and replicate studies because of dissimilar criteria throughout the world, creating a need for a standardized recording protocol. Allan Rechtschaffen and Anthony Kales, known as *R&K,* developed a sleep "scoring" manual in 1968 titled *A Manual of Standardized Terminology, Techniques and Scoring System for Sleep Stages of Human Subjects.*[27]

Scoring involves the identification of various recording parameters that occur during sleep, such as sleep staging, respiratory events, movements, cardiac dysrhythmias, and EEG arousals. The resulting report enables a sleep physician to objectively interpret the events during sleep to diagnose a potential sleep disorder.

With the establishment of a sleep scoring system in place, researchers began following the same sleep scoring criteria when conducting research. The manual was widely used for years, but with continued advancements and discoveries in sleep medicine, the manual became inadequate.

American Academy of Sleep Medicine (AASM)

Although the R&K manual described normal sleep, it did not address the all-important abnormal sleep events, such as arousals, unusual behaviors during sleep, respiratory differences, body movements, cardiac rates and rhythms, or other pathologic sleep behaviors. As a result, in 2007 the American Academy of Sleep Medicine (AASM) published a new manual titled *The AASM Manual for the Scoring of Sleep and Associated Events.*[28] This new manual included rules and recommendations for a number of sleep parameters that had been established after the R&K manual was originally published. The *AASM Manual* was most recently updated in October 2012.[29]

In 1975 researchers interested in the diagnosis and treatment of sleep disorders organized the Association of Sleep Disorders Centers (ASDC), and in 1978 the ASDC created the medical journal *Sleep* to publish research studies and articles. The ASDC, along with the fledgling Clinical Sleep Society, reorganized to form the American Sleep Disorders Association in 1987. In 1999, following significant growth and development, the organization changed its name to the American Academy of Sleep Medicine. The AASM is the primary professional society dedicated exclusively to the medical subspecialty of sleep medicine. The AASM sets standards and promotes excellence in health care, education, and research.[30]

Narcolepsy Research

In 1964 William Dement's interest in narcolepsy led him to place an advertisement in the *San Francisco Chronicle* newspaper soliciting narcoleptics in the area to participate in new sleep research on the condition. Narcolepsy is a sleep disorder in which sudden sleep attacks occur without warning. Jean Baptiste Edouard Gélineau, who gave narcolepsy its name,[31,32] described the unique characteristics of this sleep disorder as early as 1880. Until the early 1960s, very little was known about narcolepsy; it was believed to be a psychiatric disorder associated with the patient sleeping excessively due to a repression of feelings.[33]

More than 100 people responded to Dement's newspaper request. Dement studied and treated these patients per insurance criteria, but insurance payments eventually stopped and the experiment failed. In the 1970s, this endeavor did, however, pave the way for the creation of a specialized sleep clinic at Stanford University.

BOX 1-1

William C. Dement, MD, PhD—"Father of Sleep Medicine"

1928 Born in Washington state.

1950 Medical student at University of Chicago under Dr. Nathaniel Kleitman.

1955 Discovered cyclic nature of sleep of NREM and REM sleep with Dr. Kleitman.

1958 Discovered REM sleep in animals.

1961 Co-founded the Sleep Research Society.

1963 Joined the Psychiatry Department at Stanford University; for the past 40 years he has continued his studies on neurochemistry of sleep.

1964 Established the first sleep disorders center for narcoleptics at Stanford University.

1970 Founder of the Stanford Sleep Disorders Clinic and Research Center.

1971 Began teaching popular Stanford University course "Sleep and Dreams." Stopped teaching in 2003, but by student demand, began teaching the course again in 2007 and still teaches it.

1974 Wrote *Some Must Watch While Some Must Sleep.*

1975 Co-founded American Academy of Sleep Medicine, and held position of President for the first 12 years; influenced creation of National Center on Sleep Disorders Research at the National Institutes of Health.

1977 Founding co-editor-in-chief of *Sleep*, 1977-1997.

1977 Developed the multiple sleep latency test, with Dr. Mary Carskadon, to diagnose narcolepsy.

1978 First doctor to receive certification in clinical polysomnography from the American Board of Sleep Medicine.

1980 Co-authored *Sleep and Aging* (with L. Laughton and E. Miles).

1989 Co-edited *The Sleepwatchers.*

1992 Wrote *The Sleepwatchers.*

1990 Served as chairman for 3 years of the National Commission on Sleep Diagnosis Research mandated by Congress; its final report led directly to the creation of a new agency within the National Institutes of Health, the National Center on Sleep Disorders Research.

1999 Wrote *The Promise of Sleep.*

2004 Co-authored *Sleep Disorders for Dummies* (with Christian Guilleminault).

2004 Awarded the Farrell Prize from Harvard Medical School "in celebration of the work of William C. Dement, creative giant of sleep research and founding father of sleep medicine, on whose broad shoulders the entire field rests."

1996 Created and operates the Sleep Well website through Stanford University (http://www.stanford.edu/~dement/)

INTERESTING FACTS

- Recipient of more than 50 prestigious awards for outstanding service and academic and scientific achievement
- Professor at Stanford University since 1953. Currently the Lowell W. and Josephine Q. Berry Professor of Psychiatry and Behavioral Sciences at the Stanford School of Medicine, Psychiatry and Behavioral Sciences—Sleep Disorder/Sleep Center
- Author of more than 530 scientific publications, including books, authoritative textbooks for medical professionals, and scientific research articles
- A jazz musician who plays bass; jammed with Quincy Jones, befriended Ray Charles, and played with Stan Getz
- Dr. Dement has a sense of humor: "Dreaming permits each and every one of us to be quietly and safely insane every night of our lives." Newsweek, 1959

Data from Curriculum Vitae of William Charles Dement (website): http://www.talkaboutsleep.com/conference/2006/speaker-detail/dr-dement-cv.pdf and *The Promise of Sleep.*

Sleep testing at the Stanford clinic expanded to include other sleep disorders. Other universities and hospitals opened sleep clinics across the country (Box 1-1, Figure 1-2). Throughout the 1970s, continued sleep research by William Dement and by Mary Carskadon at Stanford led to the development of the **multiple sleep latency test (MSLT)**, an objective measurement of daytime sleepiness used for diagnosis of narcolepsy.[34]

Obstructive Sleep Apnea Research

A high percentage of patients seen in sleep testing laboratories have **obstructive sleep apnea (OSA)**. OSA is characterized by cessation of breathing caused by a partial or complete obstruction of the airway. OSA was first described, not by a scientist, but by Charles Dickens in his work *Posthumous Papers of the Pickwick Club*.[35]

It wasn't until 41 years later in 1877 that Henry Broadbent described the clinical features of OSA as **snoring**, interspersed between periodic breathing stops.[36]

In 1956, Albert G. Bickelmann and C. Sidney Burwell dubbed the clinical characteristics the **Pickwickian syndrome**, after Dickens fictitious character, following observed symptoms in a patient with snoring, obesity, muscular twitching, and hypersomnolence.[37] Until 1975, OSA was known as *Pickwickian syndrome.*[9]

European researchers led the way with OSA research by conducting all-night recordings using electrodes to obtain the EEG and **electrooculogram (EOG)**, body movement sensors, respiratory effort belts, and airflow sensors. Between 1964 and 1968, three unassociated European sleep researchers, Carl Jung, Henri Gastaut, and Elio Lugaresi, described the sleep apnea syndrome in Pickwickian patients.[38-40]

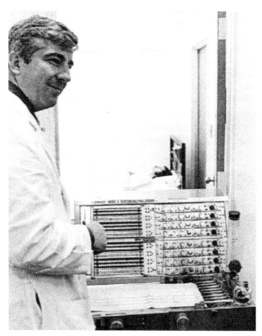

FIGURE 1-2 William Dement near analog machine. He was involved in numerous sleep discoveries and started one of the first sleep clinics at Stanford University. *From Sleep Medicine Clinics, Volume 4, Issue 3, Pages 313-321, September 2009 © Elsevier Inc.*

In 1972, Christian Guilleminault, who had been studying OSA in Europe, moved to the United States and began working with William Dement at Stanford University. Guilleminault introduced the use of respiratory and cardiac monitoring to Stanford studies.[41] The additional data provided by these monitoring parameters demonstrated the disordered breathing associated with OSA, as well as associated cardiac dysrhythmias. These discoveries ignited voluminous sleep research and, in 1975, Guilleminault introduced the terminology change from *Pickwickian syndrome* to *obstructive sleep apnea.*

During the next year, the first American sleep symposium on OSA was held and the papers presented at that symposium were published in the book *Sleep Apnea Syndrome.*[42]

Early Treatment of OSA

At the time, physicians often treated OSA surgically with tracheotomy, the creation of a stoma in the trachea below the larynx, to allow the patient to breathe unobstructed. In 1981, as part of a research study, Colin Sullivan developed an air-blowing device with an attached snout-like mask for treating OSA in dogs.[43] A human patient with severe OSA, who refused a tracheotomy, agreed to try Sullivan's air pressure machine. Sullivan fashioned a primitive continuous positive airway pressure (CPAP) device from a vacuum cleaner engine, a hose, and a diver's mask. Sullivan gradually increased the air pressure until the patient's airway was held open, or splinted open, allowing the patient to

breathe without obstruction. The patient reported the first good night's sleep in years and the CPAP device was invented for noninvasive treatment of OSA.

Early Sleep Study Data Collection

OSA was not the only major sleep disorder. In 1979 the ASDC published the first widely used classification manual, titled *Diagnostic Classification of Sleep and Arousal Disorders.*[44] Ten years later, Meir Kryger, William Dement, and Thomas Roth wrote a comprehensive textbook on basic sleep research and clinical sleep medicine, *The Principles and Practices of Sleep Disorders Medicine.*[45] Several editions of this text have been produced as it is frequently revised to keep up with the rapid rate of research discoveries.

Between the mid-1970s and the mid-1990s, sleep study data were collected via analog polysomnographs. These early analog machines, with their refrigerator-sized amplifiers and writer units, used ink pens and paper to record the data. Studies were recorded on $12'' \times 16''$ paper at a paper speed of 10 mm/sec.

With studies consisting of more than 8 hours of sleep, the recording process generated huge piles of paper. Because most regulatory agencies required that sleep studies be saved, storage space and cost became a big problem. Other limitations of analog recording equipment included the lack of channel diversity and capacity, messiness from the use of ink pens, time-consuming daily calibrations and mechanical adjustments, manual upkeep of analog amplifiers, and the laborious task of flipping through reams of folded paper to score events and calculate data. In the early 1990s, monitor resolution and other computer hardware, along with software adequate for recording and scoring sleep studies, became available. At this point, digital technology began replacing the cumbersome pen-and-paper analog devices.

PHYSIOLOGY FOR RECORDING SLEEP-RELATED PARAMETERS

CIRCADIAN VARIATIONS RELATED TO WAKE AND SLEEP

Early on, sleep research centered on circadian rhythms. A circadian rhythm is a daily cycle of biological activity influenced by regular variations in the environment, such as the alternation of night and day. Modern research has determined that circadian rhythms occur cyclically every 25 hours within the human body; however, because sunlight resets the brain, biological systems run on a 24.2-hour cycle rather than the human internal 25 hour cycle.[46]

Zeitgeber, a German word meaning "time giver," is any exogenous factor that influences and resets the

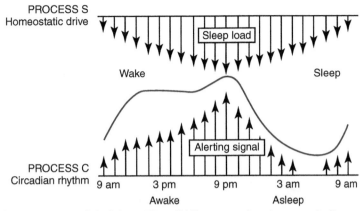

FIGURE 1-3 Opponent model of sleep. The solid line separating the *arrows* indicates sleep-wake propensity. Both sleep load builds (from Process S—homeostatic drive) and the alerting signal increases (from Process C—the circadian rhythm signals) during the waking hours. As the alerting signal diminishes in late evening, sleep occurs and the sleep load is reduced. Note that a dip in the alerting signal occurs at approximately 4-6 pm and alerting signals are at their lowest between 4-6 am. *Modified from Berry RB:* Fundamentals of sleep medicine, *St Louis, 2012, Elsevier.*

human biological clock to the external environment. The most powerful zeitgeber is light. Other external environmental zeitgebers include meal times, clock alarms, traffic noise, and many other everyday common occurrences.

Early theories suggested sleep was a passive state, unrelated to wakefulness and something akin to death in which the human system rested dormant with no activity occurring. Modern research has demonstrated that sleep is anything but passive. Sleep is now understood to be a highly complex state, with biochemical, physiologic, and neurologic processes intertwining at different times of the sleep period to physically, emotionally, and mentally restore the body and mind for optimal performance during wakefulness.[47] Sleep and wakefulness are related in an intricate balance, with each affecting the other, depending on the time of day and the need for sleep.[48]

Opponent Process Model of Sleep

Achermann and Borbely,[49]and Borbely and Tobler,[50] proposed a two-process model of sleep regulation to explain wake-sleep regulation: Process S, the homeostatic drive as sleep load; and Process C, the alerting circadian rhythm. This was later identified as the **opponent process model of sleep** by Edgar and Dement.[51]

Figure 1-3 shows that Process S represents the homeostatic drive as sleep load, which increases through the waking hours. The longer the time from the previous sleep period, the stronger the homeostatic drive. Process C represents the alerting circadian rhythm. The circadian rhythm also continues to increase to maintain an alert state during this time.

The alerting signals diminish with the reduced light from the setting sun. At approximately 9:00 pm, the **suprachiasmatic nucleus (SCN)** initiates the release

of **melatonin**, a hormone secreted by the pineal gland that promotes sleep. The alerting signal continues to decrease until it is at its lowest point between 4:00 am and 6:00 am. Melatonin continues being released, peaks in the middle of night, then declines and returns to miniscule daytime levels around 9:00 am, leaving the sleep debt at a minimum.

Humans are naturally alert during the day and sleep at night because of the alerting circadian drive and relatively low homeostatic sleep load pressures. The period between 4:00 am and 6:00 am is the most difficult time of the night for sleep technologists to maintain alertness because the sleep load is not being satisfied and only a minimal alerting signal is present.

HOW THE BODY CHANGES BETWEEN SLEEP AND WAKE

Several structures in the brain influence the sleep-wake regulation, including the thalamus, medulla oblongata, hypothalamus, pons, SCN, midbrain, spinal cord, raphe nuclei, basal forebrain, hippocampus, and **reticular formation** neurons (Figure 1-4).

Following are the most important structures involved in the sleep-wake process. The ARAS, located in parts of the pons, midbrain, medulla, hypothalamus, thalamus, and controls the homeostatic drive. The ARAS, losely connected with circadian rhythms and has powerful influences over sleep and wake. Its activation promotes wakefulness and its inhibition allows sleep.

The SCN sits above the optic nerve and controls most circadian rhythms. Light impulses coming through the retina travel through the optic nerve and into the SCN in the anterior hypothalamus. The SCN promotes both wakefulness and sleep. It produces alerting circadian rhythms from sunlight during the day, and initiates sleep-promoting

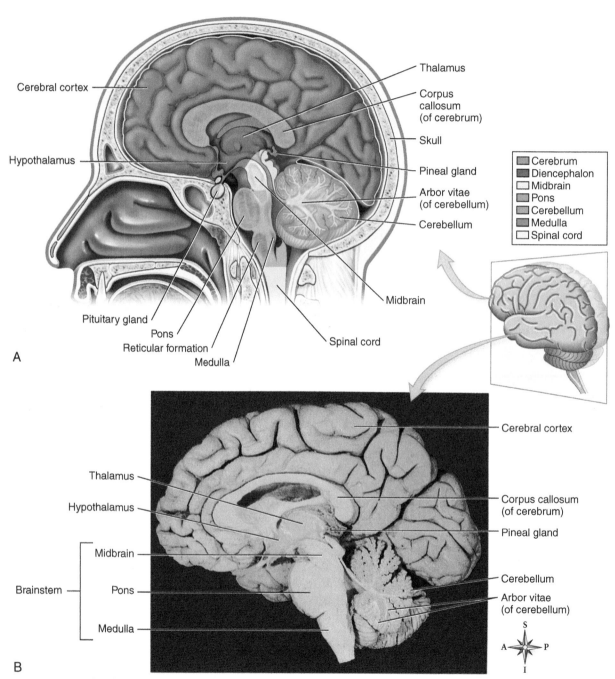

FIGURE 1-4 Structures of the brain. *From Thibodeau GA, Patton KT:* Structure and function of the body, *ed 14, St Louis, 2012, Elsevier.*

signals through melatonin secretion during the dark cycle.[52] The SCN is considered the "circadian pacemaker."[53]

The thalamus has a powerful influence over the sleep process. It has major pathways to the cerebral cortex and acts as a gatekeeper, altering and blocking information transmission from the brainstem and ARAS to the cerebral cortex. The thalamus blocks signals during sleep, filters and modifies sleep spindles coming from the midbrain, and inhibits arousals. As the drive to sleep reduces, the ability of the thalamus to block signals going to the cerebral cortex is reduced and wake occurs.

The cerebral cortex is responsible for most aspects of the sleep-wake drive and the circadian rhythms; however, input from the thalamus, basal forebrain, and hypothalamus determine much of the cerebral cortex activity. Because the thalamus controls the input that the cerebral cortex receives, the ARAS cannot influence the cortex activity. An increase in brainstem activity occurs on waking from NREM sleep, followed by increasing cerebral cortex activity.

NEUROTRANSMITTERS

The initiation of sleep is an extremely complex and active process mediated through chemical and neuronal activity. The characteristics of sleep are functions of diverse brain activities and neurocircuitry.

Several **neurotransmitters** act on the brain to initiate and terminate NREM and REM sleep. A neurotransmitter is a chemical that transmits neurologic information to another nerve, muscle, organ, or other tissue. The sleep "on-switch" is thought to be located in the anterior hypothalamus at the ventrolateral preoptic nucleus (VLPO). This nucleus inhibits arousals of the brain by releasing inhibitory neurotransmitters. Cells in the VLPO are very active during all sleep stages.

The reticular formation is the most influential component of the reticular activating system. It is an extremely complex web of interconnecting neurons in the brain stem that promote arousals. The reticular formation produces the main neurotransmitters involved in the regulation of sleep and wakefulness, including serotonin and acetylcholine (ACh).

Acetylcholine is the neurotransmitter thought to play the largest role in sleep. ACh-producing cells are situated in the forebrain and cerebral cortex and cause stimulation and arousal, resulting in wake. Although reticular formation functions maintain wakefulness, they are also involved in REM sleep. ACh release in the cortex is highest during both wakefulness and the REM sleep state.

In the peribrachial area of the pons, ACh-producing cells play an important part in activating REM sleep. These are called *REM-on cells* because they fire a minute before the onset of REM sleep and produce specific waves called ponto-geniculo-occipital (PGO) waves, the first indicators of REM sleep. PGO waves are phasic electrical bursts that move through the hypothalamus into the primary visual cortex located in the occipital area. The occipital area controls visual information, visual processing, and eye movements.

The peribrachial area could be called REM sleep headquarters because it initiates low-voltage desynchronization, rapid eye movements REMs, and skeletal paralysis (all activities related to REM sleep). Serotonin, norepinephrine, and histamine are neurotransmitters that inhibit ACh-producing cells and act as "REM-off" cells, terminating REM sleep.

SLEEP PHASES AND STAGES

A night of human sleep is divided into NREM and REM phases, depicting the characteristic changes in eye movements noted in sleep stages. These two distinct phases occur in a pattern of three to five rhythmic cycles throughout the sleep period.

NREM sleep composes approximately 75% of a total night's sleep and is divided into three distinct stages: stage N1, stage N2, and stage N3. The remaining 20%-25% of sleep is composed of REM-phase sleep, also known as *stage R,* (Table 1-1).

Typically, adult sleep begins with light sleep, advancing into deeper sleep, and then lightening again with REM sleep occurring every 90-110 minutes. The length of REM sleep increases during the night and is most prominent in the last third of the night. The first REM cycle may last only a few minutes, with the final

TABLE 1-1
Phases and Stages of Sleep

NREM Phase		
Stage of Sleep	**Type of Sleep**	**Percentage of TST**
Stage N1	Light, transitional sleep	3%-8% of TST
Stage N2	Stable sleep, defined by sleep spindles and K complexes	45%-55% of TST
Stage N3	Deep, slow wave sleep	15%-20% of TST
REM Phase		
Stage R	Desynchronized, REM sleep	20%-25% of TST

NREM, Non–rapid eye movement; *REM,* rapid eye movement; *TST,* total sleep time.
Data from Chokroverty S: *Sleep disorders medicine,* Philadelphia, 2009, Saunders; Mattice C, Brooks R, Lee-Chiong T: *Fundamentals of sleep technology,* Philadelphia, 2012, Wolters Kluwer Lippincott Williams & Wilkins.

REM cycle at the end of the sleep period lasting an hour or longer.

A **histogram** is a graphical display of the sleep stages and sleep-related events along a time axis. Figure 1-5 illustrates a histogram of a normal adult sleeper and an older adult sleeper. Although a histogram is sometimes called a **hypnogram,** by true definition, the hypnogram is a graphical display of the **sleep architecture,** or sleep stages, only along a time axis depicting a sleep session.

Sleep architecture does change throughout the life span. An older adult's sleep shows an increase in stages N1 and N2, a decrease in N3 and REM sleep, and a significant degree of fragmented sleep, or wake bouts throughout the night.

Determining Sleep Stages Using Electroencephalography

Hans Berger's groundbreaking work capturing human brain activity in an EEG was the first step toward modern sleep studies. Along with brain wave activity collected via the electrodes placed on the head, eye movement activity is collected via an EOG, and muscle activity is collected via an **electromyogram (EMG).** Sleep studies are displayed on the computer screen in standard 30-second segments known as **epochs,** historically recorded at a paper speed of 10 mm/sec on an analog polysomnograph.

Wakefulness (stage W) is considered a part of the sleep cycle process and is characterized by alpha and beta activity (Table 1-2) with voluntary blinking or "reading" eye movements seen in the EOG channels.

Dement and Kleitman[26] and Rechtschaffen and Kales[27] defined the first stage of sleep as a decrease of alpha waves slowing into theta activity over 50% of the epoch, with slow rolling eye movements and vertex waves seen near the transition to a more stable stage of sleep.

Stages N1-N2 Sleep

Most adults enter sleep through stage N1. Stage N1 sleep continues until a **K complex,** described as a well-delineated negative sharp wave immediately followed by a positive component standing out from the background EEG. Total duration is ≥ 0.5 seconds and is usually maximal in amplitude when recorded using frontal derivations, or a **sleep spindle** is noted.

A sleep spindle is initiated by the thalamus and is defined as a train of distinct waves with frequency 11-16 Hz (most commonly 12-14 Hz) and with a duration ≥ 0.5 seconds, usually maximal in amplitude in the central derivations. K complexes and/or sleep spindles interspersed between a low-amplitude, mixed-frequency background EEG indicate the sleeper has entered stage N2 sleep.

Stage N3 Sleep

Stage N3 sleep is identified when slow-wave activity occupies at least 20% of an epoch. The waves have frequency of 0.5-2 Hz and peak-to-peak amplitude > 75 μV as measured over the frontal regions. During NREM sleep stages, blood pressure, respiratory rate, heart rate, and muscle tone are fairly stable, similar to values in the resting wake state.

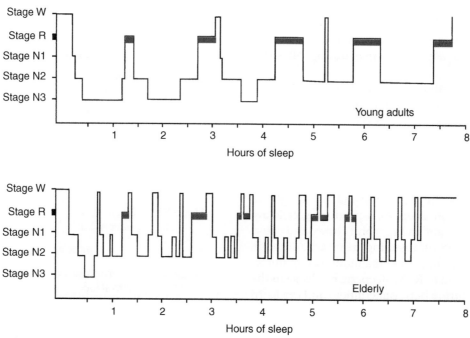

FIGURE 1-5 Histograms of young adults and older adults. *Modified from* Am Fam Physician. *1999 May 1;59(9):2551-2558.*

TABLE 1-2
Wave Frequencies and Characteristics

Type of Wave	Frequency or Duration	Characteristics	Maximal Brain Activity
Delta	0.5-4 Hz	Definitive of stage N3	Frontal region
Theta	3-7 Hz	Indication of sleep	Central region
LAMF	Predominantly 4-7 Hz during N1 sleep	Wake eyes open, N1, REM, and N2 background	Predominantly Theta
Alpha	8-13 Hz	Indication of wakefulness	Occipital region
Beta	13+ Hz	Indication of wakefulness Not typically seen on sleep EEG except interspersed within LVMF pattern When seen in sleep in trains/bursts – medication effect benzodiazepines and barbiturates	Frontal region
K Complex	≥ 0.5 sec duration	Definitive of stage N2	Frontal region
Sleep Spindle	Trains of 11-16 Hz (most often 12-14 Hz) with ≥ 0.5 sec duration	Definitive of stage N2	Central region
Vertex Wave (V wave)	< 0.5 sec duration	May be seen at end of stage N1	Central region
Sawtooth	2-6 Hz	May be seen in stage R	Central region

Data from Berry R, Brooks R, Gamaldo C, Harding S, Marcus C, Vaughn B: *The AASM manual for the scoring of sleep and associated events: rules, terminology and technical specifications, Version 2.0,* Westchester, Ill, 2012, American Academy of Sleep Medicine.

REM Sleep

REM sleep is characterized by a tonic pattern of low-voltage, mixed-frequency brain wave activity very similar to wakefulness, but with the appearance of rapid eye movements and a significant reduction in skeletal muscle tone. **Sawtooth waves** (2-6 Hz) appear almost immediately before rapid eye movement REM activity when the patient is often dreaming.

Unlike NREM sleep, during stage R sleep the body temperature drops because of a lack of thermoregulation, and the heart rate, respiratory rate, and blood pressure become variable and chaotic. REM sleep, during which skeletal muscles are paralyzed except for the diaphragm, is sometimes known as **paradoxical sleep** because the brain is very active in a paralyzed body.

PHYSIOLOGICAL PARAMETERS EVALUATED BY POLYSOMNOGRAPHY

A **polysomnogram (PSG)** is a record of many different sleep parameters. *Poly* means "many," *somno* means "sleep," and *gram* means "record." A sleep study is made up of various physiologic parameters of recorded data from different body parts that are affected by wakefulness and sleep. A minimum of three channels of EEG data are required to effectively differentiate sleep from wake and the substages of sleep.[28]

The EEG represents the electrical activity generated by the brain and recorded from the scalp using surface electrodes. Additionally, two EOG channels derived from electrical potential changes as the cornea moves toward or away from the recording electrode, and one channel of chin muscle activity are recorded.

Monitoring Vital Signs

Safety is a major concern in a sleep laboratory, and monitoring vital signs is essential. Two **electrocardiogram (ECG)** electrodes are attached using a modified lead II placement to monitor heart rhythm, and a sensor placed on the finger is connected to a **pulse oximeter**. An ECG is a recording of the electrical conduction through the heart and represents the heart's mechanical activity. An oximeter is a noninvasive device for recording the percentage of oxygen saturation obtained by pulsatile data (SpO_2) via wavelengths of light.

Snoring and breathing are both very important parameters and must be monitored. Snoring is the noise produced by the airway's soft tissues vibrating as air is forced through a partially obstructive airway. A **snore sensor** is applied to record snoring vibration or sound, and **respiratory belts** are placed over the chest and abdomen for respiratory effort.

A **thermal airflow sensor** is a small device positioned directly below the nose and in front of the mouth that responds to alterations in temperature with a change in output voltage. The output voltage of a thermal sensor is recorded as an airflow signal from which apneas are easily identified. An apnea is defined as the complete cessation of airflow.

A **nasal pressure transducer** detects pressure changes during breathing through a cannula placed at the nares. This device is more accurate than a thermal sensor for the identification of hypopneas and is able to detect flow limitation typically missed completely using a thermal sensor. A **hypopnea** is a reduction of 30% or more on the airflow signal obtained using a nasal pressure sensor.

EMG electrodes are placed 2-3 cm apart along the belly of the anterior tibialis muscle group of each leg, or one-third its length whichever is shorter. All electrode wire and sensors are plugged into a jack box or head box from which they are routed to the recorder by various electronic means.

Special Considerations

Physicians may order additional equipment or sensors on particular patients.

- For patients with a suspected seizure disorder, additional EEG electrodes may be placed for recording additional derivations from which the potential for identifying epileptiform activity is greater than from derivations routinely recorded for sleep identification.
- For patients with possible **parasomnias**, which are abnormal behaviors during sleep, additional limb sensors may be placed to record arm movements, and additional EEG electrodes may be placed as above to differentiate this activity from possible seizure activity.
- If a patient has a chronic obstructive pulmonary disease, the primary care physician, pulmonologist, or sleep specialist may order **capnography** to noninvasively monitor CO_2 levels. Capnography is a graphical display and recording of the flow curve obtained by end-tidal carbon dioxide monitoring.

The sleep technologist should explain the purpose of each piece of equipment to the patient to enhance understanding and acceptance of the procedure. This interaction may also allow the patient to relax and better cooperate. Patients often believe that they cannot sleep with all the equipment attached and need reassurance from the technologist.

Patients who are suspected of having OSA should receive education about sleep-disordered breathing and potential treatments, the CPAP device, and various masks and other interfaces. Prefitting of interfaces will facilitate a good fit and exposure to positive pressure prior to the study provides a period of adaptation for the patient should PAP therapy be required.

The technologist should allow the patient and family members an opportunity to ask questions.

Thorough patient education will increase the likelihood the patient will accept therapy and participate in his or her own success with therapy.

THE SLEEP TECHNOLOGIST

PROVISION OF HEALTH CARE

When the field of sleep medicine was in its infancy, sleep researchers and clinicians conducted sleep studies on research subjects; however, once sleep disorders were recognized and hospitals and clinics opened all-night laboratories to serve the public, sleep clinicians and doctors could not conduct both day consultations and sleep studies at night. As a result, a new allied health profession, known as *polysomnographic technology* and later *sleep technology,* was established. Initially, respiratory therapists and electroneurodiagnostic technologists who were already working in health care facilities learned on-the-job how to attach electrodes, or "hook up" patients, operate recording equipment, and monitor the sleep study. As the demand for sleep testing increased, more night technologists were needed to perform the studies.

In 1978, a group of technologists gathered and created the Association of Polysomnographic Technologists (APT). The APT later changed its name to the American Association of Sleep Technologists (AAST). Their initial mission was to unite sleep professionals as a group, offer continuing education, and promote the sleep professions at the national level.

TYPICAL ROLES AND DUTIES OF A SLEEP TECHNOLOGIST

To become a sleep technologist, specific educational and training requirements are essential. There are four categories of sleep technology workers:

- The polysomnography student is someone currently enrolled in an accredited polysomnographic technology program and as part of the clinical training requirement provides limited sleep-related services under the direct supervision of a physician, Registered Polysomnographic Technologist (RPSGT), Registered Sleep Technologist (RST), or respiratory therapist.
- The polysomnographic trainee—a new classification to the field of sleep medicine—works in a sleep center under the direct supervision of a physician, RPSGT, RST, or respiratory therapist. This individual may have earned the Certified Polysomnographic Technologists national credential through the Board of Registered Polysomnographic Technologists (BRPT).
- The polysomnographic technician works under the direct supervision of a physician, RPSGT, RST, or respiratory therapist in preparation to sit for the BRPT certification examination to become registered.

- The polysomnographic technologist has earned national certification as a sleep technologist from the BRPT, American Board of Sleep Medicine, or the National Board for Respiratory Care.

Table 1-3 lists duties of a sleep technologist, adapted from job descriptions for the sleep technology profession prepared by the American Academy of Sleep Medicine and the American Association of Sleep Technologists.

TRAINING AND CERTIFICATION

As the number of sleep technologist positions increased, it was necessary to ensure that training was adequate to accurately and safely conduct the various diagnostic and therapeutic sleep tests. In 1979, the BRPT, then a subcommittee of the APT, administered the first examination for the competency assessment of sleep technologists. The first tests were multilayered with numerous parts assessing instrument review, partial sleep study scoring, a 100-question multiple-choice examination, a physician critique—sometimes including multiple physicians—and an intensive 4-hour practical performance of a sleep study.

There were several reiterations of the examination format over the years, and in 1989, the APT made a decision to invest in the development of a standardized examination format. The first Exam Development Committee was formulated as a subcommittee of the BRPT. Working closely with a nationally recognized competency testing organization, the process of developing and transforming the previous examination into a legally defensible format began.

The first Job Task Analysis for sleep medicine technology was administered in 1990 and survey results were used to develop an up-to-date credentialing examination within a professionally administered examination format. Because of the high number of applicants, it became increasingly difficult to administer the practical portion of the examination and a decision was made to delete the practical portion of the examination process. In 1996, the BRPT moved to a 200-item multiple-choice question examination format administered as a written examination. By 2006, BRPT credentialing examinations were administered only by computer in designated testing centers. As of August 2012, there are more than 18,000 RPSGTs throughout the world.

In 2008, the National Board for Respiratory Care established the Sleep Disorders Specialty (SDS) designation for Registered Respiratory Therapists and Certified Respiratory Therapists who wish to enter the sleep field. The competency domains for the RPSGT and SDS examinations are similar; however, the RPSGT examination emphasizes performance of sleep study competencies more than the SDS examination. The SDS examination emphasizes pretesting information, administration of the sleep center, and patient treatment support.[54]

In November 2011, The American Board of Sleep Medicine (ABSM) conducted their first examination for sleep technologists who wished to become certified as an RST under the ABSM's credentialing process. The ABSM developed this examination to test job readiness skills and to determine the level of education taught in formal sleep technology programs.

The demand in the field of sleep medicine technology has also resulted in the development of higher education programs. There are numerous 1- and 2-year hospital-based, technical college, and community college educational programs accredited by the Commission on Accreditation of Allied Health Education Programs (CAAHEP) through the Committee on Accreditation for Polysomnographic Technologist Education (CoA PSG) or the Commission on Accreditation for Respiratory Care (CoARC), with one graduate-level PSG program offered at the university level.

SCOPE OF PRACTICE

According to the AAST and the AASM, sleep technologists are allied health professionals who work under the supervision of a licensed physician to assist in the education, evaluation, treatment, and follow-up of patients with sleep disorders.[55] The scope of practice includes analyzing, monitoring, and recording physiologic data during sleep and wakefulness. Duties fall under six general categories: instrumentation, performance of polysomnography, professional education, patient care and education, communication, and additional tasks.[56]

Instrumentation

Sleep technologists must be proficient in the use of specialized instruments used to record a variety of parameters during both wake and sleep. They must determine placement of EEG electrodes for application to the patient in accordance with the International 10-20 System of Electrode Placement and placement of electrodes to monitor EOG, EMG, and ECG, along with other sensors used to record a sleep study, in compliance with The AASM Manual for the Scoring of Sleep and Associated Events.

In addition to proper electrode placement, a minimally competent sleep technologist must be knowledgeable about the proper application, function, safety, care, disinfection, and capabilities of sensors for recording the following: both thermal and pressure-based nasal and oral airflow, PAP device-generated airflow, snoring, respiratory inductance plethysmography, intercostal and diaphragmatic EMG, end tidal CO_2, transcutaneous CO_2, esophageal pressure, SpO2 by pulse oximetry , esophageal pH, wrist actigraphy, and body position.

Performance of Polysomnography

The sleep technologist is responsible for initiation and completion of overnight and daytime PSGs, as

TABLE 1-3

Duties and Requirements of a Sleep Technologist

Position Summary	Works under the supervision of a clinical director or designee to provide comprehensive evaluation and treatment of sleep disorders, which may involve polysomnography, diagnostic and therapeutic services, and patient care and education. A technologist has earned certification from the American Board of Sleep Medicine or another certification body. Can perform the duties defined for a polysomnographic technician. May supervise other staff.
Gather and Analyze Patient Information	Collect, analyze and integrate patient information to identify and meet patient needs and determine final testing parameters and procedures in conjunction with physician or clinical director. Complete and verify documentation. Explain pretesting, testing, and posttesting procedures to the patient.
Testing Preparation Procedures	Prepare, calibrate, and check equipment. Apply electrodes and sensors. Perform appropriate physiologic calibrations. Perform PAP mask fitting.
Polysomnographic Procedures	Perform MSLT, MWT, parasomnia studies, PAP, titration, O_2 titration. Follow "lights out" procedures to establish and document baseline values. Perform PSG data acquisition while monitoring study-tracing quality. Document routine observations. Implement appropriate interventions. Follow "lights on" procedures to verify integrity of collected data and complete the data collection process. Demonstrate knowledge and skills necessary to provide care, assessment, and education of neonatal, pediatric, adolescent, adult, and geriatric patients. Oversee and perform difficult and unusual procedures and therapeutic interventions.
Service Management and Professional Issues	Comply with applicable laws, regulations, guidelines, and standards. Perform routine and complex equipment care and maintenance. Evaluate sleep study–related equipment and inventory. Maintain current CPR certification. Demonstrate effective written and spoken communication skills. Demonstrate appropriate social skills. Provide appropriate information to procedural-related inquiries. Demonstrate the ability to analyze complex situations and apply policy. Comply with standards of conduct.
Polysomnographic Record Scoring	Score sleep/wake stages by applying professionally accepted guidelines. Score clinical events according to center-specific protocols. Generate accurate reports.
Education and Experience	Successful completion of an accredited educational program leading to an associate degree with an emphasis in polysomnography OR Successful completion of a PSG program of at least 1 year's duration associated with a state licensed or a nationally accredited educational facility or equivalent plus experience and documented proficiency at all competencies required of a polysomnographic technician AND Certification by the ABSM as an RST or equivalent.

ABSM, American Board of Sleep Medicine; *BCLS,* basic cardiac life support; *CPR,* cardiopulmonary resuscitation; *MSLT,* multiple sleep latency test; *MWT,* maintenance of wakefulness test; *PAP,* positive airway pressure; *PSG,* polysomnogram; *RST,* registered sleep technologist.
Data from Technologist resources, American Academy of Sleep Medicine (website): http://www.aasmnet.org/traineedescription.aspx. Accessed August 30, 2012.

well as the MSLT and maintenance of wakefulness testing (MWT). Performance duties include:

- Ensuring instrumentation is properly functioning.
- Complete required equipment and patient calibrations at the beginning and end of the sleep study.
- Run continuous polysomnographic monitoring.
- Respond to, and correcting any equipment malfunction.
- Recognize and correct, artifacts.
- Document sleep stages and note events including EEG arousals, variations in respiratory effort and airflow, cardiac rate and rhythm, periodic limb movements, body movements, vocalization, and other behavioral events.
- Ensure patient wakefulness and accurately indicate sleep stages during MSLT and MWT. Maximize patient comfort and safety.
- Recognize document, and respond appropriately to epileptiform activity.
- Respond appropriately to the physical manifestations of a seizure, monitoring the cardiac rhythm.
- Identify, and appropriately respond to, non-lethal and potentially lethal cardiac dysrhythmias, O_2 desaturations, chest pain, dyspnea, anxiety, confusion, disorientation and combativeness, potentially violent and injurious behaviors, and other medical emergencies. Perform cardiac resuscitation and activate the emergency response system.
- Apply and titrate supplemental O_2 with or without PAP, continuous PAP, bilevel PAP with and without a backup rate, adaptive servoventilation, and average volume-assured pressure support.

Professional Education

Education is necessary to effectively complete one's professional duties. These include having a working knowledge of pathophysiologic conditions and behavior changes associated with sleep and arousal disorders, understanding the sleep-induced changes in the various body systems, and possessing a working knowledge of the effects of medications on sleep and physiology.

Completion of an accredited training program is recommended, and will be required in the future. Certification by the BRPT or another credentialing organization to demonstrate competency is strongly recommended, as is participation in continuing education each year to maintain and document continued competency; educating other sleep technologists, technicians, and trainees; participation in programs of self-assessment, quality assurance, and quality improvement; and completing a course in, and maintaining certification in, cardiopulmonary resuscitation.

Patient Care and Education

The sleep technologist should first review the physician's order and ensure proper patient identification, then obtain the patient's vital signs if the patient's laboratory orders include those parameters. It is essential that the sleep technologist understands the patient's sleep-related and medical history, including current issues and current medications, to provide proper patient care.

Educating the patient about what the sleep study entails, the process of sensor application, the need for audiovisual monitoring, the use and purpose of CPAP and O_2, and proper sleep hygiene, are all necessary for enhanced patient understanding and attitude regarding the procedure. In addition, increased cooperation during testing and acceptance of therapy may increase future compliance.

Communication

The sleep technologist communicates with physicians, patients, nighttime co-workers, and other medical staff. Clear understanding is essential to perform the proper type of study, and to inform the physician of findings and other pertinent information from the study that is needed for proper diagnosis. Communication with patients informs them of the process, answers their questions, puts them at ease, gains their trust, and allows the technologist an opportunity to update information related to their medical conditions. Communication with other nighttime co-workers helps to resolve recording or intervention issues, and communication with other daytime workers informs them of patient status and significant findings when daytime staff take over the study. Sleep technologists must also maintain confidentiality in compliance with the standards set by the Health Insurance Portability and Accountability Act.

Additional Tasks

Sleep technologists may perform other duties according to the needs of the sleep center such as:

- Schedule patients
- Order supplies
- Supervise staff
- Develop policies and procedures
- Manage billing
- Conduct preventative maintenance and data management
- Develop and implement an out-of-center testing program, performing quality assessment in data collection, reporting mechanisms, trending, and other administrative functions
- Track patient compliance and conduct clinical training
- Raise public awareness
- Facilitate support groups for patients with a sleep disorder
- Conduct clinical research.

The sleep technologist's duties continue to change as technology and sleep medicine change. Technology in the last few years has produced home sleep apnea testing (HSAT) devices for OSA. Some insurance companies are now requiring HSAT for patients suspected of mild or moderate OSA. In the past, these patients would have been referred for an overnight study at a sleep center; now they are tested in their homes. This has decreased the number of overnight-attended sleep studies, but actually increased the number of titration studies conducted in some sleep centers. An increasing number of sleep technologists are now needed during the day to show patients how to apply the HSAT devices and to score the home sleep apnea study results when the patient returns the recorder.

The duties of sleep technologists are specialized and multifaceted. Well-developed skills and education are necessary to perform the varied duties related to sleep testing and the provision of outstanding patient care.

CONCLUSION

Nathaniel Kleitman wrote the first comprehensive book on sleep in 1939. Some sixty years later in 1993, the National Institutes of Health recognized the sleep medicine field by establishing the Center for Sleep Disorders Research, and in 1996 the American Medical Association recognized sleep medicine as a specialty. The field of sleep medicine has come a long way and will continue to discover new information and better ways to care for patients with sleep disorders, including improved prevention of associated comorbidities.

As testing and treatment options emerge, practitioners must remain cognizant of a society that continues to become more obese, the social implications of having OSA and requiring chronic care, and the financial costs to the patient and the healthcare system that are related to sleep testing and the treatment of sleep disorders. As the gatekeepers to the field of sleep technology, sleep technologists have an obligation to evolve and, more importantly, to initiate change when appropriate.

The correct use of home sleep testing in the hands of qualified professionals has the potential for reducing the costs of sleep-disordered breathing testing and treatment, and facilitates the testing of more patients in earlier stages of disease. The more training one has in anticipation of performing these tests and follow-up of patients for aftercare, the better the job opportunities will be. According to the history of other allied health specialties that faced significant change, the more educated and well-rounded technologists who are willing to change and grow with the profession will likely improve both their professional and financial standing. Conversely, those who are opposed to the changing face of technology, or who resist formal training, may be doing something else for a living in the future.

As the profession moves forward, it will be necessary for all practitioners working in this specialty field to remain open to change and maintain up-to-date competency. As consistent with any growing and changing field, those who are not proactive will be left behind. Sleep technologists of the future will likely need more training in areas of knowledge and the performance of

duties historically attributed to the role of the sleep medicine expert, rather than the sleep technologist. For these reasons, it is necessary to rethink outdated pathways into the field and increase the number of highly trained technologists. Whether this is accomplished through formal education or by way of a highly disciplined self-directed study, keep in mind that pathways outside of formal training will eventually close.

CHAPTER SUMMARY

- The prerequisite knowledge for understanding sleep accumulated over the centuries through brain wave activity experiments and circadian rhythm and nervous system function studies. EEG brain wave studies conducted on human beings laid the foundation for sleep medicine, which began in the 1950s.
- Analog pen and paper recording machines were retired with the introduction of digital computer software.
- Groups of like-minded scientists and technologists established organizations to administer standardized protocols, manuals, and textbooks.
- Internal sleep drive and external alerting signals interact in an intricate balance to dictate the propensity for wake and sleep. Sleep-wake regulation is influenced by several brain structures and neurotransmitters, which play a part in the initiation and termination of the sleep phases.
- Sleep is divided into NREM and REM sleep. NREM sleep is divided into three stages. NREM-REM stages occur in three to five cyclic patterns throughout the night. EEG signals measure brain activity, whereas other sensors measure additional biological parameters. All of these parameters record the data, which cumulatively creates a PSG.
- The first sleep technologists were respiratory therapists and EEG technicians.
- Sleep technology workers include the polysomnographic student, the sleep technician, and the sleep technologist. Education and experience enable a person to advance through the ranks, becoming credentialed by a nationally recognized organization.
- Duties and scope of practice for sleep technologists include gathering and analyzing patient information, applying electrodes and performing CPAP mask fittings, calibrating equipment and monitoring the study, handling patient needs, scoring sleep studies, and educating patients regarding sleep hygiene and sleep apnea treatment.
- With the sleep medicine field just a half-century old, a great deal of information has been gathered and technology has kept pace, but vast amounts of sleep-related knowledge still await discovery.

References

1. Theoi Green Mythology: *Hypnos* (website). www.theoi.com/ Daimon/Hypnos.html. Accessed August 19, 2012.
2. Lindemans M: Encyclopedia Mythica, *Somnus* (website). www. pantheon.org/articles/s/somnus.html. Accessed August 19, 2012.
3. Silverberg R: *The dawn of medicine*, New York, 1975, Putnam.
4. Willis T: *The practice of physick*, London, 1692.
5. Jones WHS: *Trans Hippocrates on dreams*, Cambridge, 1923, Harvard University Press.
6. MacNish R: *The philosophy of sleep*, New York, 1834, D. Appleton.
7. Eknoyan G: Santorio Sanctorius (1561-1636)—founding father of metabolic balance studies, *Am J Nephrol* 19(2):226-233, 1999.
8. University of Minnesota: *Biological Rhythms* (website). http://cda.morris.umn.edu/~meeklesr/clock.html. Accessed August 18, 2012.
9. Pollak C, Thorpy M, Yager J: *The encyclopedia of sleep and sleep disorders*, New York, 2010, Facts On File.
10. New York Times Company: *Luigi Galvani* (website). http://inventors.about.com/library/inventors/bl_Galvani.htm. Accessed August 18, 2012.
11. Nobelprize.org: *Life and discoveries of Camillo Golgi* (website). www.nobelprize.org/nobel_prizes/medicine/laureates/1906/golgi-article.html. Accessed August 18, 2012.
12. Passouant P: Historical note: Doctor Gelineau, narcolepsy centennial, *Sleep* 3:241, 1981.
13. Freud S: *The interpretation of dreams (1900)*, translated by J. Strachey. In *The standard edition of the complete psychological works of Sigmund Freud*, vols 4 and 5, London, 1953, Hogwarth Press.
14. Legendre R, Pieron H: Le probleme des facteurs du sommeil: resultats d'injections vasculaires et intracerebrales de liquids insomniques, *C R Soc Biol* 68:1077, 1910.
15. Pieron H: *Le probleme physiologique du sommeil*, Paris, 1913, Masson.
16. Lavie P: The sleep theory of Constantin von Economo, *J Sleep Res* 2(3):175-178, 1993.
17. Nobelprize.org: *Life and discoveries of Walter Rudolph Hess* (website). www.nobelprize.org/nobel_prizes/medicine/laureates/1949/hess-bio.html. Accessed August 18, 2012.
18. Moruzzi G, Magoun H: Brain stem reticular formation and activation of the EEG, *Electroenceph Clin Neurophysiol* 1:445, 1949.
19. Caton R: The electric currents of the brain, *Br Med J* 2:278, 1875.
20. Berger H: Uber das elektroenkephalogramm des menschen, *J Psychol Neurol* 40:160, 1930.
21. Kryger M: History of sleep medicine and physiology, *Atlas of physical sleep medicine: expert consult*, St Louis, 2009, Elsevier.
22. Loomis A, Harvey E, Hobart G: Cerebral states during sleep as studied by human brain potentials, *J Exper Psychol* 21:127, 1937.
23. Kleitman N: *Sleep and wakefulness*, Chicago, 1939, University of Chicago Press.
24. Blake H, Gerard R, Kleitman N: Factors influencing brain potentials during sleep, *J Neurophysiol* 2:48, 1939.
25. Aserinsky E, Kleitman N: Regularly occurring periods of eye motility, and concomitant activity during sleep, *Science* 118:273, 1953.
26. Dement W, Kleitman N: Cyclic variations in EEG during sleep and their relation to eye movements, body motility, and dreaming, *Electroenceph Clin Neurophysiol* 9:673, 1957.
27. Rechtschaffen A, Kales A: *A manual of standardized terminology, techniques and scoring system for sleep stages of human subjects*, Los Angeles, 1968, Brain Information Service/Brain Research Institute University of California.
28. Iber C, Ancoli-Israel S, Chesson A et al: *The AASM manual for the scoring of sleep and associated events: rules, terminology and technical specifications*, Westchester, Ill., 2007, American Academy of Sleep Medicine.
29. Berry R, Brooks R, Gamaldo C, Harding S, Marcus C, Vaughn B: *The AASM manual for the scoring of sleep and associated events: rules, terminology and technical specifications, Version 2.0*, Westchester, Ill., 2012, American Academy of Sleep Medicine.
30. American Academy of Sleep Medicine: *About the American Academy of Sleep Medicine* (website). www.aasmnet.org. Accessed August 26, 2012.
31. Gélineau J: De la narcolepsie, *Gazette des hôpitaux* 53:626, 1880.
32. Gélineau J: De la narcolepsie. Surgères, Charente-Inférieure: *Imprimerie de Surgères* 64, 1881.
33. Switzer RE, Berman AD: Comments and observations on the nature of narcolepsy, *Ann Intern Med* 44(5):938-957, 1956.
34. Carskadon M, Dement W, Mitler M, et al: Guidelines for the multiple sleep latency test (MSLT): a standard measure of sleepiness, *Sleep* 9:519, 1986.
35. Dickens C: *The posthumous papers of the Pickwick club*, London, 1836, Chapman and Hall.
36. Broadbent H: *The Lancet* 142:3645, 102, 1893.
37. Bickelmann AG, Burwell CS, Robin ED et al: Extreme obesity associated with alveolar hypoventilation; a pickwickian syndrome, *Am J Med* 21(5):811-818, 1956.
38. Jung R, Kuhlo W: Neurophysiological studies of abnormal night sleep and the pickwickian syndrome, *Prog Brain Res* 18:140, 1965.
39. Gastaut H, Tassinari C, Duron B: Etude polygraphique des manifestations episodiques (hypniques et respiratoires) du syndrome de Pickwick, *Rev Neurol* 112:568, 1965.
40. Tassinari C, Lugaresi E: Obstructive sleep apnoea-hypopnoea syndrome, *Rev Neuro* 123:267, 1970.
41. Kryger M, Roth T, Dement W: *Principles and practice of sleep medicine*, Philadelphia, 2005, Saunders.
42. Guilleminault C, Tilkian A, Dement W: The sleep apnea syndromes, *Ann Rev Med* 27:465, 1976.
43. Sullivan C, Issa F, Berthon-Jones M et al: Reversal of obstructive sleep apnoea by continuous positive airway pressure applied through the nares, *The Lancet* 1:862, 1981.
44. Dement W, Guilleminault C, editors: Diagnostic classification of sleep and arousal disorders, *Sleep* 2:1, 1979.
45. Kryger M, Roth T, Dement W: *Principles and practice of sleep medicine*, Philadelphia, 2010, Saunders.
46. Czeisler C, Duffy J, Shanahan T, et al: Stability, precision, and near-24-hour period of the human circadian pacemaker, *Science* 284:2177, 1999.
47. Avidan A, Barkoukis T: *Review of sleep medicine*, Philadelphia, 2012, Elsevier.
48. Johns M: Rethinking the assessment of sleepiness, *Sleep Med Rev* 2:3, 1998.
49. Achermann P, Borbely AA: Mathematical models of sleep regulation, *Front Biosci* 8:683, 2003.
50. Borbely AA, Tobler I: *Brain mechanisms of sleep*, New York, 1985, Raven Press.
51. Edgar DM, Dement WC, Fuller CA: Effect of SCN lesions on sleep in the squirrel monkey: evidence for opponent processes in sleep-wake regulation, *J Neurosci* 13:1065, 1993.
52. Cassone VM, Chesworth MJ, Armstrong SM: Entrainment of rat circadian rhythms by daily injection of melatonin depends upon the hypothalamic suprachiasmatic nuclei, *Physiol Behav* 36:1111, 1986.
53. Reppert SM, Wever DR: Coordination of circadian timing in mammals, *Nature* 418:935, 2002.
54. American College of Chest Physicians: *Sleep technician training and credentialing: an update* (website). www.chestnet.org/accp/article/chest-physician/sleep-technician-training-and-credentialing-update. Accessed August 25, 2012.
55. American Association of Sleep Technologists: *The scope of practice for sleep (polysomnographic) technologists*, A2Zzz September 2011.
56. American Association of Sleep Technologists: *Job Descriptions—Sleep Technologist* (website). http://www.aastweb.org/Job Descriptions.aspx#Technologist. Accessed September 1, 2012.

REVIEW QUESTIONS

1. Alpha signals are characterized by which of the following:
   a. 8-13 cps, most prominent in the occipital region
   b. 8-13 cps, most prominent in the frontal region
   c. 11-16 cps, most prominent in the central region
   d. 12-14 cps, most prominent in the occipital region

2. Who was the first to argue for the existence of a center for regulation of sleep?
   a. Moruzzi and Magoun
   b. Loomis and Hobart
   c. Kleitman and Aserinsky
   d. Constantin von Economo

3. Who discovered the cyclical pattern of NREM and REM sleep?
   a. Kleitman and Aserinsky
   b. Kleitman and Dement
   c. Michel Jouvet
   d. Moruzzi and Magoun

4. Who is considered the father of sleep research?
   a. Nathaniel Kleitman
   b. William Dement
   c. George Zeitgeber
   d. Christian Guilleminault

5. Which of the following provides a measure of SpO_2?
   a. Pulse oximeter
   b. Snore sensor
   c. Respiratory belts
   d. Capnography

6. Zeitgebers are associated with:
   a. Narcolepsy
   b. Sleep-related breathing disorders
   c. Circadian rhythms
   d. Sleep terrors

7. Which of these statements is true about melatonin?
   a. Melatonin is released at approximately 9:00 pm.
   b. Melatonin is released in stressful situations.
   c. Melatonin is released by the cerebral cortex.
   d. Melatonin is released at approximately 9:00 am.

8. In which time range are the alerting signals the lowest?
   a. 1:00-3:00 am
   b. 4:00-6:00 pm
   c. 4:00-6:00 am
   d. 9:00-11:00 am

9. The opponent process model of sleep states the cause of sleep is the result of the interaction of two opposing forces. What are the two opposing forces?
   a. Sleep load versus alerting signals
   b. Circadian rhythm versus alerting signals
   c. Sleep load versus homeostatic drive
   d. Non-REM versus REM sleep

10. Which structure is known as the *circadian pacemaker*?
    a. Heart
    b. SCN
    c. ARAS
    d. Thalamus

Chapter 2

Classification of Sleep Disorders

Jackie Compton

CHAPTER OUTLINE

LEARNING OBJECTIVES

After reading this chapter, you will be able to:
1. List the different sleep disorders and their basic characteristics.
2. Identify of the insomnias and potential causes.
3. Identify each of the insomnias and potential causes of each.
4. Describe the disorders of hypersomnia.
5. Identify the circadian rhythm sleep disorders.
6. Explain the parasomnia sleep disorders.
7. Describe the sleep-related movement disorders.
8. Define the different breathing patterns.

KEY TERMS

actigraphy
adjustment insomnia
behavioral insomnia
cataplexy
fatal familial insomnia
hypercapnia
hypersomnia
hypnagogic hallucinations

hypoventilation
hypoxemia
idiopathic insomnia
inadequate sleep hygiene
microsleep
overlap syndrome
paradoxical insomnia
periodic limb movements (PLMs)

psychophysiologic insomnia
primary insomnia
secondary insomnia
sleep attacks
sleep log
sleep paralysis
sleep state misperception
ventilation

The sleep technologist must have a basic understanding of sleep disorders to assist in decision making for sleep testing purposes. Reading the patient's history and being aware of potential sleep disorders and existing sleep disorders will enable the technologist to perform a quality sleep study and aid in the diagnostic process. As many of these patients present with a complexity of sleep-related breathing disorders, diagnosis and treatment is extremely important and the sleep technologist plays a significant role.

The *International Classification of Sleep Disorders: Diagnosis and Coding Manual,* second edition (ICSD-2) lists more than 80 sleep disorders.[1] The vast majority of these sleep disorders are classified in the following six categories:

- Insomnias
- Sleep-related breathing disorders
- Hypersomnias of central origin
- Circadian rhythm disorders
- Parasomnias
- Sleep-related movement disorders

THE INSOMNIAS

Although not normally studied in the sleep testing laboratory, insomnia is the most common sleep disorder.[1] Approximately 33% to 50% of US adults report insomnia or sleep difficulties at least a few nights a year, and 9% suffer from chronic insomnia with resulting interpersonal relationship problems, moodiness, and memory and attention-deficit problems.[2] Women,, individuals with psychiatric illnesses, and shift workers suffer from insomnia more often than the general public.[3] Sleep technologists who work the night shift frequently suffer from insomnia because of fragmented sleep resulting from their work cycle. Acquiring quality daytime sleep is difficult because the circadian rhythm alerting signal is at its peak during the day.

There are many types of insomnia (Table 2-1). Insomnia, in general, is defined as difficulty initiating sleep (sleep-onset insomnia), maintaining sleep (sleep-maintenance insomnia), and waking too early (terminal insomnia). These conditions occur despite an adequate amount of time or opportunity to sleep

TABLE 2-1

Types of Insomnia

Type	Alternate name	Primary or Secondary	Description
Adjustment insomnia		Secondary	Acute insomnia characterized by a change from the patient's normal sleep pattern caused by a stressor in the person's life. This condition can lead to psychophysiologic insomnia.
Psychophysiologic insomnia	Learned insomnia, conditioned insomnia, chronic insomnia	Secondary	Chronic condition characterized by the patient ruminating about not sleeping.
Paradoxical insomnia	Sleep state misperception, subjective insomnia, pseudoinsomnia	Secondary	Chronic insomnia in which the patient complains that he or she is sleeping very little or not at all; however, despite this perception of sleeplessness, a PSG often demonstrates normal sleeping patterns and an actigraphy study may indicate sleep during the time the person states he or she was awake.
Idiopathic insomnia	Childhood-onset insomnia	Primary	A rare, chronic, lifelong insomnia. Onset occurs during infancy or childhood with no identifiable cause; patient is unable to initiate or maintain adequate sleep in his or her entire lifetime.
Fatal familial insomnia		Primary	Extremely rare, neurologic disorder with onset in adulthood that ends in death on average 18 months after onset. It is characterized by progressively severe insomnia with sleep deprivation symptoms of panic attacks, phobias, paranoia, hallucination, and dementia.
Inadequate sleep hygiene		Secondary	Caused by a person voluntarily avoiding sleep and is the most common insomnia in the general population.

PSG, Polysomnogram.

and are accompanied by poor-quality and nonrestorative sleep, tiredness, memory problems, accident-proneness, lethargy, stomach complaints, and other physical or mental impairment.[1]

Insomnia is considered a clinical diagnosis and is based on subjective information from the patient. A polysomnogram (PSG) is usually not performed to diagnose insomnia.[4] A PSG may be ordered if the patient exhibits a comorbid medical or physical condition, if there is the possibility of another sleep disorder, or if behavioral or pharmaceutical treatment for insomnia has not been successful.

Primary insomnia indicates that poor sleep is due to a conditioned aversion to the bedroom or from subclinical emotional/cognitive/physiologic turmoil, whereas **secondary insomnias** are sleep problems that occur as the result of a primary medical, psychiatric, or substance/medication use condition, including other sleep disorders.

PRIMARY INSOMNIAS

Idiopathic Insomnia

Idiopathic insomnia, also known as *childhood onset insomnia,* is a rare, chronic, lifelong insomnia.[1] Onset occurs during infancy or childhood with no identifiable cause. The sufferer is unable to initiate or maintain adequate sleep throughout his or her entire lifetime. There may be an inherited neurochemical imbalance that affects the arousal system or sleep-inducing and maintenance system.

Fatal Familial Insomnia

Fatal familial insomnia is a very rare neurologic disorder with onset in adulthood that ends in death on average 18 months after onset; it has been discovered in fewer than 40 families worldwide.[1] Although no cause has been determined, protein mutation and loss of neurons in the thalamus have been implicated. The disorder is characterized by progressively severe insomnia with sleep deprivation symptoms of panic attacks, phobias, paranoia, hallucination, and dementia.

SECONDARY INSOMNIAS

Adjustment Insomnia

Adjustment insomnia is an acute insomnia characterized by a distinct change from the patient's normal sleep pattern caused by a stressor in the person's life.[1] Stressors can include divorce; a death; loss of a job; being a victim of a crime; neighborhood noise; pain; or effects of medication or other physiologic, psychological, or environmental factors. Once the stressor is resolved, the insomnia ceases. If the patient worries about the insomnia, the adjustment insomnia may turn into **psychophysiologic insomnia.**

Psychophysiologic Insomnia

Psychophysiologic insomnia, also known as *learned insomnia, conditioned insomnia,* and *chronic insomnia,* is a chronic condition characterized by the patient ruminating about not sleeping.[1] There is excessive focus and heightened anxiety about sleeping, and there may be heightened arousal as the time for planned naps and bedtime approaches, and when the person is in his or her own bed. Intrusive thoughts and the perceived inability to sleep may prohibit sufficient relaxation to allow sleep to occur. The person may not have any trouble falling asleep during monotonous activities, when not intending to sleep, or in a different sleeping environment, such as in a hotel.

Paradoxical Insomnia

Paradoxical insomnia, also known as **sleep state misperception**, *subjective insomnia,* and *pseudoinsomnia,* is a chronic insomnia in which the patient will complain that he or she is sleeping very little or not at all during most nights, and produce **sleep logs** that average well below normal amounts of sleep.[1] A sleep log is a diary kept for a 1-week period or longer that tracks bed times, wake times, and daily activities. Despite the patient's incorrect perception of sleeplessness, a PSG often demonstrates normal sleeping patterns, and an **actigraphy** study may indicate sleep during the time the person states he or she is awake. An actigraphy study is the process of recording gross body movements over time using a small device worn on the wrist similar to a watch, known as an actigraph (Figure 2-1). The insomniac's reported daytime impairment is often not consistent with a truly sleep-deprived individual's daytime impairment.

Inadequate Sleep Hygiene

Inadequate sleep hygiene is caused by a person voluntarily avoiding sleep; it is the most common insomnia in the general population.[1] With our 24/7 society, humans have developed poor habits that impair good-quality sleep. Consuming caffeine and staying up late to continue daily activities does not allow time for adequate, rejuvenating sleep. During the day the individual suffers the symptoms of sleepiness, which affects daytime alertness. Improvement in sleep hygiene can be achieved by following the proper sleep hygiene principles listed in Box 2-1.

Behavioral Insomnia

Behavioral insomnia of childhood is differentiated into two major categories: sleep onset–association disorder and limit-setting disorder.[1]

Sleep-onset association occurs when the child needs a specific item (such as a doll), activity (such as being read a story), or environmental condition (such as the light being on) to fall asleep.[1] Falling asleep is an extended process and both initial sleep onset and

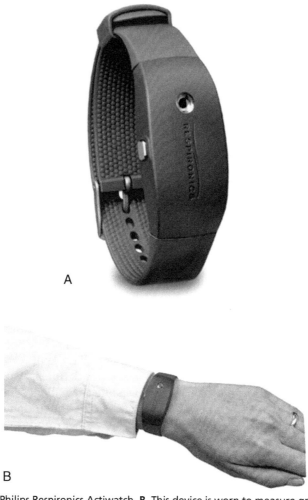

A

B

FIGURE 2-1 **A,** Philips Respironics Actiwatch. **B,** This device is worn to measure gross motor movements for extended periods. *Courtesy Philips Respironics, Inc.*

BOX 2-1
Proper Sleep Hygiene

- Maintain regular bedtime and wake time, even on days off.
- Use bed for sleeping and sex, not as a place to watch TV, call friends, or use the computer.
- Establish relaxing presleep rituals.
- Go to bed when you feel drowsy.
- Make bedroom comfortable and conducive to sleeping: block out sound and light.
- Exercise regularly; avoid heavy exercise within 6 hours of bedtime.
- Avoid stimulants (e.g., caffeine and/or nicotine) 6 hours before bedtime.
- Avoid alcohol at bedtime; alcohol causes sleep disruption.
- Eat a healthy diet.
- Avoid eating full meals too close to bedtime.
- Maintain a regular schedule.
- If you must nap, do it at the same time every day.

- Sleeping pills should be used conservatively and with a doctor's advice.
- Avoid unnecessary stress when possible.

PROPER SLEEP HYGIENE FOR OLDER ADULTS

- Decrease time in bed awake.
- Rise at the same time every day.
- Exercise daily (but not close to bedtime).
- Eat a light snack before bedtime.
- Avoid caffeine, alcohol, and tobacco, particularly after lunch.
- Avoid frequent use of sedative-hypnotics.
- Get out of bed if not able to sleep, especially if feeling tense, angry, or frustrated.
- Limit any naps to 30 minutes in the early afternoon.
- Spend more time outdoors to increase light exposure, particularly later in the day.

Data from Chokroverty S: *Sleep disorders medicine,* Philadelphia, 2009, Saunders; Mattice C, Brooks R, Lee-Chiong T: *Fundamentals of sleep technology,* Philadelphia, 2012, Wolters Kluwer Lippincott Williams & Wilkins.

returning to sleep following awakening are delayed in the absence of the associated item, activity, or condition. Nighttime awakenings require caregiver intervention for the child to return to sleep.

Children with limit-setting disorder push the caregivers' boundaries by avoiding bedtime and insisting on staying awake.[1] Behaviors include screaming, begging, asking for water, and leaving the bedroom.

Both sleep onset–association insomnia and limit-setting association insomnia intimately involve the parent-child relationship, and resolution of the insomnia depends on the caregivers' behavior.

SLEEP-RELATED BREATHING DISORDERS

Sleep-related breathing disorders are characterized by abnormal breathing during sleep. These disorders are classified in the ICSD-2 as central sleep apnea (CSA) syndromes, obstructive sleep apnea (OSA) syndromes, sleep-related hypoventilation and hypoxemic syndromes, and sleep-related hypoventilation and/or hypoxemia caused by a medical condition. These are the sleep disorders most commonly seen in the sleep testing facility.

CENTRAL SLEEP APNEA (CSA) SYNDROMES

Primary CSA is characterized by a cessation of both airflow and respiratory effort in an intermittent or cyclic fashion resulting from central nervous system dysfunction.[1] The cyclical interruption may result in fragmented sleep and frequent nocturnal awakenings, both of which contribute to excessive daytime sleepiness. The patient may wake with shortness of breath. The individual who has CSA may have increased carbon dioxide (CO_2) levels during the day and abnormal oxygen (O_2) desaturations during sleep.

Cheyne-Stokes

Cheyne-Stokes breathing pattern, also known as periodic breathing and Cheyne-Stokes respiration (CSR), is characterized by apneas or hypopneas recurring between waxing and waning hyperpnea.[1] CSR typically occurs in older men during the transition from wake to non–rapid eye movement (NREM) sleep. This is a neurologic system disorder associated with congestive heart failure, stroke, or renal failure. Atrial fibrillation may be present. These patients often arrive at the sleep testing facility with high acuity presentation. Treatment can be quite challenging as they present with a complexity of sleep-related breathing disorders.

High-Altitude Periodic Breathing

High-altitude periodic breathing occurs with an ascent to very high altitudes.[1] The individual experiences periods of hypopnea and apnea with no respiratory effort. There is often a sensation of suffocation, but adaption will occur if the individual remains at the high altitude.

Drug-Related CSA

Patients who have been on long-acting opioids regularly for at least 2 months, may experience CSA due to drug or substance.[1] Patients taking methadone, time-release morphine, or hydrocodone may also experience this disorder. Other respiratory patterns, such as obstructive hypoventilation, Biot breathing pattern, and periodic breathing, may also be observed.

OBSTRUCTIVE SLEEP APNEA (OSA) SYNDROMES

OSA in adults is characterized by obstruction in the upper airway.[1] This obstruction can be caused by a number of structures located in the nasopharynx, oropharynx, or laryngopharynx, also known as the hypopharynx. Complete or partial airway obstruction causes apneas, hypopneas, and snoring. Sleep disruption, fragmented sleep, and blood O_2 desaturations are common with OSA. Patients may complain of excessive sleepiness, and can be a danger to themselves and others when working or driving.

Several serious medical conditions are associated with OSA, including cardiovascular disease, myocardial infarction, high blood pressure, stroke, coronary heart disease, metabolic syndrome, and depression.[5] A laboratory sleep study or a home sleep apnea test are recommended when OSA is suspected. Continuous positive airway pressure (CPAP) is considered the gold standard treatment.

Pediatric OSA

Signs and symptoms of OSA in pediatric patients include snoring and labored breathing, apneas, and hypopneas.[1,6] Large tonsils and adenoids can block the airway passage and cause loud snoring and apneic activity. The primary therapy for pediatric OSA is an adenotonsillectomy.

SLEEP-RELATED HYPOVENTILATION AND HYPOXEMIC SYNDROMES

Hypoventilation is defined as a significant reduction in normal tidal breathing, or normal resting breathing, and results in **hypercapnia** (increased levels of CO_2 in the blood) combined with **hypoxemia** (reduced O_2 levels in the blood). **Ventilation** is a function of the precise regulation of pH, O_2, and CO_2 in the blood. O_2 is inhaled on inspiration and CO_2 is exhaled upon expiration. Breathing patterns during the day are robust and stable, but during sleep breathing can fluctuate in efficiency and stability. Several sleep disorders involve the inadequate exchange of O_2 and CO_2.

Patients who have hypoventilation with normal lung function and no identifiable cause are typically diagnosed with the sleep-related nonobstructive alveolar hypoventilation, idiopathic disorder. They present with a decreased tidal volume associated with hypercapnia and hypoxemia.[1]

SLEEP-RELATED HYPOVENTILATION/ HYPOXEMIA DUE TO MEDICAL CONDITIONS

Chronic obstructive pulmonary disease (COPD) patients suffer from sleep-related hypoventilation and hypoxemia as a result of lower airways obstruction caused by chronic bronchitis or emphysema.[1] Sleep disorder testing facilities are seeing an increase in patients with comorbid conditions of COPD and OSA, commonly referred to as **overlap syndrome**.

The increased CO_2 and decreased O_2 commonly seen with patients having sleep-related hypoventilation/hypoxemia due to neuromuscular and chest wall disorders are the result of weak or dysfunctional ventilatory muscles or a neuromuscular disease, such as muscular dystrophy.[1] Obesity increases the burden on these muscles and worsens symptoms of the disorder. When a neuromuscular or chest wall disorder coexists with OSA, added burden is placed on the ventilatory system because of the combined effect of upper airway obstruction and muscular weakness.

HYPERSOMNIAS OF CENTRAL ORIGIN

Hypersomnia is characterized by excessive sleepiness or daytime sleepiness. It is not caused by nighttime sleep disturbances or circadian rhythm disorders. Hypersomnia results in drowsiness, **microsleeps** (falling asleep for a moment then awakening), and unintentional napping. Diagnostic tools for hypersomnia include the multiple sleep latency test, which is a series of four or five trials performed to measure the tendency to fall asleep.

NARCOLEPSY

Patients with narcolepsy are subject to **sleep attacks**, often in rapid eye movement (REM) sleep. The patient falls asleep during everyday activities, including eating, driving, or conversing.[1] Patients with narcolepsy frequently have **cataplexy**, which is a sudden loss of muscle tone and can be triggered by strong emotion such as anger or laughing. Cataplexy can range from very minor, such as a head drop or facial sagging, to a complete loss of muscle tone and physical collapse. Obviously, the sudden onset of REM sleep can pose grave physical dangers to an individual, including head injuries and fractures. Cataplectic attacks usually only last a few minutes and the person recovers completely.

Other symptoms of narcolepsy include excessive daytime sleepiness, sleep paralysis, and hypnagogic hallucinations, which, along with cataplexy, make up the Narcolepsy Tetrad. Disrupted sleep maintenance and automatic behaviors are also associated with narcolepsy. **Sleep paralysis** occurs when the patient cannot move immediately upon awakening. **Hypnagogic hallucinations** are vivid, dreamlike sensations that occur at sleep onset. The sensations are often fear-driven with someone or something threatening the person.

RECURRENT HYPERSOMNIAS

Recurrent hypersomnias include Kleine-Levin syndrome and menstrual-related hypersomnia.[1]

Kleine-Levin syndrome usually begins during adolescence and is more common in males. This neurologic disorder is characterized by recurring periods of excessive sleeping, binge eating, and hypersexuality. At episode onset, the individual becomes drowsy and sleeps most of the day and night. When awake, patients have an altered personality. The individual with Kleine-Levin may appear aggressive, confused, disoriented, or depressed. Understandably, in this state the individual cannot attend school or work during episodes. Between episodes, the patient has normal alertness, cognitive function, and behavior.

Menstrual-related hypersomnia usually begins within the first months after menarche. A hormone imbalance is the suspected cause of this hypersomnia.[1]

SECONDARY HYPERSOMNIA

Hypersomnia due to drug or substance is a secondary condition that occurs when a patient complains of excessive nocturnal sleep, excessive daytime sleepiness, or excessive napping that is due to alcohol, or prescription or street drug use.[1] Narcolepsy is not a condition of this particular disorder.

CIRCADIAN RHYTHM DISORDERS

Circadian rhythm disorders deal with sleep disturbances that are out of rhythm with the 24-hour clock. There will be a persistent recurrent pattern of sleep disturbance caused by alterations of the circadian time-keeping system, or by misalignment between the circadian rhythms and factors that affect the timing and duration of sleep. This alteration leads to insomnia, excessive daytime sleepiness, or both, and the disorders cause social and/or occupational functional impairment.

Patients suffering from irregular sleep-wake rhythm have a lack of clearly defined circadian sleep and wake rhythm.[1] Sleep and wake periods are variable throughout the 24 hours, which causes chronic insomnia and excessive daytime sleepiness. There is limited knowledge of the pathophysiologic characteristics of this disorder. Most patients are usually studied in facilities that have long-term monitoring capabilities over a 72-hour period.

DELAYED SLEEP PHASE DISORDER

Delayed sleep phase disorder is characterized by the sleep-wake cycle being delayed in relation to the desired clock time, so that drowsiness and sleep occur several hours later in the night than normal.[1] This results in symptoms of sleep-onset insomnia or difficulty in waking at the desired time. This disorder is more common in adolescents and young adults and can cause social and mental impairment, affecting both school and home life. Refreshing, restorative sleep is achieved when patients are allowed to sleep at their body's natural rhythm, going to bed late and rising late in the morning.

ADVANCED SLEEP PHASE DISORDER

Advanced sleep phase disorder occurs frequently among older adults. The major sleep episode is advanced in relation to the desired clock time, resulting in symptoms of compelling early evening sleepiness, early sleep onset, and awakening in the morning earlier than normal sleepers.[1] Individuals are usually in bed before 8:00 p.m. and are ready to awaken around 4:00 a.m. to begin their day. There is less negative influence on social or work life with this disorder compared with delayed phase type.

FREE-RUNNING

Free-running is a rare, nonentrained type of circadian rhythm disorder in which there is a steady pattern composed of 1- to 2-hour daily delays in sleep onset and wake times.[1] More than half of all totally blind individuals have free-running type. The lack of sight and the ability of light cues to be given to the brain prevent synchronization of the sleep-wake cycle by the suprachiasmatic nucleus.

Actigraphy data on these patients demonstrate a sleep-wake cycle of 25 hours a day. This extended sleep-wake cycle causes the patient to fall incrementally out of phase for many days of the month. If the patient attempts to synchronize his or her sleep and wake time with normal society, he or she will obtain progressively less sleep and develop excessive daytime sleepiness, interfering with social and work obligations.

JET LAG

Jet lag is a common problem in this global environment. This disorder is caused by a temporary mismatch of the sleep-wake cycle when flying over more than two time zones.[1] Complaints include insomnia or excessive daytime sleepiness. The more time zones one crosses, the more severe the jet lag. Flying eastward is more difficult to adjust to than flying westward. There may be impairment during daytime functioning, a general malaise, and gastrointestinal disturbance within 1 to 2 days after travel. It generally takes 1 day per time zone to make the adjustment back to the normal sleep-wake cycle.

SHIFT WORK DISORDER

Many sleep technologists suffer from shift work disorder, a circadian rhythm disorder associated with a recurring work schedule that overlaps the usual time for sleep.[1] Sleep disturbance is most common in "graveyard shift" night workers and early morning shift workers. Shift workers encounter bouts of insomnia or excessive daytime sleepiness that occur in relation to work schedules. Patients complain of unrefreshed sleep, insomnia, fatigue, impaired mental ability, reduced alertness, gastrointestinal distress, social life disruption, and poor work performance. Safety becomes an issue, especially when driving home after a night shift.

CIRCADIAN DISORDER DUE TO MEDICAL CONDITIONS

Circadian disorder due to medical or neurologic condition is a secondary disorder. Disruptions of sleep-wake patterns can vary from minor phase changes to irregular sleep-wake patterns depending on the primary condition causing the circadian disturbance.[1] Examples of primary conditions are dementia, Alzheimer disease, Parkinson disease, hepatic encephalopathy, and blindness.

PARASOMNIAS

Parasomnias are undesirable physical events or experiences that occur while falling asleep, during sleep, or during arousals from sleep. These experiences are the result of central nervous system activation being transmitted to the skeletal muscles via the autonomic ("fight or flight") mechanism. Parasomnias can occur in both NREM and REM sleep.

NON-RAPID EYE MOVEMENT (NREM) SLEEP PARASOMNIAS

Parasomnias in NREM sleep usually occur during the first one third of the sleep period and typically in stage N3 sleep. NREM parasomnias include disorders of arousal (such as confusional arousals), sleepwalking, and sleep terrors.[1]

Confusional Arousal

Confusional arousals are exhibited by mental confusion or confusional behavior during or after arousals from sleep.[1] The patient may move slowly, mumble, moan, be unresponsive, exhibit automatic behavior, or become agitated if someone tries to help. Patients usually do not remember the event when they wake in the morning.

Sleepwalking

Sleepwalking includes ambulation while asleep. This usually occurs in children ages 8-12 and spontaneously stops around puberty.[1] Sleepwalkers can be difficult to arouse and may be confused when awakened. They usually do not remember the event in the morning. Safety is an issue and households with a sleepwalker should make the environment as safe as possible.

Sleep Terrors

During a sleep terror, the patient wakes from stage N3 sleep crying or screaming and displaying signs of intense fear. During this state, they are inconsolable and will not respond to caregivers. They do not usually remember the event in the morning. In most cases, this parasomnia also spontaneously stops during the teen years.[1] Both sleepwalking and sleep terrors can be familial in nature.

RAPID EYE MOVEMENT (REM) SLEEP PARASOMNIAS

Parasomnias in REM sleep usually occur during the latter half of the sleep period. REM parasomnias include nightmare disorder, sleep-related groaning (catathrenia), recurrent isolated sleep paralysis, and REM sleep behavior disorder (RBD).[1]

Nightmare Disorder

Nightmare disorder develops from recurring nightmare experiences.[1] A nightmare has disturbing visual dream sequences involving fear, anger, or other strong emotions that wake the patient from sleep. There is no confusion on awakening; the patient is alert and can remember the nightmare, but there may be a delay in falling back to sleep caused by the disturbing dream mentation following an episode.

Catathrenia

Patients with sleep-related groaning (catathrenia) emit monotonous sounds when exhaling during REM sleep.[1] The patient is unaware of the phenomena, but the bed partner complains and encourages the patient to get help.

REM Sleep Behavior Disorder (RBD)

Normally during REM sleep, the patient's muscles are paralyzed, prohibiting movement and the acting out of dreams. REM sleep behavior disorder (RBD) occurs when there is a lack of skeletal muscle paralysis and the patient is able to move and act out his or her dreams.[1] Patients often remember their dream on awakening. This disorder is more common in men older than 60 years of age, and is often associated with an underlying neurologic disorder—particularly Parkinson disease or narcolepsy. This disorder is also seen during alcohol withdrawal with an accompanying intense REM sleep rebound. Antidepressants can also trigger RBD. Serious safety issues occur with RBD. Injury to the individual or the bed partner is common.

OTHER PARASOMNIAS

Sleep-Related Dissociative Disorder

Sleep-related dissociative disorder occurs in patients who have a corresponding daytime dissociative disorder. These patients are mostly females and are often victims of sexual or physical abuse or posttraumatic stress disorder who have exhibited self-mutilating behaviors or attempted suicide, and have had psychiatric hospitalizations.[1] During sleep, the patient may scream, run, attempt to self-mutilate, or engage in other violent behaviors. The onset of this sleep disorder typically occurs in childhood to middle adulthood.

Sleep Enuresis

Sleep enuresis, also known as *nocturnal bedwetting* or *enuresis nocturia,* occurs in patients older than 5. Sleep enuresis is classified as primary or secondary.[1] Primary sleep enuresis is diagnosed when recurrent involuntary voiding occurs during sleep at least twice per week in a patient who has never been consistently dry. Secondary sleep enuresis is diagnosed when recurrent involuntary voiding begins to occur at least twice a week, following a period during which the subject was consistently dry during sleep for at least 6 months.

Sleep-Related Eating Disorder (SRED)

Sleep-related eating disorder (SRED) is characterized as recurrent episodes of involuntary "out of control" eating and drinking during arousals from sleep.[1] Recall of the event can vary from no recall at all to substantial recall. Patients may consume peculiar substances such as cat food and salt sandwiches, coffee grounds, raw bacon, or buttered cigarettes. Safety becomes an issue when the individual attempts to cook. Other problems include weight gain and obesity, digestive tract disorders, morning anorexia, and sleep disruption. SRED can be associated with sleepwalking, OSA, irregular sleep-wake type disorder, dissociative disorder, and restless legs syndrome (RLS). In the sleep testing environment, it is important that food be made readily available to assist in the diagnosis of this parasomnia.

Parasomnias Related to Drug or Substance Use

Parasomnia caused by drug or substance use is a secondary disorder.[1] Disorders of arousal, SRED, and RBD are the parasomnias most associated with medications or substances. Antidepressant medications such as tricyclic antidepressants and large amounts of caffeine and chocolate have been known to trigger this disorder. It is imperative that the sleep technologist have full knowledge of all medications taken by the patient before and during sleep testing.

Testing for Parasomnias

The sleep testing process for the parasomnias involves detailed video and audio recordings in addition to the routine polysomnography montage. In fact, an extended electroencephalogram (EEG) montage may be needed if a sleep-related seizure is suspected in the manifestation of the parasomnia. Without an extended EEG montage and quality audio and video monitoring, it may be difficult to differentiate nocturnal seizure activity from activity seen during a parasomnia since overlap exists during the events. The sleep technologist must also keep detailed records of unusual behaviors, motions, and activities by the patient during the sleep test. The correlation of these activities, combined with audio and video recording and physiologic data, is essential for accurate diagnosis.

SLEEP-RELATED MOVEMENT DISORDERS

Sleep-related movement disorders are conditions in which body movements delay sleep onset or disrupt sleep. Sleep disturbance or excessive daytime sleepiness is a requirement for a diagnosis of a sleep-related movement disorder. Movements are repetitive and stereotypical, unlike parasomnia movements. This category includes the following disorders: restless leg syndrome (RLS); periodic limb movement disorder (PLMD); sleep-related leg cramps; sleep-related bruxism; sleep-related rhythmic movement disorder; sleep-related movement disorder, unspecified; sleep-related movement disorder resulting from drug or substance use; and sleep-related movement disorder caused by a medical condition.[1]

RESTLESS LEG SYNDROME (RLS)

Restless leg syndrome (RLS), also known as *Willis-Ekbom disease*, is a clinical syndrome based on patient history. A PSG is not needed for diagnosis unless the patient complains of other sleep problems. RLS is a medical condition that occurs while the patient is awake; however, it is closely related to PLMD and is included in the movement disorders category.

RLS usually involves a strong, nearly irresistible urge to move the legs, trunk, or arms accompanied with an unpleasant sensation of tingling, vibration, or pins and needles, particularly in the legs.[1] Symptoms are worse in the late afternoon and evening, and are less prominent in the morning. Lying down or sitting may make the symptoms worse; walking or stretching temporarily relieves the symptoms.

Involuntary jerking or twitching of the legs and the accompanying unpleasant sensations may cause sleep onset delay and maintenance insomnia when the person wakes up in the night. RLS often results in a reduction in sleep time and nonrestorative sleep. Daytime fatigue or excessive daytime sleepiness is a requirement for diagnosis.

Women are more affected than men, and there may be a genetic link. Symptoms can occur at any age, and may be intermittent, but gradually get worse. Secondary RLS can be caused by iron deficiency, pregnancy, severe kidney failure, and certain medications.

PERIODIC LIMB MOVEMENT DISORDER (PLMD)

RLS is closely associated with periodic limb movement disorder (PLMD). Eighty-five percent of people with RLS experience PLMD. PLMD is a condition characterized by very stereotypical **periodic limb movements (PLMs)** that occur during sleep. A PSG is needed to diagnose PLMD.

SLEEP-RELATED BRUXISM

Sleep-related bruxism involves strong repetitive jaw muscle contractions in a grinding or clenching fashion, usually associated with arousal.[1] This behavior leads to abnormal wear of teeth; broken, loose, or painful teeth; jaw pain; and headache. Bed partners may complain about the grinding noise and a dental examination may bring attention to tooth destruction. There may be a family history, and bruxism may also be associated with other disorders such as Parkinson disease, RLS, OSA, dementia, and depression.

SLEEP-RELATED RHYTHMIC MOVEMENT DISORDER

Sleep-related rhythmic movement disorder is characterized by repetitive, stereotypical, rhythmic movements in large muscle groups that begin in drowsiness or sleep.[1] This disorder can display as body rocking, head banging, head rolling, body rolling, and leg banging. These behaviors interrupt sleep, and cause daytime function impairment and self-inflicted bodily injury.

CHAPTER SUMMARY

- Insomnia is the most common sleep disorder and is characterized by difficulty falling asleep, staying asleep, or waking too early.
- Sleep-related breathing disorders exhibit as abnormal breathing during sleep, fragmenting sleep and resulting in negative cardiovascular effect.
- Sleep-related hypoventilation and hypoxemic syndromes result in higher than normal CO_2 and decreased O_2 in the body.

- Hypersomnias are disorders of excessive sleepiness or the excessive need to sleep.
- Circadian rhythm disorders result from misalignment of the patient's sleep-wake cycle with the natural circadian cycle.
- Shift work disorder is diagnosed when insomnia, excessive daytime sleepiness, and physical discomfort occur as the result of one's work schedule being misaligned with the circadian cycle.
- Parasomnias are undesirable events that occur while falling asleep, during sleep, or during arousals from sleep.
- Sleep-related movement disorders are conditions in which stereotypical movements are disruptive to the patient's sleep or the bed partner's sleep.

References

1. *International classification of sleep disorders: diagnosis and coding manual*, ed 2, Westchester, Ill., 2005, American Academy of Sleep Medicine.
2. Roth T, Ancoli-Israel S: Daytime consequences and correlates of insomnia in the United States: results of the 1991 National Sleep Foundation survey: II, *Sleep* 1:22 Suppl. 2 S354-S358, 1999.
3. Roth T, Roehrs T: Insomnia: epidemiology, characteristics and consequences, *Clin Cornerstone* 5(3):5-15, 2003.
4. Chesson A, Hartse K, Anderson WM, et al: Practice parameters for the evaluation of chronic insomnia. *Sleep* 23(2):237, 2000.
5. Punjabi NM, Shahar E, Redline S, Gottlieb DJ, Givelber R, Resnick H: Sleep heart health study investigators: sleep-disordered breathing, glucose intolerance, and insulin resistance: The Sleep Heart Health Study. *Am J Epidemiol* 160(6):521, 2004.
6. American Thoracic Society: Standards and indications for cardiopulmonary sleep studies in children, *Am J Respir Crit Care Med* 153:866, 1996.

REVIEW QUESTIONS

1. What is the gold standard treatment for obstructive sleep apnea of adulthood?
   a. Tracheotomy
   b. CPAP
   c. Weight loss
   d. Adenotonsillectomy

2. What is the most common sleep disorder or group of disorders?
   a. Hypersomnia
   b. Narcolepsy
   c. Sleep apnea
   d. Insomnia

3. A person who has recently been a victim of a crime has adjustment insomnia and begins to ruminate. Which of the following is most likely to develop?
   a. Restless legs syndrome
   b. Psychophysiologic insomnia
   c. Paradoxical sleep
   d. Paradoxical insomnia

4. Which of the following represents a habit of good sleep hygiene?
   a. Drink a glass of wine before bed to relax.
   b. Go to bed at the same time every night.
   c. Exercise one hour before bedtime.
   d. Watch TV in bed to relax

5. Which of the following is *most* commonly associated with congestive heart failure, stroke, and renal failure?
   a. CSR
   b. OSA
   c. COPD
   d. OHS

6. COPD is most often associated with which of the following?
   a. Apneas
   b. Hypopneas
   c. Bronchitis
   d. Obesity

7. Sleep walking and sleep terrors most often occur during which sleep-wake state?
   a. N1
   b. N2
   c. Stage R
   d. N3

8. Which population is most likely to experience recurring hypersomnia?
   a. Infants
   b. Adolescents
   c. Middle-aged adults
   d. Elderly adults

9. What is the primary treatment for childhood OSA?
   a. Tracheotomy
   b. CPAP
   c. Adenotonsillectomy
   d. Weight loss

10. Which of the following conditions is most likely to present with complex breathing disorders during the sleep testing process?
    a. Seizures
    b. Neuromuscular disease
    c. Pediatric snoring
    d. Narcolepsy

Chapter 3

Electronics and Electricity

James T. Mitchum

CHAPTER OUTLINE

LEARNING OBJECTIVES

After reading this chapter, you will be able to:
1. Define electricity.
2. Explain the fundamental laws that describe the behavior of electricity.
3. Record observations of electronic circuitry.
4. Identify the components of a circuit.
5. Define current flow.
6. Identify the forms of electricity and their generation.
7. Define conductors, resistors, and insulators.
8. Identify two forms of electrical transmission and their differences.
9. Demonstrate how electricity is used in a sleep laboratory setting.
10. Record grounding and patient isolation techniques.
11. Define the units and prefixes used in describing electrical charge, current, and potential differences.
12. Demonstrate an understanding of electromotive force.
13. Identify the general concepts of thermoelectric effect, piezoelectric effect, and static electricity.
14. Define Ohm's law.
15. Demonstrate a basic understanding of leakage currents.
16. Demonstrate a conceptual understanding of ancillary equipment used in polysomnography.

KEY TERMS

alternating current (AC)
ampere
closed circuit
conductor
conservation of charge
Coulomb's law
current flow
direct current (DC)
electrochemistry
electromagnetic induction
electronic circuit

ground
hertz (Hz)
impedance
leakage current
negative charge
net charge
Ohm's law
open circuit
photoelectricity
photon
piezoelectric effect

positive charge
power isolation
resistance
Seebeck effect
static electricity
thermoelectric effect
voltage

INTRODUCTION TO ELECTRICITY

The effects of electricity are evident everywhere. The lightening in the skies, the train crossing the countryside, the sound emanating from concert speakers, and even the familiar green lines tracing a patient's cardiac activity across a screen are all the resulting actions of electrical activity; otherwise, electricity is not tangible, at least no more than gravity. There is no color, no texture, no smell that defines electricity, and this intangible nature requires a great deal of imagination if one is to thoroughly understand it. Yet, electricity is used every day. Eyes are sensitive to electromagnetic waves in the visible light spectrum, sending electrical pulses to the visual cortex of the human brain. These pulses do not stop there, but send off a ripple of responses, allowing us the ability to orient, predict, and understand the information sent in high definition in less than one tenth of a second. Understanding the theories and laws that govern electrical phenomena promotes not only a better understanding of the technology used in polysomnography, but also a better understanding of the human body and its functions.

This chapter imparts some of the basic concepts needed to understand how electricity works and how it is generated. Physical concepts such as charge, current, conduction, and resistance are introduced thoroughly enough to grasp a basic understanding of how electrical circuits work, which relates directly to the recording amplifiers and sensors used by polysomnographic technologists every night. These goals may feel distant when starting with the elementary knowledge needed to move forward in this topic, but taking a path of least resistance will lead to a poor understanding of future concepts such as recording artifacts, amplifier filters, and patient safety.

Through experimentation, scientists piece together the rules under which electricity operates, and often these theorems and laws are named for the scientist who validated the theory. Terms like *ohms, watts,* and *volts* were named for the scientists who described these concepts first. The term *electricity* comes from the early discovery that rubbing pieces of amber with fur generated an attracting force. The same observation is made by rubbing an air-filled balloon against a head of hair. *Elektron* is the Greek word for "amber." The attraction demonstrated between the balloon and hair, the fur and amber, is the starting point for understanding electricity.

A word of caution: The study of electrical concepts examines how charged objects behave in proximity to each other. Asking *why* electrical phenomena occur is philosophical and is answered by science no more completely than asking why the universe exists. Not knowing why an electrical charge behaves the way it does has not prevented the extensive use of electricity in any way, and simply understanding how charge behaves is sufficient and beneficial to a polysomnographic technologist.

FORMS OF ELECTRICITY

Electricity arises from several sources and each of them participates in technology and nature in unique ways. Forms of electricity may be a bit misleading at first, but the important differences are clarified. The type of energy being converted defines a form of electricity.

- **Static electricity** is the electrical energy created by the interaction of charged objects in close proximity, as in a balloon that has been rubbed against fur.
- **Electrochemistry** is the conversion of chemical energy into charge and is the form of electricity generated by batteries.
- **Photoelectricity** is the conversion of light into electricity, a process used in modern solar panels.
- **Piezoelectric effect** is a form used commonly in medical sensing equipment, including sensors used by polysomnographic technologists, and it arises from the mechanical strain put on certain types of crystals.

- The **thermoelectric effect** is also used in polysomnography and is the conversion of temperature differences into electricity, typically used for airflow monitoring.
- Nuclear electricity is the conversion of the energy that binds the nucleus of atoms together into electrical charge, either by breaking the atom apart—fission—or combining atoms together—fusion.
- **Electromagnetic induction** uses the motion of magnets in close proximity to wires to convert mechanical energy into electricity, and is used widely for power generation on both a large and small scale. Examples of this use include a car's alternator and the hydroelectric turbines of a dam. The line frequency that provides power to electrical outlets in our homes and polysomnography recording equipment is electromagnetically generated.

Static Electricity

Although several forms of electrical generation exist, static electricity, in some sense, is a good starting point for introducing several basic and important concepts about electricity such as charge, polarity, voltage, and the **conservation of charge**. As such, this form of electricity is covered in more detail than the others as a foundational beginning for understanding.

Static electricity was the first observed form of electrical activity. It is the build-up of static electricity in the clouds that eventually results in lightning, the shock between a fingertip and a metal doorknob, and the cling found in clothes after a hot tumble in the dryer. All of these phenomena can be traced to the behavior of electrons and protons, and their interactions with one another.

Charged Particle Interactions

Benjamin Franklin described two types of charges and labeled them positive and negative. **Negative charges** result from the build-up of electrons and **positive charges** are the result of a build-up of protons. Electrons are subatomic particles that orbit the nucleus of the atom. Protons and neutrons form the nucleus and give the atom its atomic weight. In general, the number of electrons orbiting the nucleus is equal to the number of protons in the nucleus giving the atom a balanced, or neutral, **net charge**. Net charge is the sum of all electrical charges present in a system. The common convention for identifying positive charge is with a plus (+) sign and the common convention for identifying negative charge is with a minus (−) sign.

The Greek philosopher Thales of Miletus reported that after rubbing amber with fur, the amber could attract and deflect small objects, either pushing them away or pulling them toward the amber. Negative charges, when brought into close proximity, are repelled, as are positive charges when brought close to other positive charges (Figure 3-1). When a positive charge is in proximity to a negative charge, the attraction that results causes them to attempt to move toward one another (Figure 3-2). The separation of charges at some distance creates a **voltage**, or a potential difference in the energy between the charges. The symbol for volts is V.

To clarify this relationship, a simple experiment with balloons and furs demonstrates several of these concepts. When a balloon, *A*, is vigorously rubbed against a fur, *B*, balloon A rubs electrons off of fur B, and the electrons distribute themselves on the surface of balloon A. The fur, having given up some of its electrons, now has a positive charge and the balloon, having gained electrons, has a negative charge. If balloon A is brought close to fur B, the fur will point in the direction of the balloon. In fact, the balloon is also being pulled to the fur, but the physical force is small enough that a person would not notice the pull. But a balloon left near the fur may appear

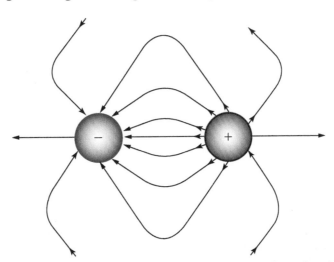

FIGURE 3-1 Electric field represents the interactive forces between charged particles. The closer the lines are to each other, the stronger the interaction. Opposite charges pull the field lines toward each charge.

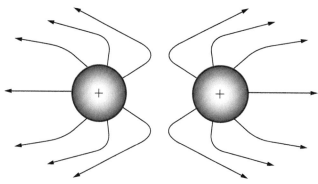

FIGURE 3-2 Similar charges repel each other, and the lines of the electric field bend away from similar charge.

to stick strong enough to overcome the force of gravity below it. To take this concept a bit further, the electrons that were evenly distributed on the surface of balloon A will gather to the side nearest the fur when the charges are close enough to interact.

Now another balloon, C, is introduced and another fur, D, is vigorously rubbed against it. Balloon A and balloon C both are negatively charged. Bring them together and a repelling force pushes them away in opposite directions. Bring fur B close to fur D and the hairs of the fur will push away, attempting to lie down and away from each other. The closer the charged objects are to each other, the stronger the interaction. In general, the interaction continues as long as these objects are held in proximity.

Over a longer period, and with the interaction of other objects, the balloons and furs will return to a neutral charge. However, as long as negative and positive charges are built up and in close range of each other, static electricity is at work and the positive and negative charge will remain on the objects.

Coulomb's Law

How close the objects need to be for an interaction is based on the strength of the charges. This was described by Charles Coulomb in what is now known as **Coulomb's law**:

$$F = k_e \frac{q_1 q_2}{r^2}$$

For the purpose of understanding electrical interactions, describing all of these symbols in detail is avoided, but this formula reflects the discussion of static electricity thus far. The force, F, which can be thought of for now as the strength of attraction or repulsion of two charged objects, is equal to the absolute value of charge on object 1 times the absolute value of charge on object 2, divided by the square of the distance between the two charges. Coulomb's constant, k, results from experimentation is not important for this discussion. What is important is that the greater the charges (q_1 and q_2), the greater the attraction or repulsion between

the two objects. Similarly, the greater the distance between the objects, the weaker the attraction or repulsion is between the objects. Calculating this force is beyond the needs of a technologist, but the formula neatly reflects the behaviors observed in nature and experimentation.

A balloon and fur interact within inches of space, but lightning forms miles from the opposing charges. The amazing power of the lightning bolt is directly related to the separated charges from which it is born.

Conservation of Charge

Charge is always conserved. Charge can neither be lost nor created in a system, but it can be rearranged. As negative charge moves in one direction, positive charge is exchanged in the opposite direction. As neutral charge atoms give up electrons, the atoms become positively charged. Atoms and molecules may attract electrons beyond the balance of protons and thus become negatively charged.

Consider the balloon and fur once again: The balloon gains electrons while the fur loses them. Bound strongly in the nuclei of the various atoms that form the fur's structure, protons are unable to cross over with the electrons they have lost. Consequently, the fur gains a positive charge and electrons shift their concentration to the balloon.

Electrochemical Electricity

Electrochemical electricity is the conversion of chemical energy into electrical energy. This exchange of energy is how batteries allow for the simple transportation and use of electricity in objects such as pacemakers, portable monitoring equipment, remote controls, and almost any portable electronic device (excluding ones that run from photoelectric, or solar, electricity). Regarding human physiology, neuronal firing in the brain and throughout the nervous system would not be possible without the conversion of chemical energy in the body into electrical charge.

Cells in the body generate electrical energy by controlling the quantity of positively charged sodium ions and negatively charged potassium ions

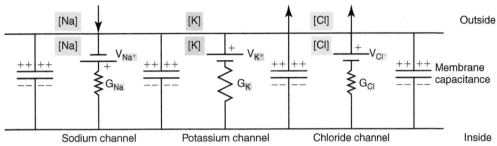

FIGURE 3-3 Electrochemical electricity. *Modified from Kasap, SO: Thermoelectric effects in metals: thermocouples, Kasap, 2001, McGraw-Hill e-booklet.*

inside and outside the cell membrane. Although this mechanism is highly complex, the basic concept is simple. In a resting state, the cell has a small negative charge difference, but not enough to evoke an electrical impulse. At the necessary time, the cell membrane allows sodium and potassium ions to flow freely through the cell membrane, driven by charge and a concentration gradient. As the negatively charged sodium ions move to the outside and the positively charged potassium ions move to the inside, the negative charge accumulates to the outside of the cell until an impulse is generated, sending an electrical signal away from the cell (Figure 3-3).

Several chemical reactions lead to the production of electricity, and all of them involve the generation of positive and negative molecules. Sodium ions (Na^-) are prevalent enough in bioelectrical generation that sweat on the surface of the skin is able to create voltage differences between recording electrodes and produce an artifact in the recording.

Photoelectricity

The photoelectric effect is a relatively complex way to generate electricity. The behavior of light garnered the attention of such scientists as Albert Einstein, and his observations of light would become part of the foundation of quantum theory while earning him the Nobel Prize in Physics in 1921. Light behaves simultaneously as a particle flying through space and like a radio wave transmission.

The particle in a light wave is called a **photon**, which is massless and has a neutral charge. When photons are absorbed by the electrons in a material, the energy of the material is increased. If enough energy is absorbed, the bonds holding electrons to their respective atoms are broken and the electrons are freed. The stronger the intensity of the light source, the greater the increase is in the energy being delivered to the material. The photoelectric effect is the driving concept behind solar panels and light sensors.

Thermoelectric Effect

Thermoelectric effect arises from the difference in temperature across a charge-carrying medium, such as aluminum. Just as photons can increase the energy

of electrons, a change in temperature is a measure of the change of energy in the medium. If a medium is heated unevenly, so that one area is warmer than another, the free electrons from the warm side move to the cooler area and create a voltage difference between the two sides. This outcome, called the **Seebeck effect**,[1] works in both directions. If a voltage difference is applied across the same medium, it will warm the medium.

The thermoelectric effect is used in polysomnography to record air temperature changes in front of a person's nose and mouth with a thermocouple.

Piezoelectric Effect

The piezoelectric effect comes from the deformation of certain types of crystals. When a crystal of quartz is deformed, or squeezed, the material generates a voltage, or electrical energy. This relationship is reversible as well. Applying a voltage to either side of a crystal will deform the crystal's shape.

ELECTRONIC CIRCUITS

Generating and capturing electricity is only as useful as the ability to apply the stored energy to some useful purpose. Today, the uses of electricity are so numerous that the methods employed to use it effectively are often taken for granted. **Electronic circuits** are a combination of conductive materials and electronic components that are assembled to perform one or more functions. A simple example of an electronic circuit is a light bulb (electronic component), copper wire (conductive material), and battery (electrical source) connected in a loop.

OPEN, CLOSED, AND SHORT CIRCUITS

In the previous example, when the circuit's wires, battery, and light bulb are connected, the light glows and the circuit is said to be **closed** (Figure 3-4). If a wire is disconnected, or the light bulb is pulled from the circuit, the current pathway is disrupted, the light bulb no longer glows, and the circuit is said to be **open** (Figure 3-5).

A special case of a closed circuit is a short circuit. A short circuit occurs when the loop is closed before

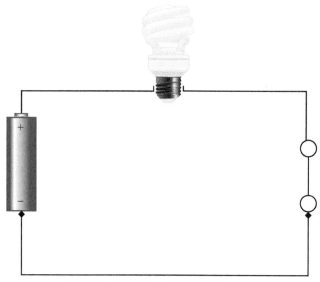

FIGURE 3-4 A closed circuit diagram.

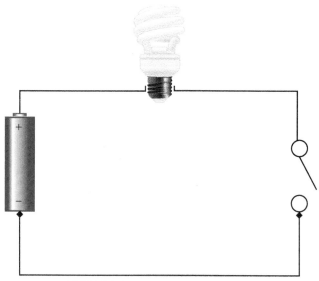

FIGURE 3-5 An open circuit diagram.

the current can travel through all the intended elements of the circuit; thus the intended path has been shortened (Figure 3-6).[2]

Observe that the terms *closed* and *open* describe the connections of the electrical components themselves. This is a departure from the analogy to the current of fluids, where an open valve allows fluid to flow, and a closed valve stops fluid.

The light bulb circuit is very simple and performs only one function; however, a computer, traffic light system, and smartphone are all examples of much more complex circuits capable of performing a large quantity of functions. In performing polysomnographic testing, both simple and complex circuits are in place.

Understanding the fundamentals of electronic circuits requires the introduction of several concepts. One must understand how electrical energy moves and what can be done to alter the movements of this energy. Answers to these questions will help the technologist both understand the basic function of recording devices and sensors, and the signals being obtained from the patient's body.

CURRENT FLOW

For a moment, consider the dynamics of fluids, such as water. The shape and motion of water is not always easy to discern. A calm lake surface may seem smooth and without motion and yet a slow and gentle current moves the lake from its source river to a dam that

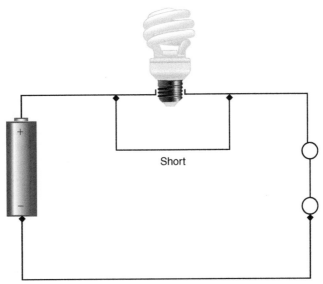

FIGURE 3-6 A short circuit diagram.

spills out some quantity of water downstream. This motion is due to the interaction between the earth and water by gravitational force. The terminology used in describing river motion also reflects the difference in altitude from one point to another. Upstream is at a higher elevation than downstream, and the river flows from the higher elevation where greater pressure is exerted on the body of water to an area of lower elevation and pressure, always taking the path of least resistance.

Current flow is the motion of charged particles through a conductive medium. In electronics applications, current is the motion of electrons through a conductive medium moving from a lower voltage to a higher one. The voltage difference is the motivating force for electron flow and is also known as electromotive force, or EMF.

Principles of Current

Early experimenters, including Benjamin Franklin who first described positive and negative charges, thought of and described electricity as a type of fluid. Indeed, many observations of the behavior of electricity share similarities to fluids, and this comparison to fluid is both helpful and misleading. The flow of electricity from positive to negative is one area in which comparing electricity to fluid can be misleading. With conventional flow, we have learned throughout our lives that a liquid or gas moves from positive to negative, or at least lower pressure. This is also referred to as "the path of least resistance." With a battery, however, the flow of electrons is from the negative terminal of the battery to the positive terminal. Protons are strongly bound to other protons and neutrons in the atomic structure by nuclear forces much stronger than the affinity electrons have for orbiting a nucleus from

afar, and so moving protons to generate current is much less likely to occur.

When the voltage potential remains the same across a given circuit, such as with a battery connected to a light bulb in a closed circuit, then the current is described as **direct current (DC)**. The electrons flow in a single direction in the circuit (Figure 3-7). DC electricity flows in only one direction and is either on or off. Current will flow as long as the power source and circuit are available and no components are placed in the circuit, causing the signal to decay.

Alternating current (AC) is created by the constant alternation of positive and negative terminals in a circuit. This alternation of voltage is often created by electromagnetic induction, when a magnet is spun inside a coil of conductive wire. Think of a cyclist pedaling both feet on a bike. Professional cyclists attach the soles of their feet to the pedals so they can simultaneously push down on one side while pulling up on the other side. While the motion of the feet is always in opposing directions, the cyclist generates power. As the magnet rotates, the positive and negative terminals switch polarity in a waveform called a *sinusoid*.

The time it takes for one rotation is called a rotational period, often denoted as *T*. The number of rotations in a given time frame is the frequency of rotation and is often denoted as cycles per second, or **hertz (Hz)**.

Power stations in the United States have agreed on a single frequency, or line frequency, standard of 60 Hz, whereas most European power stations use 50 Hz. A consistent frequency is required for reliable power delivery to avoid spikes and drops in power and allow for more reliable electronics that use the AC source for power. If line frequency varied, every electronic device would require extra circuits to normalize the current within the device.

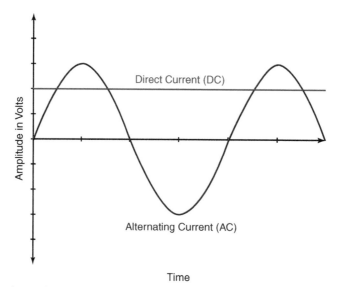

FIGURE 3-7 Alternating current versus direct current. The *Y* axis represents volts. The actual current through a given circuit is known when the combined resistive and capacitive elements are taken into account, according to Ohm's law.

Units and Prefixes

An electron and proton both have the same value of charge, but opposite signs. This unit of charge is based on the coulomb, named for Charles Coulomb who described the relationship of charged particles, distance, and the force between them. The symbol for coulombs is the capital letter *C.* A proton has 1.602×10^{-19} C of charge. Such a small number is difficult to put into perspective, but a bolt of lightning contains enough charged particles to equal roughly 15 C. If 1 positive coulomb (+1 C) charge was placed 1 meter (1 m) apart from another positive coulomb (+1 C) charge, the repulsing force between the two charges would be equivalent to 920,000 metric tons on earth.

The unit of current is the **ampere**, named after André-Marie Ampère, and its symbol is *A.* Electrical current is denoted by *I,* which originates from the French when current was known as *intensité de courant,* meaning "current intensity." Likewise, the International System of Units with 29 base and derived units, among others standardized for use in the sciences, is abbreviated as SI, the first two initials of its French name *Système International d'Unités.*

Current (I) is measured in amperes (A). One ampere (1A) is equal to 1 coulomb (1C) passing through a point in an electric circuit in 1 second (1 s):

$$1A = \frac{1C}{s}$$

Metric Prefixes

The SI prefix modifies a basic unit of measure and also offers a symbol prefix to SI units. *Kilo-* is commonly used to modify *gram* and a *kilogram* is 1000 g, or 1 kg. A *kilometer* is 1000 m, or 1 km. Other prefixes modify the unit of measure into smaller quantities. Volts (V) are rarely noted in human physiology, but the resting potential of a neuron is −70 microvolts (μV), or −0.00007 volts.

INTRODUCTION TO ELECTRICAL COMPONENTS

CONDUCTORS

A **conductor** is any material that permits the flow of electrons. Without a conductive pathway, a current of electrons is without a path to travel, and so there is no current. The more readily a material allows electrons to pass through, the greater that material's conductance. Metals are often excellent conductors because they willingly accept and give up electrons (Figure 3-8). Water is a poor conductor unless some form of salt is introduced, in which case the solution then becomes a terrific conductor. Metals such as copper, lead, silver, and gold are used extensively in electronics as conductors. Electrons move surprisingly slowly in copper wire at a rate of −1 m/s (the negative symbol shows that the electrons move toward the positive terminal), or approximately a normal walking pace for an average adult. The velocity of the electrons, however, is not as important as the quantity that can pass through at any given time.

Insulators often surround conductors, and are materials that do not allow the passage of electrons. Rubber, glass, and plastic are all examples of insulators.

RESISTANCE

Resistance is the ability of a material to impede the flow of electrons. It is denoted by the symbol *R* and measured in Ohms, after the German physicist

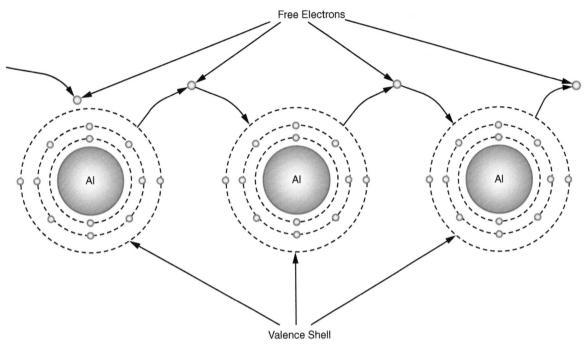

FIGURE 3-8 Atoms that readily give up and receive 'free' valence shell electrons make the best conductors.

George Ohm. Conductance and resistance are two sides of the same idea. A good conductor is a very poor resistor and a poor conductor is a very good resistor.

Ohm's Law

Named after George Ohm, who described this relationship in 1827, **Ohm's law** describes the relationship between voltage, V, current, I, and resistance, R, in a circuit:

$$V = I * R$$

This law is used to establish the **impedance** values of electrodes attached to a patient. Impedance is similar to resistance in that the value of impedance describes the opposition to the flow of electrons. In fact, the unit for impedance is Ohms, although the symbol is Z. Resistance applies to DC power sources and impedance applies to AC power sources. A circuit's resistance is the same at any given time, whereas a circuit's impedance changes based on the frequency of the power source applied to the circuit. Impedance is the term used in polysomnography because biological signals are most similar to an alternating power source. Furthermore, the impedance values are found by sending a small alternating current from one electrode to another.

Ohm's law does not change significantly for impedance, but the mathematical concepts involved do and are beyond the scope of an introduction. What remain the same are the relationships between voltage, impedance, and current. The graphical representation of brain activity is a timed record of local potential differences, or voltages. Some value of impedance is necessary, as a zero value would mean that no voltage changes would ever be detected on the graph. Conversely, too large of an impedance value restricts current flow to the amplifier, and external artifacts become more prominent in the recording.

LEAKAGE CURRENT

Leakage current is a common phenomenon related to electrical components in which current is lost or generated by various properties of the circuit itself. Often, this leakage is considered undesirable, but in some cases it's a necessary byproduct. For example, circuit designs that limit the recorded frequency range are called filters and these filters generate leakage current. The AC from a wall plug is transformed into DC before being used in the amplifier; however, some AC is bound to make its way through the process and is considered a leakage current. Proper grounding techniques direct this unwanted current away from the patient while preserving the integrity of the recording.

GROUND AND POWER ISOLATION

Ground

A **ground** is a point in an electric circuit with an assumed potential value of zero. Ground wires were originally paths that ended in the earth itself, but now refer broadly to a return point for current in any circuit. Grounds provide intentional and safe paths of departure for current in a circuit. When a metal enclosure, such as a computer case, is used as a grounding point, it is referred to as a chassis ground. In computer repair, it is common for a repair technician to wear a metal bracelet with a wire clipped to the chassis of the computer under repair. The bracelet allows excess charge from the repair technician to be safely discharged away from the components of the computer. This also helps to prevent the technician from becoming a ground point and thus helps to prevent shock to the technician.

In polysomnography, grounding occurs in at least two places: the earth ground wire in the three-wire plug from the wall outlet to the amplifier, and a chassis ground on the patient's scalp. The earth ground helps ensure any excess current in the amplifiers is discharged away from the patient. The chassis ground that is attached to the patient provides a complete circuit for the recording and protects the patient from any excess discharge that *might* occur from within the amplifier. It is important the patient have only one ground lead attached to prevent multiple current paths through the patient.

Power Isolation

Another technique used to protect the patient and the equipment is **power isolation**. Through induction, a phenomenon described by British scientist Michael Faraday, current from a coil of wire can induce a current in a nearby but physically separate coil of wire (both circuits must be closed). If both coils of wire have the same number of rotations, the current in both circuits is nearly equal. However, if the number of coils in either wire is greater or lesser, then the amount of current passed on is either stepped up or stepped down in the receiving circuit. This basic configuration of coils describes a transformer, which is used ubiquitously in power applications. A transformer box steps down the high voltage from the power plant to a usable 120 V in homes, for example.

Power isolation also helps to prevent unwanted noise in a circuit. Leakage currents and 60 Hz noise from the wall outlet are minimized or removed in the transformer as long as both circuits have a separate ground. This is the reason for both a chassis and earth ground on the typical sleep laboratory recording equipment setup.

AN OVERVIEW OF ANCILLARY EQUIPMENT

Ancillary equipment encapsulates any device incorporated into sleep testing in addition to that needed for detecting physiologic sleep. The founding technology for monitoring sleep was electroencephalogram (EEG) equipment that was used for research applications. As the field evolved, and later sleep-disordered breathing was identified for what it is, additional

parameters began to be recorded in conjunction with the EEG, electrooculogram (EOG), and electromyogram (EMG) needed for recording sleep architecture. The sensors and additional pieces of equipment that are interfaced with a modern sleep recording system are all considered ancillary devices.

Pressure transducers and thermocouple devices are used to monitor airflow, respiratory-induced plethysmography and piezoelectric belts can be used to monitor respiratory effort, and devices using piezo technology can be used to determine the presence of snoring. The oximeter probe uses a mixture of photoelectric and plethysmographic devices to determine the oxygen level in the blood.

Most ancillary sensors represent a type of transducer, a device that converts one form of energy into another. Transducers are most commonly used in sensing technology, allowing otherwise nonelectric phenomena to be converted into an electrical form for the purpose of recording. Ancillary recorders, or monitors, such as the pulse oximeter and end tidal carbon dioxide monitor are typically interfaced with the recorder via a DC amplifier input.

The discussion that follows is an introduction to equipment used in polysomnography with a focus on the electrical properties that allow them to operate. A more thorough treatment of ancillary equipment is offered later in this text.

DEVICES USED TO MONITOR AIRFLOW

Airflow in polysomnography refers to the inhalation and exhalation patterns of the patient. The airflow signal is a qualitative representation of the patient's ability to move air in and out of the nose and mouth, and is not monitored in terms of actual volume of air. Presently, airflow is monitored by at least two devices: a thermal sensor and a pressure transducer.

Thermal Sensor

A thermocouple makes use of the thermoelectric effect by which a junction of two dissimilar metals will create a voltage that is proportional to the temperature applied to the metals.[2] As the patient exhales, the metal conductors warm and a voltage develops between the hot junction of the two conductors near the mouth or nose and the cold junction away from the source of heat. This voltage potential also generates a current, because the thermocouple is a closed circuit and the recording equipment is able to digitize and produce an image based on these voltages. If the cold junction has a temperature slightly more than room temperature, but less than body temperature, then the voltage difference switches positive and negative sides as the patient exhales and inhales. If the cold junction is at body temperature, only the cooler temperatures produce a voltage potential.

Pressure Transducer

Pressure transducers detect the air pressure (or vacuum) produced by airflow at the nares. Several technologies exist for converting gas pressure into an electrical signal. One solution includes a thin film of metal or bonded metals that are deformed from air pushing on them, like a balloon being filled, but with a much more subtle deformation. As the film stretches, the metal becomes more resistive to current flow. This is called the piezoresistive effect. With a changing value of resistance, all that is needed is either a constant current moving through the metal film, or a constant voltage across the metal film. Ohm's law states that if the voltage across the film is constant, as with a battery for example, then any change in resistance will have an inverse change in current. In other words, if the resistance becomes greater, then the current decreases and the basis for an electric signal is set.

OXYGEN SENSORS

Pulse oximetry is the indirect monitoring of a patient's oxygen level by the use of sensors that detect light wave absorption. Varying colors of the light spectrum are absorbed or reflected more readily by different materials. Oxygenated blood, for example, absorbs infrared light more than deoxygenated blood. Deoxygenated blood absorbs more red light than oxygenated blood. These two variations of light can be detected on respective photoreceptors. As photons of the appropriate wavelength come into contact with the photoreceptor material, electrons are freed from the material and a voltage is generated. These voltages are compared to help identify an approximation of the patient's blood oxygen level.

It is worth observing that the blood has also gained energy, although the conversion of the photon's energy is most commonly into heat; hence the probe often seems to warm the skin. Energy is always conserved.

SNORE MICROPHONES

Standard diaphragm microphones have been used in the past for polysomnography recordings, but have many shortcomings. Ideally, the snore microphone should detect the patient's snoring; however, typical condenser and dynamic microphones depend on a moving diaphragm, which responds to any pressure wave strong enough to move the diaphragm back and forth. By using a piezoelectric device touching the skin of the patient, the mechanical vibration of snoring or vocalization is much stronger than the background noise of the sleep testing environment. The mechanical motion of the skin itself provides the mechanical energy that the piezoelectric material will convert to a voltage change.

POSITION SENSORS

The recording technologist is often responsible for determining and tracking the patient's orientation in the bed. The patient's orientation can be tracked visually, by way of video monitoring or the more manual method of looking in the room. These methods are prone to error, however, as bedding and pillows often obscure the patient position, or the low resolution of some video systems provides insufficient contrast for determining a reliable position.

Position sensors resolve these issues. Determining the position of a patient can be done in a variety of ways, and solutions provided by vendors are often proprietary. However, a simple liquid mercury model should demonstrate the principle well. Mercury is a liquid at room temperature and a conductor of electricity as a metal. If a sphere, made from an insulating material such as plastic, is filled halfway with mercury and several conductive wires are inserted through the plastic into the cavity, then it is possible to determine the position of the mercury at any given point by measuring the voltage across any two (or more) wires. As the patient rotates in bed, the liquid mercury moves within the ball, leveling itself with the surface of the earth, and the measurement of observable voltage shifts from one set of wires to another.

This model is clunky as it only detects changes in perfect 90-degree rotations. If the patient is resting in between a lateral and supine position, this particular design may not detect any position at all. Also, mercury is toxic to work with and creates a risk to the patient should the ball break open or a hole develop around the conductive wires. Several digital devices have come into the field of medical and consumer electronics, improving safety and precision of the sensor.

An accelerometer is a device that measures the acceleration of objects. Acceleration, in physics, occurs whenever an object experiences a change in direction or speed (or both). An accelerometer, in principle, makes use of a test weight, a spring, and a piezoelectric or piezoresistive device. The spring and weight, when no acceleration is occurring, is at a steady state. As the patient moves, the spring deforms under the acceleration of the test weight by either stretching or compressing under the changing direction. The compression or stretching of the spring deforms the piezoelectric device and a voltage change is detected.

CHAPTER SUMMARY

- Electricity involves the study, science, and technology associated with the flow of electric charges. Similar to gravity, electricity is understood through observable interactions.
- Static electricity involves the interactions of charged particles in close proximity to each other. Charges are described as being either *positive* or *negative*, which relates directly to the charges of protons and electrons, respectively, in atoms.

- Like-charged particles repel each other whereas oppositely charged particles attract each other. The strength of this attraction or repulsion varies proportionally to the amount of charge on each particle and inversely to the distance between the two particles. This relationship is described mathematically in Coulomb's law.
- Charge can be generated in several ways, but is most often generated from electromagnetic induction (generator motors) and electrochemistry (batteries). No matter how the charge is generated, it is always conserved. In other words, in any isolated system, charge cannot be created nor destroyed.
- Electronic circuits take advantage of the behavior of electricity through different elements to perform one or more functions. These elements are connected by a conductive medium, often a copper wire surrounded by an insulated medium.
- *Current* is the flow of electrons from a relatively negative origin to a relatively positive destination and is measured in amperes. This is opposite of conventional flow.
- Voltage is the potential difference in electrical energy from one point to another. The greater the voltage, the greater the force on charged particles. When voltage is transmitted through conductive wires at a constant rate it is called *direct current,* and when it continually switches between positive and negative values it is called *alternating current*
- Resistance is the impediment of current flow, both of which are related to voltage in Ohm's law. When an alternating sensing current is sent between two electrodes to measure opposition to current, the measure is called *impedance.*
- Earth grounding and power isolation are for patient safety. Grounding involves the connection of a circuit to a potential that is considered zero, the earth ground. Power isolation grounds the patient separately from the ground coming from the main power supply.
- All devices connected to the main recorder are collectively referred to as ancillary equipment.

References

1. Fitzgerald MJT: *Clinical neuroanatomy and neuroscience,* ed 5, Philadelphia, 2007, Elsevier.
2. Kasap SO: *Thermoelectric effects in metals: thermocouples,* Kasap, 2001, McGraw-Hill e-booklet.

REVIEW QUESTIONS

1. In regard to atomic structure, negative charges are associated with:
   a. Electrons
   b. Protons
   c. Neutrons
   d. Coulombs

2. In regard to atomic structure, positive charges are associated with:
   a. Electrons
   b. Protons
   c. Neutrons
   d. Coulombs

3. Current flow is the movement of:
   a. Lower voltage to higher voltage
   b. Higher voltage to lower voltage
   c. Electrons to protons
   d. Neutrons to protons

4. Which of the following produces an opposing force when brought together?
   a. Positive charge near a positive charge
   b. A positive charge near a neutral charge
   c. A positive charge near a negative charge
   d. A neutral charge near a neutral charge

5. Which of the following describes an open circuit?
   a. A circuit in which not all components are connected
   b. A circuit with access to a negative charge
   c. A circuit with compact electrical components
   d. A circuit in which the electrical element is bypassed

6. In polysomnographic testing, a ground is necessary to:
   a. DC toward the patient
   b. direct current away from the patient
   c. Keep the circuit patent
   d. Keep the circuit closed

7. A typical car battery operates using:
   a. Static electricity
   b. Electrochemical electricity
   c. Photoelectricity
   d. Piezoelectricity

8. A thermocouple works by:
   a. Measuring the piezoresistive effect
   b. Recording the resistance of two dissimilar metals
   c. Measuring the temperature of the ambient air
   d. Recording air vibrations

9. Hertz is defined as the number of:
   a. Rotations in a given time frame
   b. Electrical charges in a circuit
   c. Vibrations per second
   d. Electrons in an atom

10. Ohm's law is used in polysomnography to measure:
    a. Impedance
    b. Signal voltage
    c. Ground currency
    d. Electrode placement

Chapter 4

Frequency, Voltage, and Morphology of Signals

*Kristine Servidio • Buddy Marshall •
Bonnie Robertson • Margaret-Ann Carno*

CHAPTER OUTLINE

LEARNING OBJECTIVES

After reading this chapter, you will be able to:
1. Explain concepts related to bioelectric signals recorded on the polysomnogram.
2. Explain other physiologic signals of interest to the sleep technologist.
3. Describe the process of obtaining and recording physiologic parameters.
4. Inspect the effect of instrumentation and technologist action on study quality.
5. Examine waveform components related to data analysis and interpretation.
6. Observe waveform patterns representative of changing sleep-related variables.
7. Adjust instrumentation controls for optimal recording quality.

KEY TERMS

action potential
alternating current (AC)
  electricity
alternating current (AC)
  amplifier
amplitude
analog-to-digital converter
ancillary devices and
  equipment
artifacts
attenuate
bandwidth
baseline
biphasic
bipolar derivation
bipolar electrode board
bipolar inputs
bipolar jack box (see *bipolar
  electrode board*)
bipolar montage
bipolar recording and recorder
cannula
capacitance
common mode rejection
common mode signal
common referential montage

cycle
decay time constant
depolarize
derivation
differential amplifier
direct current (DC) amplifier
duration
electrode
electrode board
electrode lead or wire
electromyogram (EMG)
esophageal manometry
exploring electrode
frequency
gain
GIGO
graded potential
gradient
ground electrode
high-frequency filter (HFF)
impedance meter
inductance
international nomenclature
intrathoracic pressure - (see
  esophageal manometry)
low-frequency filter (LFF)

monophasic
montage.
morphology
notch filter
numerical nomenclature
outlet ground
paper speed
peak
polarity
polyphasic
potential difference
reference electrode
referential recorder and
  recording
resting potential
rise time constant
sampling rate
sensitivity
sinusoidal
system reference electrode
time base
transducer
triphasic
trough
WYSIWYG Technology

The word polysomnogram (PSG) with its derivatives breaks down to *poly,* meaning "many"; *somno,* meaning "sleep"; and *gram,* meaning "writing" or "recording." The term polysomnography was first used in 1974 by Holland and colleagues to describe the recording, analysis, and interpretation of multiple concurrent indicators of sleep physiology.[1] A polysomnograph recorder is a series of devices connected in sequence to sample, integrate, amplify, record, manipulate, store, and print a representation of physiologic data.

Analog polygraphs have almost exclusively been replaced by digital recorders that are remarkably similar to their predecessors. It is difficult to discuss the modern digital acquisition system without making reference to the analog recorder. This is particularly true when analog polygraphs are still in occasional use and the digital controls of current recorders were designed to mimic the analog controls of the past. Before a discussion of polysomnography can occur, the basic concepts of frequency, amplitude, and terminology related to waveforms need to be discussed.

ESSENTIALS OF PHYSIOLOGIC WAVEFORMS

FREQUENCY AND DURATION

Timing is a distinguishing characteristic of the waveforms recorded on a sleep study, and must be well understood. **Frequency** refers to the number of events observed to occur within a particular period, whereas **duration** is defined as how long a particular event lasts. On sleep recordings, the duration of physiologic parameters is measured in milliseconds, seconds, minutes, and hours. Duration is measured from **trough** to trough along the x-axis (horizontally).

The term band or band width is used to describe the range of frequencies associated with particular signals of interest, from lowest to highest. For example, the bandwidth of a sleep spindle typically includes frequencies of 12-14 **cycles** per second or hertz (Hz). Likewise, the overall bandwidth of an electroencephalogram (EEG) is made up of the frequencies from delta-range to beta-range activity, or 0.5 Hz to approximately 30 Hz, respectively. Frequency and duration have a reciprocal relationship, which can be beneficial toward both the understanding of concepts related to timing and analysis of very quickly and very slowly changing data.

Using D to denote the duration, in seconds (s), of a sine wave, similar to data measured during recording of physiologic parameters; and f to denote the frequency of waves in Hz, we can state the reciprocal relationship between average duration and frequency as:

$$f = 1 \div D \text{ and } D = 1 \div f$$

Calculation of Duration (D) and Frequency (f)

The average duration of one cycle making up a spindle burst is 0.07 seconds.

$$\text{(spindle } f = 14 \text{ Hz)} \quad 1 \div 14 = 0.07 \text{ s}$$

The average frequency of a cycle with a 4 seconds' duration is 0.25 Hz (Figure 4-1).

$$\text{(respiratory waveform } D = 4 \text{ s)} \quad 1 \div 4 = 0.25 \text{ Hz}$$

Measuring the exact duration of a fast waveform can be very difficult. In this case, assessment of the waveform frequency may be the best way to determine its timing. In Figure 4-1 a sine-wave calibration signal is generated by the calibration circuit of the recorder. Three complete cycles clearly occur in 1 second for a frequency of 3 Hz. Dividing 1 by the frequency of 3 Hz yields an average duration of 0.33 seconds. It is easy to see in this example that one cycle completes every ⅓ second.

When the frequency of a group of waves is 12 Hz, the reciprocal of 12 is calculated to determine the average waveform duration, 0.08 s. In a more easily calculated example, what if the frequency is 10 Hz? Simply divide 1 by 10 Hz for an average duration equal to 0.1 seconds. The accuracy of this calculation depends on the rhythmicity of the waves; if the width of individual waves varies, the estimation of

average duration will be skewed. For very rhythmic data, however, the calculated value of average duration can be quite accurate. This method of calculating average duration is of most benefit when assessing signals of very fast frequency such as epileptiform spikes. Alternatively, when signals are slower than one cycle per second, frequency can be difficult to conceive and duration may be the best choice for determination of this variable. When the duration of data is 1 second or longer, it is simple to measure.

As outlined previously, the reciprocal of duration is frequency. Consider a slow wave that lasts 3 seconds: $1 \div 3 \text{ s} = 0.33 \text{ Hz}$. In this example, one third of a cycle completes every second for an approximate frequency of 0.33 Hz. A waveform with duration of 10 seconds has an approximate frequency of 0.1 Hz, because $1 \div 10\text{s} = 0.1 \text{ Hz}$. In this example one tenth of a cycle occurs each second. Measuring duration and dividing by its value is most helpful when dealing with very slow frequency signals such as those associated with respiratory parameters. Figure 4-2 and Box 4-1 list and define the components of a waveform.

AMPLITUDE

Amplitude is the vertical height of a waveform, or the distance between the most positive and the most negative part of a wave. A negative signal produces an upward deflection on the polygraph, whereas a positive signal produces a downward deflection. This response to positive and negative signals is the result of the input selection. In the world of biopotentials, this has historically been described as **peak**-to-peak amplitude, although it is actually trough-to-peak amplitude with the amplitude being measured from the lowest point on the graph to the highest point at its immediate right (refer to Figure 4-2). Electrical brain biopotentials are measured in the range of microvolts (μV), which are one millionth of 1 volt.

Signal amplitude displayed on the PSG is an index of the voltage responsible for producing the deflection. According to the way in which data were obtained, the

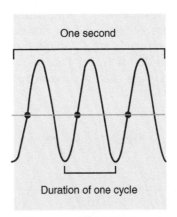

One second

Duration of one cycle

FIGURE 4-1 Recording of a machine-generated 3-Hz sine-wave signal of 1-second duration.

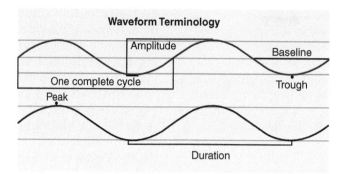

FIGURE 4-2 Components of a waveform.

BOX 4-1
Waveform Terminology

Peak: The highest point a wave reaches just before it begins to descend.

Trough: The lowest portion of a wave just before it rises.

Baseline: A horizontal plane that runs through the center of a wave.

Amplitude: The vertical distance, or height, of a waveform measured from a trough to the following peak; represents signal voltage.

Cycle: Identified as any point on a wave through its corresponding point as the wave repeats (e.g., peak to peak, trough to trough, or a rise from baseline to peak followed by a drop to trough and a return back to baseline). For physiologic data, the number of cycles is determined by counting the number of peaks.

Frequency: The number of cycles that occur within a specific timeframe (e.g., 1 second).

Duration: The time that it takes in seconds for a cycle to complete, as measured from trough to trough.

amount of voltage arising from the patient's body can be determined by measuring amplitude. For the most basic interpretation of frequency, duration, and voltage, the scale must be known. The two fundamental measures of scale required for evaluation of polysomnographic data are vertical height representative of a known voltage, and a horizontal distance equal to time in seconds. It is possible to have data of great vertical height that was actually derived from a low-voltage signal. Unless the

way in which the data were acquired or a physical scale to measure these data is known, the actual voltage, frequency, or duration of the physiologic data cannot be determined. Because amplitude is an index of voltage, if the amplification of the displayed signal is known, the signal's original voltage can be deduced. The polygraph controls responsible for increasing amplitude are the gain and sensitivity, which are discussed later.

MORPHOLOGY

The shape and number of phases that make up a waveform are known as the signal **morphology**. Along with morphology, additional characteristics, including frequency, amplitude, and polarity, influence a waveform's overall appearance. In Figure 4-3, 2 seconds of data containing perfectly rhythmic, machine-generated, sinusoidal (sine) waves are depicted at a frequency of 3 Hz. The 100 μV input signal resulted in an amplitude of one horizontal gridline to the next, referred to as one division. The recorder was calibrated to display 100 μV/division.

A waveform may be **sinusoidal** (s-shaped), irregular, **monophasic** (one phase), **biphasic** (two phases), **triphasic** (three phases), or **polyphasic** (many phases). A sinusoidal sleep spindle is s-shaped with a frequency of 12-14 cycles per second, whereas a delta wave is monophasic with an amplitude greater than 75 μV and frequency of 0.5 to 2 Hz. The low-amplitude, mixed-frequency EEG signal is polyphasic because it is composed of waves with several phases and varying amplitudes and frequencies. Figures 4-3 through 4-7 illustrate the multitude of waveform morphologies that exist.

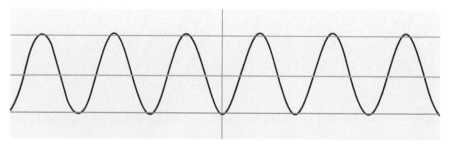

FIGURE 4-3 Sinusoidal (sine) wave.

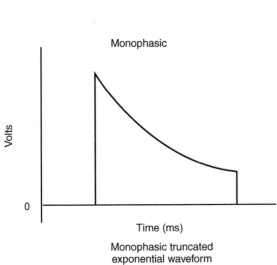

Monophasic

Monophasic truncated
exponential waveform
FIGURE 4-4 Monophasic waveform.

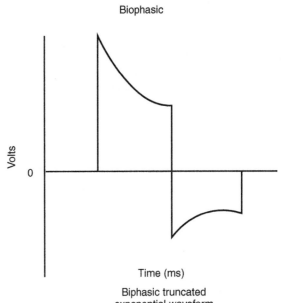

Biophasic

Biphasic truncated
exponential waveform
FIGURE 4-5 Biphasic waveform.

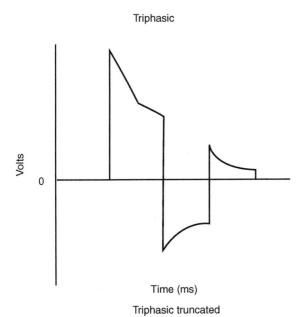

Triphasic

Triphasic truncated
exponential waveform
FIGURE 4-6 Triphasic waveform.

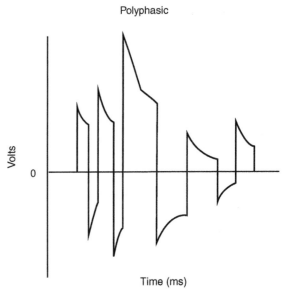

Polyphasic

Polyphasic truncated
exponential waveform
FIGURE 4-7 Polyphasic waveform.

BIOELECTRICAL SIGNALS

Electrical signals produced from living tissues are called **biopotentials**. Biopotentials are sampled using two electrodes connected to an amplifier via an input box. Biopotentials change in polarity, frequency, amplitude, and shape as cells **depolarize** or **repolarize** and as the cell membrane potential changes. As part of a sleep study, the overall patterns, including morphology, frequency, polarity, and amplitude of many summed bioelectric signals are recorded as the electroencephalogram (EEG), electrocardiogram (ECG), electrooculogram (EOG), and the **electromyogram (EMG)**.

The cell membrane does more than separate the intracellular fluid from the extracellular fluid. It defines the conditions under which the potential is measured.[2] Cell membrane permeability to potassium and sodium ions changes when a stimulus is introduced.

Resting Potential

The **resting potential** is the point when the amount of potassium leaving a cell is very close to the amount of potassium entering a cell. The cell membrane is considered depolarized when the membrane is less negative than the resting membrane potential. It is hyperpolarized when the membrane is more negative than the resting membrane potential. To keep potassium inside the cell and sodium outside the cell and not allow their **gradients**, or the difference between the two levels, to fall too low, the cell membrane has a "pump." The membrane sodium pump uses cellular energy to move excess sodium out of the cell and potassium back in.

Graded Potential

When a stimulus such as heat causes part of the membrane to change potential, it is called a **graded potential**. As current flows through the cell's cytoplasm, ions begin leaking out along the way because of membrane permeability to ions. These currents fizzle out within a few millimeters of the potential origin like water trickling through a leaky hose. This type of membrane potential does not lead to cell depolarization. Graded potentials play an important role in nerve activity, but action potentials create the "big bang" in physiology.

Action Potential

Action potentials are different from graded potentials in that they occur when a stimulus leads to a rapid change in cell membrane potential. During this 1-millisecond period, the cell membrane changes from $-70\ \mu V$ to $+30\ \mu V$ and then returns to its resting potential. Only nerve and muscle cells can excite the cell membrane enough to create an action potential.

During an action potential, the cell membrane becomes hundreds of times more permeable to sodium ions. As sodium ion with a positive ionic charge (Na^+) rushes into the cell, the intracellular fluid becomes more positive than the extracellular fluid. Sodium entry is greater than the amount of potassium, a negatively charged ion (K^-), exiting the cell. This point is called the **threshold**. Then, as membrane permeability is quickly turned off, the membrane permeability to potassium increases. Sodium entry slows down, potassium moves out of the cell, and repolarization to **baseline** occurs. After depolarization, it takes time for the cell membrane to return to its baseline permeability for sodium and potassium. During this refractory period, another stimulus is not likely to trigger another action potential until the cell can recover. The refractory period is similar in length to the depolarizing membrane changes.

Action potentials in nerve cells are usually initiated at the cell receptors and travel in one direction, along the nerve cell body to the axon terminals. Current flows away from the stimulus and to other neurons in close proximity similar to an electrical relay system. Action potentials that occur in skeletal muscle are initiated in the middle and spread in two directions, causing muscle contractions. Because potentials are so small, networks of cells with summed charges, called **potential fields**, are measured.[2,3] The recorded signals of a polysomnograph are composed of constantly changing electrical voltages.

POLARITY

Polarity can be defined as having oppositely charged poles (dipoles), one positive and one negative. Polarity determines which direction a current flows. Cortical cells line up in a row and behave like the poles of a magnet. Current generated by these rows of cells flows from the relatively positive to the relatively negative poles, creating a sinusoidal rhythm resembling **alternating current (AC) electricity.**

The voltages from the patient's body are measured using electrodes that are directly attached to the surface of the skin. Small insulated wires connect the electrodes to special amplifiers with the purpose of increasing or amplifying the size of the signal so it can be visualized by the naked eye. The signal is also filtered to **attenuate**, or minimize, the frequencies that are above and below the frequency range of the particular data being recorded for the purpose of reducing unwanted waveform interference, or **artifacts**. In this way, signals unrelated to the particular parameter being observed can be minimized. Artifacts can arise from the body, the environment, or the recording circuit itself.

In respect to circuit artifact, both stray **capacitance** and **inductance** can develop within the recording circuit and cause unwanted current to flow. Capacitance is the ability of a body, or capacitor, to store a charge. When conductive plates are separated by insulators, such as the three wires in the recorder power cord, current can be generated and recorded as artifact. Inductance occurs as the result of the electromagnetic properties of alternating current (AC) electricity. When a circuit such as the patient input cable lies in close proximity to another circuit that is carrying AC electricity, an AC current with opposing polarity can develop (be induced) in the circuit not previously carrying it. This is particularly true when the cables run parallel to one another. When this occurs, the ground wire cannot effectively carry unwanted electrical noise away from the recorder and artifact appears on the recording. More importantly, the equipment ground wire and building ground are unable to direct current (DC) away from the patient in the event of excessive electrical leakage current. Electrical safety is covered in detail in Chapter 6.

RECORDING EQUIPMENT, CONTROLS, AND PRACTICES

ELECTRODES AND ELECTRODE BOARDS

An **electrode** is a small device, typically constructed from highly conductive metal, which provides an interface between the skin and amplifier through a small insulated wire known as an **electrode lead** or **electrode wire**. Electrodes are most often constructed from a precious metal and may be metal plate over another metal or even metal plate over plastic.

When a metal electrode is plated with another metal, as when a silver electrode is gold-plated, care must be taken not to crack or scratch the thin plating. When two metals contact one another within a recording channel, electrical potentials are generated, similar to the way a battery produces DC electricity. These electrical potentials show up as unwanted signals known as artifacts, which contaminate the recording.

Care should also be taken to avoid fracturing the small conductive wire across which data travels between the patient and the **electrode board**. These wires can be easily broken, resulting in intermittent loss of signal and artifact, or complete loss of data from the patient.

Conductive electrolyte material, typically a paste or gel, reduces resistance between the skin and the electrode and enhances the electrode's ability to detect microvolt changes at the skin's surface. Electrodes are attached to the patient and plugged into the **electrode board** at the bedside. This input receptacle may also be referred to by various other names, including the terminal box, input board, head box, and jack box. Bioelectrical signals travel from the patient electrodes to the electrode board.

Many electrode boards also act as the interface between the amplifiers and signals from the various transducers attached to the patient. Transducers used during testing may include a snoring microphone or sensor, a body position sensor, a thermal air flow sensor, respiratory inductive plethysmography belts, and pressure flow transducers. Some head boxes also allow the technologist to directly input ancillary equipment signals such as those from an oximeter, carbon dioxide (CO_2) monitor and positive airway pressure device. Other systems have a secondary amplifier or in-line signal processor to receive ancillary equipment signals.

Many current recording systems incorporate differential amplifiers, filters, and digitizers into a bedside computer. From there, processed data can be sent via wireless remote to another computer in the instrumentation room. The majority of facilities, however, route data to the instrumentation room computers via CAT-5 cable or something similar, through the ceiling of the testing room and across the facility to the instrumentation room for connection to the recorder.[4]

DATA ACQUISITION SYSTEMS

The numbers and letters on the jack box correspond to either the anatomic location at which electrodes are placed or numbers, each of which are used by the technologist to route physiologic data through the various system components and amplifiers for recording at the output. The system of organizing electrodes and associated equipment using anatomic locations is referred to as **international nomenclature**, whereas **numerical nomenclature** refers to the system of numbers used to identify these items.

In some cases, a shielded multiconductor cable runs from the jack box to preamplifiers and then to a personal computer where data are digitized. This type of system is much like an analog recorder with the exception that data are output from the amplifiers to an **analog-to-digital converter** instead of being output to galvanometers and recorded on paper. The most common digital acquisition systems in use today, however, digitize data within the electrode board before sending it to a computer. Both advantages and disadvantages exist to each of these methods of obtaining data.

Many digital acquisition systems will have one of these arrangements in use for cephalic electrodes, but use a simpler convention for transducers and signals for which input changes are only infrequently necessary or no advantage is gained by electrically tying them to a common connection, known as a **system reference electrode**. Instead of a system reference, this system uses **bipolar inputs** (not to be confused with bipolar recordings) that route two electrodes or the two cables from a transducer directly to the recording parameter's amplifier.

As an example, the nasal airflow sensor has two connections that are plugged into the electrode board. In the previously described arrangement, each of the two connectors is plugged into predetermined inputs in the electrode board. Within the recorder software, or by using another method of selecting electrodes, the two inputs are chosen for the channel where nasal airflow is to be recorded. With bipolar inputs, either numbers are assigned to the two inputs on the electrode board or they may be labeled, such as "nasal airflow." The two connectors are plugged into the "nasal airflow" input 1 and input 2, or perhaps "channel 10" input 1 and input 2. In this scenario the signals are directly routed to channel 10 where nasal airflow is intended to be recorded.

The electrode board illustrated in Figure 4-8 provides examples of various signal input types. The inputs in the top half of the interface use both international nomenclature for the head and numerical nomenclature for numbers 22 through 33. This portion of the input board relies on a common system reference electrode against which every other electrode plugged into the top of the board is recorded.

The system reference electrode is typically placed at Cz as an electrically neutral recording site, although some laboratories prefer Cz or Pz, and for some recorders a back-up reference electrode option exists. The back-up option is usually placed at Fz or Pz. While data are being acquired, each electrode is recorded tied to the electrically neutral system reference. During acquisition and during subsequent review, the data from two electrodes is linked to display a channel of data through the Input 1-Input 2 convention. When data obtained from electrode 2, tied to the system reference is subtracted from electrode 1 tied to the system reference, the system reference data are subtracted out of the equation and data from electrode 1 and electrode 2 remain. This process is referred to as a **referential recording** and the equipment that is used is a **referential recorder**.

In addition to referential inputs, the system that uses this electrode board has both bipolar input capabilities and direct DC connections. Bipolar inputs

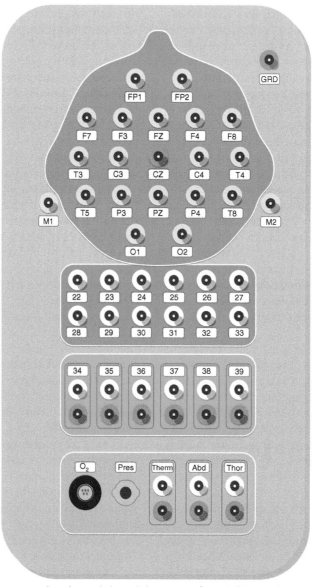

FIGURE 4-8 Representative electrode board that uses referential inputs for system referencing, bipolar input capabilities, and direct current connections at the bedside.

allow the two signals needed to make up a channel derivation to be plugged into the electrode board and directly connected to the amplifier channel on which the data will be displayed. This type of connection is ideal for signals such as those monitoring breathing that need little, if any, manipulation throughout the test aside from what is under digital control. For channels requiring derivation or polarity changes, bipolar inputs are impractical as the changes must be made by changing plugs in the electrode board. Likewise, when one input needs to be routed to more than one derivation, electrode "jumpers" must be used, which add another path for artifact to invade the recording.

Direct DC connections allow ancillary equipment, such as a pulse oximeter or end-tidal CO_2 monitor to be routed directly through the bedside input board. Most often, when these devices reside in the patient's room, an additional cable must be routed to the instrumentation room. In some cases, the pulse oximeter may be integrated with the input board, allowing direct connection of the pulse oximeter probe.

Although not widely used, recorders have been produced with a "bipolar" electrode board. In other words, each recording channel is routed to two predefined inputs in the electrode board. Whatever was to be displayed on channel 1 would be plugged into the electrode board at channel 1, input 1 and input 2, and so forth for the total number of recording channels. For recording EEG and other bioelectric signals, this method of connecting electrodes to the input board is not very practical as it limits the ability to make changes during the recording, among other issues. The bipolar inputs can, however, work well when used along with a more robust electrode board and electrode selection system. The majority of acquisition systems currently in use have some bipolar capabilities.

ELECTRODE IMPEDANCE

Resistance is measured between the electrode and scalp using an **impedance meter**. In fact, electrode **impedance** is actually the combined measure of skin resistance, electrode resistance, electrode wire resistance, and resistance within the input board. Resistance within the patient circuit is measured using an impedance meter rather than an Ohm meter for important, practical reasons.

When the impedance measure of an electrode is being tested and recorded by the impedance meter, a low-voltage AC signal is delivered to the electrode that is unlikely to be perceived by the patient. The AC signal is similar to the varying signals generated by the patient; therefore, the assessment of resistance is physiologically similar to the signal occurring during data acquisition. Most importantly, however, if a DC Ohm meter is used to measure resistance while the

electrodes are attached to the patient's skin, the electrodes will become polarized and electrochemical burns to the skin are possible. The formula for impedance also takes into consideration the effects that capacitance and inductance have on the AC circuit.

When impedance measures are low and equal within a derivation being routed to a differential amplifier, the common signals are minimized and the dissimilar signals remain as recorded data. The ability of a differential amplifier to minimize signals common at both inputs is known as **common mode rejection**. Common mode rejection is responsible for minimizing artifacts, particularly those from the surrounding environment. This is an important reason why differential amplifiers are used for physiologic testing.

RECORDING POLARITY

On the PSG, polarity refers to the upward (negative) or downward (positive) direction of most recorded signals. Recording polarity can either be changed during or after data acquisition in various ways. Early polysomnographs allowed the technologist to plug electrodes into a jack box and select each of two inputs for a given channel, via an electrode selector panel. Each channel had two dedicated rows of inputs, or grids, referred to as G1 and G2, which routed signals to its amplifier. By convention, G2 was always subtracted from G1 to yield the **potential difference** between the two input signals. Swapping these connections would reverse the signal polarity on the recording. Depending on the recording system being used, polarity may be changed by reversing the two inputs on an electrode selector panel, the insertion position of the two electrodes in a bipolar input board (jack box), input selection within recording or review software, or other means.

Typically, channels recording biopotentials are adjusted for an upward deflection in response to a negative input: the ECG channel is adjusted for an upright P wave, and respiratory channels are adjusted for an upright deflection during inspiration and a downward deflection during exhalation. On the other hand, recording channels for DC signals, like that from a pulse oximeter, are usually configured for an upright deflection in response to a positive input. This convention yields an upward deflection when oxyhemoglobin values increase and a downward deflection when values decrease.

When making changes to polarity, and other parameters on a digital acquisition system, the recording technologist must be aware of whether these are temporary "display" changes seen only during recording, or whether these are permanent "hardware" changes that will be retained for subsequent review by the scoring technologist, physician, and others.

AMPLIFIERS

Once acquired, electronic data travel to an amplifier where they are adjusted to a viewable height and the signal is filtered to minimize extraneous signals. The **differential amplifier**, common to polysomnography, retains the difference between two input signals while subtracting components simultaneously common to both inputs.

Common amplifier controls include gain or sensitivity used to adjust the amplitude, or height of the output signal. A **low-frequency filter (LFF)** is used to minimize the amplitude of signals slower than those wanted on the recording, whereas a **high-frequency filter (HFF)** is used to attenuate the amplitude of frequencies above the signals of interest. These filters allow the user to select bioelectrical signals within a discrete frequency range of most interest to the sleep technologist.[6]

A line filter may also be used to minimize the amplitude of frequencies consistent with power line noise that will contaminate the recording from any proximal source of electrical leakage current. In the United States, line current travels at a frequency of 60 Hz, requiring a 60-Hz line filter. In many other countries, the line filter is specific to 50 Hz because this is the frequency at which power travels in these areas.

Depending on how data are digitized, signals entering the electrode board will be directed to a particular amplifier either through software selection, by choosing inputs on a mechanical electrode selector panel composed of buttons or switches, or, as previously mentioned, directly through input 1 and 2 of a **bipolar electrode board**.

Direct Current (DC) and Alternating Current (AC) Amplifiers

The two types of amplifiers currently employed by all data acquisition systems used for polysomnography are the **direct current (DC) amplifier** and the **alternating current (AC) amplifier**.

Direct Current (DC) Amplifier

When current is constant and flows in only one direction through a conductor, it is called direct current (DC) electricity. DC is either on or off; there is no in-between. It does not decay and remains at full amplitude until the power source is either removed or depleted, as depicted in Figure 4-9. Devices like an oximeter and a capnometer respond to slowly changing variables, and generate an output signal that is likewise slowly changing.

The DC amplifier, designed to monitor constant or slowly changing variables, was so named because of the similarities between signals it is intended to record and the characteristics of DC electricity.[1,5] A defining characteristic of a DC amplifier is its lack of a LFF. When an amplifier has an LFF, the signal it processes will decay over time, even at the lowest settings. Without an LFF, no **fall time constant** (TC) exists and the signal will not decay. The lack of an LFF makes the DC amplifier ideally suitable for recording constant or slowly moving variables such as those mentioned previously.

If a signal, like that from an oximeter, is recorded using an AC amplifier, the signal will decay too quickly for the data to be meaningful. Although the DC amplifier has no LFF, it does have an HFF that can be used to attenuate fast-moving noise arising from external sources.[9] Because signals requiring a DC amplifier are most often directly connected rather than being routed through the input board, some technologists have referred to this type of amplifier as a *direct coupled amplifier*.

Alternating Current (AC) Amplifier

AC amplifiers were named by similar convention. The polarity of AC electricity alternates at a constant frequency of 60 Hz in the United States and 50 Hz in many other countries. AC amplifiers were so named because the data for which they are suitable to record is relatively fast, similar to AC electricity. The AC amplifier has both an LFF (high-pass filter) used to attenuate unwanted, slowly moving variables, and an HFF (low-pass filter) for attenuation of unwanted fast signals.

The EEG, EOG, EMG, and ECG signals recorded during a sleep study often exhibit rapid changes in polarity and frequency and extraneous slow components of the data need to be attenuated. The signal processing capabilities of its filters and the range of an AC amplifier make it ideal for recording these physiologic parameters. Filters are set above and below the frequencies of interest to minimize unwanted fast and slow signals without affecting the data being sampled.

Differential Amplifier

A differential amplifier has two connections for receiving electrical information. Amplifiers used to record biopotentials are called differential amplifiers because

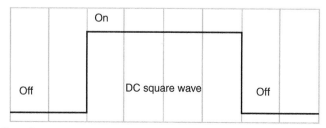

FIGURE 4-9 A direct current calibration signal with unfiltered square-wave morphology.

they measure the potential difference between input 1 and input 2. These inputs were originally called *G1* and *G2* (grid 1 and grid 2). By convention, input 2 is always subtracted from input 1. The continuously changing difference between these two inputs is processed by amplifier controls (filters; gain or sensitivity) prior to being output as data to the acquisition system.

For a fundamental understanding of this process, it is helpful to consider a single, fixed point in time. The following derivations, and their numerical values at the moment in time, exist for channels one through four using the input 1 – input 2 convention:

C4-O2 $-70\ \mu V - (-30\ \mu V)$
$$= -70\ \mu V + 30\ \mu V = -40\ \mu V$$

C4-M1 $-70\ \mu V - (50\ \mu V)$
$$= -70\ \mu V - 50\ \mu V = -120\ \mu V$$

F4-M1 $50\ \mu V - (50\ \mu V)$
$$= 50\ \mu V - 50\ \mu V = 0\ \mu V$$

M1-C4 $50\ \mu V - (-70\ \mu V)$
$$= 50\ \mu V + 70\ \mu V = 120\ \mu V$$

C4-O2: Input 1 is more negative than input 2, so there is a negative (upward) deflection.

C4-M1: Input 1 is also more negative than input 2.

F4-M1: Input 1 and input 2 are identical, resulting in no deflection.

M1-C4: Input 1 is more positive than input 2, so there is a positive (downward) deflection.

Note the difference in output from the C4-M1 and M1-C4 derivations. Reversing the inputs has reversed the polarity of the channel.

DERIVATIONS, MONTAGES, AND RECORDER TYPES

Derivations

Electrode selection is the first step the technologist takes toward choosing which data are sampled for each channel. Each channel is defined by the two input signals from which the displayed data are made up, known as the channel **derivation**. The derivation is simply a listing of input 1 and input 2 written as electrode name—electrode name 2. By convention, input 1 is always referred to as the **exploring electrode**, whereas input 2 is always the **reference electrode**. These designations have no bearing on the anatomic location or type of data being introduced to the two inputs, respectively.

It is important for EEG electrode impedances to be less than 5 K Ohms to ensure optimum amplifier performance and artifact rejection. Electrodes act like tiny antennae and pick up extraneous artifacts, including electrical leakage current from power lines, overhead lights, some appliances, and even the recorder

itself. When the exploring electrode and the reference electrode have relatively equal impedance values, the differential amplifier effectively measures the potential difference between the two. It can then amplify the difference and attenuate the common signal that arises from other sources. If the two electrodes within a derivation have imbalanced impedances, the common mode rejection feature of a differential amplifier will be ineffective for attenuating the unwanted signals.[6,7,8]

Montages

In simplest terms, a **montage** is a listing of derivations or recording channels. The montage defines, at the very minimum, the order of recording channels and the location from which data were obtained during the particular study. In reference to digital acquisition systems, the montage is a predefined configuration of channels showing how data are to appear on the computer screen.

The electronic montage consists of channel label and type, channel inputs, channel order, label and tracing color, and amplifier settings most typically used for each channel. An unlimited number of montages can be programmed for a digital recorder. In reality, only a few montages need be predefined for recording sleep diagnostic and therapeutic studies. The technologist can view the specific channels of a selected montage while recording, and while additional data are being acquired and stored for later inspection as needed. Likewise, the montage can be adjusted at any time during data acquisition. This is the main advantage of using a system reference electrode to perform a referential recording (not to be confused with a *referential montage*). Data obtained in this manner can be manipulated after the fact, or in real time, to display derivations composed of any two electrodes.

The Bipolar Montage

Along with the data typically recorded on a sleep study, additional EEG derivations, similar to what is obtained in the clinical EEG laboratory, may be requested. The ordering practitioner may request a **bipolar montage** to set up a chain of potentials for recording on separate channels.

Analog systems allowed the technologist to select a string of **bipolar derivations,** composed of exploring electrodes that overlie electrically active recording sites for both input 1 and input 2, using a mechanical electrode selector panel. This could also be accomplished using a **bipolar jack box** on which designated connections listed for input 1 and input 2 of each channel routed signals directly to the respective amplifier.

Today, the selector panel has been replaced by a digital system with software control of electrode switching. A bipolar montage is made up of bipolar derivations that allow the recording of data from electrically active recording sites on each channel. With a bipolar montage the potential for misinterpretation of an abnormality is essentially eliminated because the same field can be viewed in both positive and negative polarities. Figure 4-10, *A*, displays electrode connections for one of the bipolar montages. Figure 4-10, *B*, is an example of an EEG displayed in a bipolar montage.

The Referential Montage

Sleep study recordings are typically performed using referential derivations for the EEG and EOG channels. These channels make up a short **referential montage**. For this reason, it is said that a referential montage is employed during sleep testing, despite the fact that various channels are recorded from bipolar derivations. For a referential montage, all G1 inputs are independently selected from electrodes that overlie an electrically active area on the head. All G2 inputs are connected to either the right mastoid (M2) or left mastoid (M1) electrode. The exploring electrode, sometimes called the active electrode, is connected to input 1, and a mastoid reference, or silent electrode is connected to input 2. Theoretically, when the silent electrode potential is subtracted from input

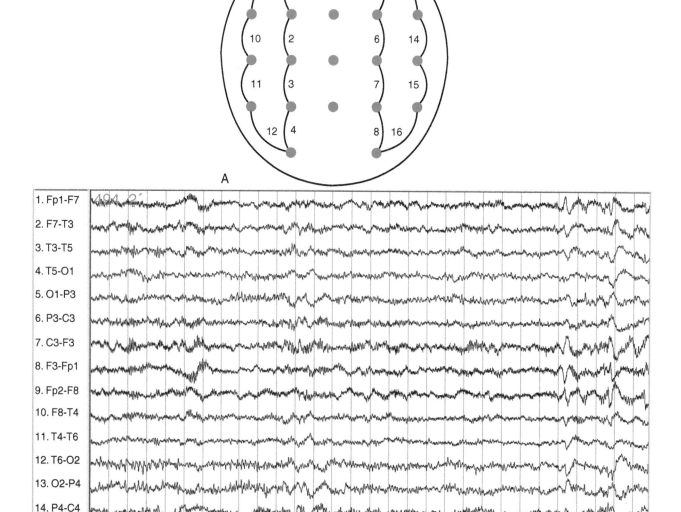

FIGURE 4-10 **A,** Represents electrode selection for a bipolar electroencephalogram (EEG) montage; **B,** EEG displayed in a bipolar montage.

1, the result is the potential from that field less any activity common to both inputs.

Figure 4-11, *A,* illustrates electrode selection for a referential montage. Figure 4-11, *B,* is an EEG displayed in a referential montage. The sleep technologist should be familiar with both bipolar and referential montages and be able to distinguish between the proper uses of each.

The following depicts the output of a referential derivation at a fixed point in time. The referential derivations that make up a referential montage yield higher voltage signals than those recorded using bipolar derivations:

$$\text{Input 1} = \text{exploring} = \text{C4} = -150 \ \mu\text{V}$$
$$-150 \ \mu\text{V} - (0 \ \mu\text{V}) = -150 \ \mu\text{V}$$

$$\text{Input 2} = \text{reference} = \text{M1} = 0 \ \mu\text{V}$$

Data Recording

Data from a referential recording can be used to display bipolar derivations, referential derivations,

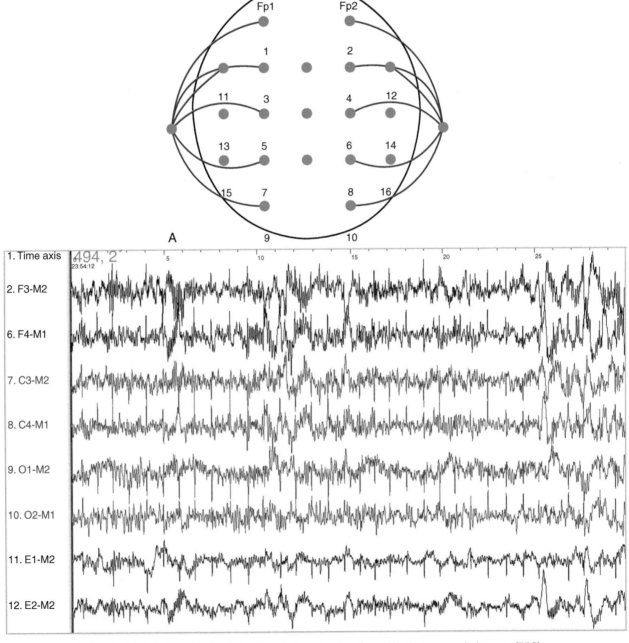

FIGURE 4-11 **A,** Represents electrode selection for a referential electroencephalogram (EEG) montage; **B,** EEG displayed in a referential montage.

bipolar montages, or referential montages. For referential recording, as opposed to **bipolar recording**, all electrodes are recorded as the exploring electrode in a derivation for which a common, system reference electrode, typically placed at Cz or Fz, is recorded in the input 2, or reference, position. These derivations are stored in the background of the recording and accessed as needed to produce a viewable derivation within a montage. By the convention known as input 1 – input 2, the system reference electrode is subtracted from the equation and what remains for display are the two electrodes originally in the *exploring* position. This is more thoroughly discussed later.

The main drawback to using a system reference electrode is that the recording relies on the patency of a single electrode. If the system reference electrode becomes faulty, all channels recorded referentially will be contaminated with artifact, requiring the technologist to disrupt sleep testing to repair or replace the electrode. Most modern systems offer the capability of placing a backup system reference electrode that can be selected within the recorder software to avoid this problem. The backup electrode is typically placed at Fz or Pz.

A *bipolar recorder* refers to the original analog recorders, now known as *polysomnographs.* Digital recorders use analog amplifiers for which data are digitized between the amplifier system and the computer. The main drawback to this type of recording is that new channel derivations cannot be viewed after the fact. Whatever is seen by the recording technologist during acquisition is the permanent record. This has been referred to as "what you see is what you get" (**WYSIWYG**) technology.

Although modern technology provides the ability to record data and to filter unwanted characteristics later, after-the-fact digital manipulation is no substitute for a clear, artifact-free study that was maintained in real time. Post-hoc manipulation of data by digital filters has limitations. When the input data quality is poor, the output will simply be filtered poor-quality signals.

Digital technology, no matter how advanced, is always limited by the acronym **GIGO**, or garbage-in-garbage-out. Furthermore, if the study is not relatively artifact-free in the first place, it can be difficult or impossible for the recording technologist to identify a new artifact when it arises or to determine whether the underlying signals are intact. Filters are only useful when the underlying signals of interest are intact. The sleep technologist must be proficient at analyzing signals during data acquisition to produce a clear, artifact-free tracing; identify and quantify sleep stages; determine the presence of pathologic conditions; and identify when therapeutic intervention is warranted.[4]

The Recorder

Paper chart recorders were, and occasionally still are, used to record bioelectrical signals. A paper chart recorder operates by having large stacks of folded paper, similar to that commonly used for a dot-matrix computer printer in the past, pulled from right to left underneath pens that move back and forth. On this type of system a galvanometer, consisting of a magnet with a wound coil of wire attached to a pen mount drove a pen for each recording channel. In response to a voltage, the coil of wire and pen mount moved. Many chart recorders contained as many as 24 pens and could, therefore, record 24 different channels of data simultaneously. These were very sophisticated machines, capable of recording signals that change even faster than a person can write. The **paper speed** was very well controlled.

When paper speed is a known constant, the time between signals or interesting parts of the signals can be determined by measuring the distance between them on the paper using a scale. Likewise, the height, or amplitude, of a signal is measured to easily determine the amount of voltage required to produce it, as long as scale is known. Paper studies from analog systems were recorded at a 10 mm/second paper speed. The technologist viewed 30 seconds of data on each 300-mm- wide sheet of recording paper.

Using computers to record physiologic data allows the technologist to record and review data at the standard 30-second epoch or in any one of various time increments. Data can be viewed in real time during acquisition or after the fact in segments lasting 1 second, 10 seconds, 30 seconds, 1 minute, 1 hour, or the entire recording. When data are compressed or stretched out so either shorter or longer segments of the study can be viewed on the screen at a time, this is referred to as changing the **time base** (Figure 4-12, *A-C*).

Using recorders of the past, studies were limited by the number of amplifiers or the number of galvanometers that the polysomnograph would accommodate. With the digital systems of today, the issue of not having enough recording channels is a thing of the past. The question that arises today relates to the number of channels that can be effectively monitored on a computer screen.

Instead of measuring amplitude distance for determination of voltage or horizontal distance to determine duration, digital acquisition system software offers options for electronically determining these parameters. How this task is accomplished varies from system to system. Most recorders, however, provide vertical gridlines or other markers that represent 1 second, 10 seconds, or some other amount of time depending on the epoch size being viewed. Typically, there is also a horizontal amplitude gridline feature or some way to visually determine amplitude and approximate voltage at a glance. In addition to these reference markers, most systems provide some form

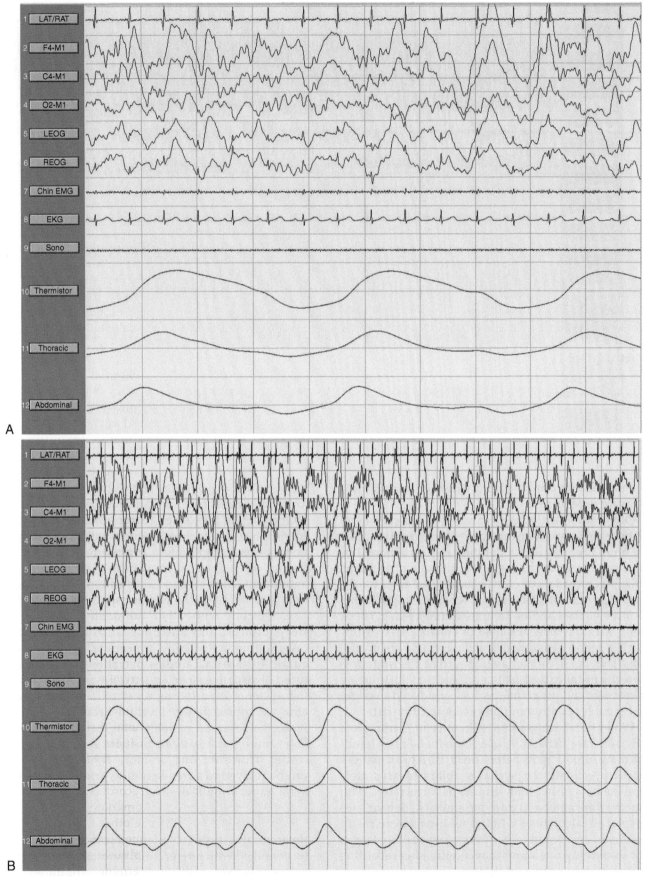

FIGURE 4-12 Views of recorded data beginning on the same second with different time base: **A,** typical display of sleep study data at 30 seconds per epoch; **B,** an expanded 1-second view of the sleep study recording;

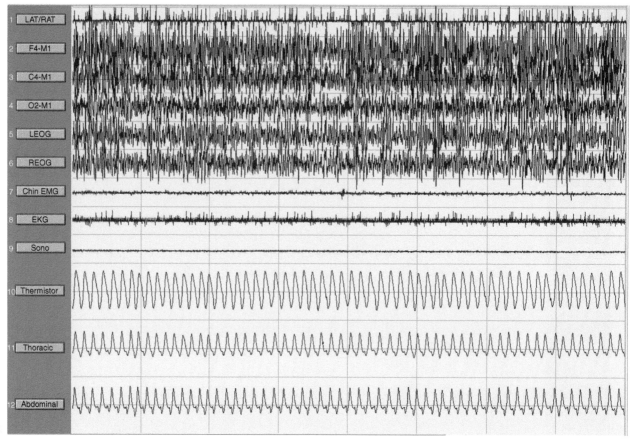

C

FIGURE 4-12, cont'd **C,** a compressed 240-second (4-minute) view of the study data.

of a cursor that can be placed when a more accurate measure is required.

Often, the exact voltage of a waveform can seemingly be seen instantaneously by simply placing a cursor on it. Likewise, exact duration can be obtained by placing a cursor at the beginning and end of an event.

Digital recorders offer many additional tools for the recording technologist, some of which help him or her be more vigilant and/or accurate during testing. These, along with the tools available to enhance sleep study scoring, report generation, and data review, are invaluable. This is, of course, assuming that the system is correctly installed and calibrated, and that the software developers and programmers have produced a system that reliably acquires and processes accurate data.

When purchasing a new system or upgrading to a new software version, it may be beneficial to hand-calculate report parameters on a variety of patient types to validate the system's ability to accurately tabulate data rather than assume its correctness. With the overlap among report parameters, one or two misplaced calculations within the software can result in drastic and potentially devastating results. This is not something one wants to recognize after recording and scoring hundreds of studies.

Despite the erroneous data that sometimes has to be found and followed up on by the end user, digital acquisition and computer-assisted manual scoring are much more efficient than the processes of the past. Unfortunately, the reliability of automated sleep study scoring has not been adequately validated for adoption by most sleep centers. Practitioners who use this feature often spend a great deal of time editing the automated sleep stage scoring and even event detection, depending on the patient type being studied.

Consistent with other automated measures of sleep, arousal, and breathing, such as pulse transit time, automated scoring appears to be the least accurate for scoring studies of patients with complicated obstructive sleep apnea (OSA).[1,9] Even some of the systems reported as most reliable may not be able to approach the level of accuracy a human scorer achieves on patients with complicated OSA.[9] Polysomnograph systems of today have no chart recorder. However, one or more time-based epochs can be relayed to a free-standing printer for producing a paper copy, if desired.

Referential Recording

Referential recording (system referencing) should not be confused with a referential montage. A referential montage is a way of displaying recorded data, whereas a referential recording is a method of acquiring data using a digital recorder. Data recorded with a system reference can be displayed after the fact in bipolar derivations, referential derivations, bipolar montages, or referential montages. Data from each exploring and reference electrode is saved independent of other recording electrodes. These data can be placed into derivations to display any combination of recording sites desired during acquisition or review of data.

In this method of data acquisition, a common or system reference electrode, typically placed at Fz or Cz, is recorded alongside each exploring and reference electrode to yield G1-ref for each electrode plugged into the digital acquisition system electrode board. Display derivations are constructed from the combination of any two G1-ref derivations recorded to computer memory. When the quantity of G1-ref is subtracted from another G1-ref, the two exploring electrodes (G1-G1) remain. With a referential recording any possible combination of electrodes can be displayed in a derivation during or after acquisition.

Recorded to computer memory:

O2-ref, M1-ref, M2-ref, C4-ref, C3-ref, O1-ref, etc.

Example display derivation:

$$O2\text{-ref} - (M1\text{-ref}) =$$
$$O2\text{-ref} - M1 + \text{ref} =$$
$$O2\text{-}\cancel{\text{ref}} - M1 + \cancel{\text{ref}} =$$
$$O2\text{-}M1$$

Differential amplifiers perform the first step in signal processing. As discussed previously, differential amplifiers have two input connections for each channel displayed as output on the monitor, known as derivations. The order in which the derivations are arranged for viewing is the montage. Sleep recordings typically use a montage that displays data in a similar order as the following, although order of recording parameters is according to laboratory preference.[10] See Figure 4-13 for the settings recommended by the American Academy of Sleep Medicine (AASM).

The EEG configuration included in the previous derivation is a **common referential montage**. The F4 electrode is located over an electrically active cephalic site. This exploring electrode is input 1 in the channel 1 derivation. The mastoid reference electrode located at M1 is connected to input 2 and is used in multiple derivations. The reference electrode is located over the bony area behind the ear where relatively little bioelectrical activity occurs. When input 2 (M1) is subtracted from input 1 (F4), most of the potential difference will be amplified producing a wave form of higher amplitude than would be present using a bipolar derivation.[3]

Annotation and Documentation

Throughout acquisition, the technologist can annotate the recording with information about study conditions, patient actions, or anything else relevant to testing at the exact moment it occurs on a digital acquisition system. In addition to this real-time annotation, information can typically be entered ahead of time so that the touch of a button or two is all that is required to document commands and comments commonly made during testing. Annotations become part of the medical record and are useful when looking back during acquisition and when reviewing the stored recording at a later date. Technologist's notes also provide the reviewer information about the recording that may not be apparent when visualizing the recorded signals.

Whenever changes are made to amplifier settings, most acquisition systems will make some form of entry into the record. In addition, the technologist should document the change being made and his or her rationale for the change. Depending on the testing facility, the technologist may be responsible for writing a narrative summary in addition to ongoing documentation.

Always be mindful that everything entered into the acquisition system becomes a part of the patient's medicolegal record, and that documentation may be the only interaction between the recording technologist and ordering practitioner.

SIGNAL SAMPLING

With traditional paper chart recorders, a continuous input signal is obtained from the patient and applied to the system as the deflecting pen makes a continuous mark on the moving paper. With digital acquisition systems, there are no paper or pens. Advanced signal acquisition theory is applied to take periodic samples of the continuous signal and store them. The samples are generally obtained at a fixed rate, called a **sampling rate**. For example, very fast signals may be sampled at 1000 times per second. For 1000 samples per second, a sample is obtained every 1 millisecond. For simplicity, this is often described as a sampling rate of 1000 Hz.[10] However, it is not a 1000-Hz signal; it is the process of obtaining 1000 samples per second. The use of Hz indicates the speed of sampling and does not imply anything about the signal.

The Nyquist-Shannon sampling theorem states that a digital copy of a band-limited signal can be completely reconstructed from samples made at a sampling rate faster than twice the bandwidth of the highest frequency of the original data. To determine the optimal sampling rate, one must determine the highest frequency of the data and double it. Sampling at a frequency above this rate will facilitate a more accurate reconstruction of the signal, particularly when it is very fast. For example, if the highest

Recommended Recording Parameters							
Physiologic parameter	Signal	Reference	High freq filter	Low freq filter	Sensitivity	Recommended storage rate	Acceptable storage rate
EEG	C_4	M_1	35 Hz	0.3 Hz	5 μV/mm	500 Hz	200 Hz
EEG	C_3	M_2	35 Hz	0.3 Hz	5 μV/mm	500 Hz	200 Hz
EEG	O_2	M_1	35 Hz	0.3 Hz	5 μV/mm	500 Hz	200 Hz
EEG	O_1	M_2	35 Hz	0.3 Hz	5 μV/mm	500 Hz	200 Hz
EEG	F_4	M_1	35 Hz	0.3 Hz	5 μV/mm	500 Hz	200 Hz
EEG	F_3	M_2	35 Hz	0.3 Hz	5 μV/mm	500 Hz	200 Hz
EOG	ROC (E_2)	M_1	35 Hz	0.3 Hz	5 μV/mm	500 Hz	200 Hz
EOG	LOC (E1)	M_2	35 Hz	0.3 Hz	5 μV/mm	500 Hz	200 Hz
ECG	Modified lead 2	Bi-polar	70Hz	0.3 Hz	Gain	500 Hz	200 Hz
EMG	Anterior tibialis	Bi-polar	100 Hz	10 Hz	Gain	500 Hz	200 Hz
EMG	Sub-mental chin	Bi-polar	100 Hz	10 Hz	Gain	500 Hz	200 Hz
EMG	Intercostal	Bi-polar	100 Hz	10 Hz	Gain	100 Hz	25 Hz
Airflow	Thermal sensor	Bi-polar	15 Hz	0.1 Hz	Gain	100 Hz	25 Hz
Airflow	Nasal pressure	DC	100 Hz	—	Gain	100 Hz	25 Hz
Snoring	Microphone or sensor	DC	100 Hz	10 Hz	Gain	500 Hz	200 Hz
Effort	Esophageal pressure	DC	100 Hz	25 Hz	Gain	100 Hz	25 Hz
Effort	Thoricic RIP	Bi-polar	15 Hz	0.1 Hz	Gain	100 Hz	25 Hz
Effort	Abdominal RIP	Bi-polar	15 Hz	0.1 Hz	Gain	100 Hz	25 Hz
Position	Position sensor	Bi-polar	See mfg spec	—	Gain	1 Hz	1 Hz
Oximetry	SpO2	DC	15	—	Gain	25 Hz	10 Hz

FIGURE 4-13 The American Academy of Sleep Medicine recommended settings for polysomnography. *Data from Berry R, Brooks R, Gamaldo C, Harding S, Marcus C, Vaughn B: The AASM Manual for the Scoring of Sleep and Associated Events, V2.0, Darien, Ill, 2012, American Academy of Sleep Medicine.*

frequency within the bandwidth of a signal is 100 Hz, it should be sampled at a rate faster than 200 Hz (samples per second). From those samples a digitized copy of the original signal can be completely reconstructed according to mathematical theory. In real-world application, the reconstructed signal is always only an approximation of the original, albeit a close approximation with adequate sampling rate.

SIGNAL RECONSTRUCTION

Reconstructing a signal is complicated by the fact that a special filter is required. A reconstruction filter captures the peaks of the signals at the given sample rate and, using an algorithm, extrapolates the data between samples turning the data into a smooth continuous signal similar to the original. If too few data points are sampled, reconstruction of the data may appear blunted or distorted.

Even with a sampling rate greater than twice the fastest recorded data, overlapping of the frequency spectrum can occur during reconstruction. This causes components to "fold back" into lower frequencies, resulting in distortion of the lower frequency signals. These distortions are known as aliases because they are not part of the original signal. Aliasing is less likely the more sampling is increased above the minimum rate specified by Nyquist and Shannon. Unfortunately, a sampling rate that is set too high will unnecessarily use more memory than required and waste valuable recorder storage space. A higher sampling rate will always increase the resolution of high-frequency signals, and will always result in larger file size.

The AASM developed two levels of recommendations for sampling rates for use on PSG channels.[10] The higher range settings significantly reduce the likelihood of signal aliasing. Because sampling rate affects file size, each facility must determine whether the cost of additional storage space is outweighed by the benefit of obtaining higher data resolution (Figure 4-14).

SENSITIVITY AND GAIN

Biopotentials from the brain are measured in microvolts (μV), which are 1000 times smaller than a millivolt and 1,000,000 times smaller than a volt. Biopotentials are assessed by the voltage, frequency, and morphology of the recorded signal. When an input signal of known voltage is applied to the amplifier to produce a deflection, the signal amplitude can be used to extrapolate the voltage responsible for other deflections. Likewise, if the recorder amplification settings are known, voltage can be determined.

SENSITIVITY

Sensitivity is a control on the polygraph used to increase or decrease the amplitude of recorded data. It has been defined as the ratio of input voltage to the output deflection. Although somewhat outdated, it is literally the amount of voltage or microunits of voltage (μV or mV), required to produce a 1-mm deflection or 1-cm deflection on the recorder. Despite adoption of gain for use with digital acquisition of data, some manufacturers continue to rely on the concept of sensitivity. Rather than expressing sensitivity in terms of microvolts per millimeter (μV/mm) or millivolts per centimeter (mV/cm), it may be defined in terms of divisions or some other scale more appropriate for a computer screen.

During recorder calibration, a known voltage is introduced to all amplifiers to ensure there is consistent response on all channels. An all-channel calibration is performed on some recorders by setting all amplifiers to like settings.

The mechanical calibration performed just before lights out, the montage calibration, is obtained using

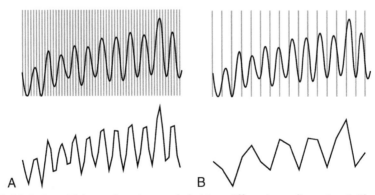

FIGURE 4-14 A sinusoidal waveform is recorded at two different sampling rates: **A,** The sampling rate is greater than twice the frequency of waveforms being sampled. This yields a true digital representation of the original data, which is at best a close approximation. **B,** The sampling rate is less than twice the highest frequency of the data and produces a false (aliased) representation of the original waveform. Under-sampling always results in aliasing and produces a lower frequency waveform compared with the original signal. *From Fisch BJ:* Fisch and Spehlmann's EEG primer: basic principles of digital and analog EEG. *Philadelphia, 2000, Elsevier.*

the amplifier settings that will be used during the study. Typically, a 50-μV calibration signal is generated and the corresponding deflections are recorded on each channel. Ideally a 10-mm or 1-cm deflection is generated for each recording channel. This means that for every 50 μV of input, there will be 10 mm of deflection. This could be expressed as the ratio 50 μV:10 mm. This could be further reduced to 5 μV:1 mm. Because ratios and fractions are one and the same, 5 μV/1 mm means the same thing, and because there is always an understood 1 in front of every unit, 5 μV/mm is an identical statement. This is the concept of amplifier sensitivity.

If the amplifier sensitivity setting is 5 μV/mm, it literally means that 5 μV of input is required (from the patient or the calibrator) to generate a 1-mm deflection on the recording (*5-μV of input per 1 mm of deflection*). The sensitivity setting of 5 μV/mm is a given here. Later, recorded data yields a 10-mm deflection. To determine the voltage that results in the deflection, the sensitivity setting must be considered. If 5 μV of input is required to produce a deflection of 1 mm, how much input was required for a 10-mm deflection? For this simple example, the answer is 50 μV. However, for a 13-mm deflection, what input would be required?

The sensitivity setting is expressed in the units of μV/mm or voltage/deflection. Using a basic expression, it could be stated that sensitivity (S) = voltage (V)/deflection (D), or S = V/D. To answer the previous question, two of the three variables are already present: the sensitivity setting of 5 μV/mm and the measured deflection at 13 mm.

S = V/D, then is 5 = V/13. To determine voltage, both sides are multiplied by 13:

(13) 5=V/~~13~~ (~~13~~/1) → 13 • 5

$$= V \rightarrow 65 = V \rightarrow V = 65 \text{ or } = 65 \text{ μV}$$

When dealing with sensitivity and two of the three variables are known, the following three versions of this expression will yield the third variable:

$$S = V/D$$
$$V = S \cdot D$$
$$D = V/S$$
$$\text{Sensitivity} = \text{input/output}$$

GAIN

Gain, which has largely replaced the sensitivity control for use in digital polysomnography, has been defined as the ratio of output deflection to input voltage. It is simply a multiplication factor that represents how many times the original signal that arose from the patient was amplified for visual display. To put gain into perspective, a typical setting for EEG is 20,000 times; the

EEG signal is amplified 20,000 times for visual display on the recorder. Compared with the concept of sensitivity, gain is quite simple:

$$\text{Gain} = \text{output/input}$$

Both gain and sensitivity must be documented (with numerical values and units) at the recording start, each time there is a change to amplifier settings, and at the end of the PSG.

COMMON MODE REJECTION

The ideal differential amplifier generates an output that is purely the difference between two input signals. When artifact is superimposed on both inputs of a recording channel, the extraneous signal is called the **common mode signal**. When both inputs of a derivation are contaminated by artifact of identical phase and equal voltage, the like components of the signal will be eliminated. This characteristic of a differential amplifier is referred to as *common mode rejection*. Because input 2 is always subtracted from input 1, signals of identical phase, polarity, amplitude, and frequency that reach both inputs, such as 60 Hz activity from electrical leakage current, will be subtracted before reaching the recorder output.

Common mode rejection is most effective when the electrodes connected to the two inputs share low and fairly equal impedance values. The amplifier retains the underlying biopotentials of different phase at input 1 and 2 and the bioelectric signal being recorded remains intact. In practice, the differential amplifier cannot completely eliminate the artifact because impedance values are rarely exactly the same and the amount of external artifact is never sensed equally at two electrode sites. Therefore the output signal always contains some portion of the common mode signal, when present.

The **common mode rejection ratio (CMRR)** is defined as the differential gain divided by the common mode gain. The higher the CMRR, the more efficient the amplifier and less common mode signal reaches the output.[11] This allows optimal recording of the pure bioelectric signal with minimal artifact. Because impedance is the resistance to an AC signal, as it increases the amplitude of the signal is reduced.

The absence of an effective patient ground electrode can also reduce the effectiveness of common mode rejection. The patient **ground electrode** establishes a universal reference for all scalp potentials. It is the baseline at which the differential amplifier begins the potential difference calculation. Without this reference point, identical electrical signals can be excluded from the differential calculation. The patient ground electrode does nothing to protect the patient from electrical shock, and when electrical safety practices are followed, it poses no appreciable risk to the patient.[8] A patent ground wire within the recorder power cord and its connection to the electrical **outlet ground**, the **building ground**, and the earth ground does protect the patient from exposure to electricity. Electrical safety is covered thoroughly in Chapter 6.

AMPLIFIER FILTERS

THE LOW-FREQUENCY FILTER AND DECAY TIME CONSTANT

Only a limited number of frequencies are of interest to polysomnography. To concentrate on these specific frequencies of interest, filters are employed to isolate them. An analog filter is made of resistors and capacitors, which slow down the time a signal has to move from peak to baseline. A digital filter takes the digitized data and passes it through programmed microchips, where algorithms attenuate signals below the filter setting, also referred to as the cut off frequency. Filters, therefore, change the characteristics of the original signal. Ideal digital filters attenuate data in a manner similar to that of analog filters.

Low-Frequency Filter (LFF)

The low-frequency filter (LFF) is also known as the high-pass filter, because it allows signals above the cutoff frequency to pass through. A LFF attenuates components below the filter setting and preserves those above it. The LFF is particularly useful when the signal of interest rides on an unwanted DC level. For example, sometimes electrodes create a DC offset voltage, known as an unstable battery effect, which is high voltage compared with the EEG signal. The DC offset can limit the amount of amplification possible because the DC offset is also amplified. This DC signal can push the EEG signal baseline up or down until it is clipped by exceeding the range of the amplifier or display. If the DC component is first minimized, the pure bioelectric signal can be amplified according to the properties of the amplifier.

The LFF is useful on EEG channels for attenuating signals below delta wave activity such as sweat artifact and respiratory artifact. Sweat artifact causes the signal baseline to slowly move up. Increasing the LFF will attenuate this wandering baseline, but care must be taken not to attenuate signals of interest. When the LFF is set to 0.3 Hz, most slow signals are attenuated but delta activity, with a bandwidth of 0.5 to 2 Hz is above the setting and unaffected. When an LFF is set too close to the low end of the EEG bandwidth of 0.5 Hz, it attenuates delta waves, and makes it difficult for the scoring technologist to properly identify stage N3 waveforms. The AASM recommends an LFF setting of 0.3 Hz on EEG channels to ensure lower delta wave frequencies are preserved.[10]

When the baseline EEG signal becomes contaminated with high amplitude, slow-wave artifact, it is most likely due to sweat, movement, or a combination of the two. If the issue is the result of sweat artifact, lowering the room temperature is the first step toward resolving this issue. If the artifact is aligned with respiratory channel excursion, multiple items may be moving in synch with breathing and may be responsible for the artifact. A later chapter covers various artifacts and potential causes more thoroughly.

When the input signal frequency is equal to the LFF setting, it is attenuated to 80% of its original amplitude.[8] As a signal with a frequency higher than the cut-off frequency progressively slows, it will begin being attenuated to between 80% and 100% of its original amplitude. As the slowing frequency moves toward the cut-off frequency, the signal's amplitude is progressively attenuated. When the frequency is reduced to exactly that of the cut-off frequency, the amplitude is exactly 80% of the original signal. As the input signal frequency drops to a value below the cutoff frequency, the amplitude drops below 80% of its original. Finally, as the signal's frequency continues to decline, the amplitude progressively drops further below 80% of its original amplitude until it can no longer be seen.

The HFF operates in the exact manner on the high end of a graphical representation of filter performance, the frequency response curve. The 80% in the previous example is specific to a particular manufacturer's amplifier filter, and is the convention most commonly used. An amplifier may, however, attenuate an input signal to 70% or even 50% of the original amplitude when the input frequency equals the filter setting. For the purposes of this text, a drop to 80%, or by 20%, of the original signal amplitude will be used as the standard for filter attenuation.

Decay Time Constant (TC)

A time constant (TC), more specifically the **decay time constant** or fall TC, is defined as the time it takes, in seconds, for a square wave to decay to 37% of its original amplitude.[11] The LFF and the decay TC are recorder controls used for the same purpose. One instrument may have an LFF control on the amplifier system, whereas an instrument from another manufacturer may use a TC control instead. For this reason, the technologist must possess a functional understanding of the relationship between these controls. On channel 1 of Figure 4-15 the input signal was recorded using a DC amplifier. Because DC amplifiers lack an LFF, the signal does not decay and the TC is equal to infinity. Decay TC values for the amplifiers used to record channels 2 through 5 are 1.03 seconds, 0.43 seconds, 0.16 seconds, and 0.033 seconds, respectively.[6] To enhance the ability to see how the various LFF settings distort slow waves, the HFF

The Effect of Various LFF Settings on a DC Square Wave

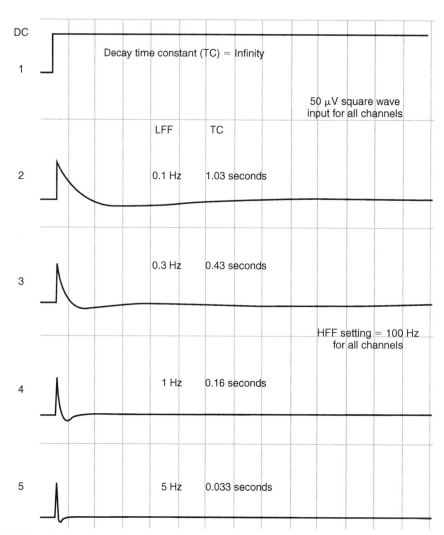

FIGURE 4-15 The effects of various low-frequency filter settings and the decay time constant associated with each.

was set at 100 Hz for all channels—high enough that there is no effect on the square-wave signals. Figure 4-15 also illustrates the relationship between the LFF and the decay TC. Note that a higher LFF (Hz) results in a shorter TC (seconds); a lower LFF setting imposes a longer TC.

Figure 4-16 displays the effect of different LFF settings on sine waves recorded at various frequencies. Here there is no DC channel. The HFF, LFF, and TC settings are identical to those used to record the bottom four channels in the previous example. The sine-wave input signals, applied to each amplifier at a frequency of 0.3 Hz, 1 Hz, 3 Hz, 10 Hz, and 30 Hz, were either allowed to pass through the amplifier because of its LFF setting, or the filter attenuated the signal by varying degrees.

The shorter the TC, the more slow frequencies will be attenuated. This is very important because while attempting to reduce slow frequency sweat or respiratory artifact, delta waves, which are similar in frequency, could also be attenuated. Attenuation of delta waves reduces the amount of stage N3 sleep on the study that can be scored. It can be helpful for the technologist to think about the inverse relationship that exists between the LFF and the fall TC, because frequency is something that can easily be counted. As one goes up, the other goes down. A relatively lower LFF corresponds to a relatively longer TC as measured in seconds. A higher LFF setting corresponds to a shorter TC.

THE HIGH-FREQUENCY FILTER

The high-frequency filter (HFF) is also known as a low-pass filter. It attenuates signal components with a frequency approaching, meeting, and surpassing the cut-off frequency, and preserves or only nominally attenuates the signal components with a frequency below the filter setting. These data, or the majority of

The Effect of LFF Settings on a Sine Wave Signal

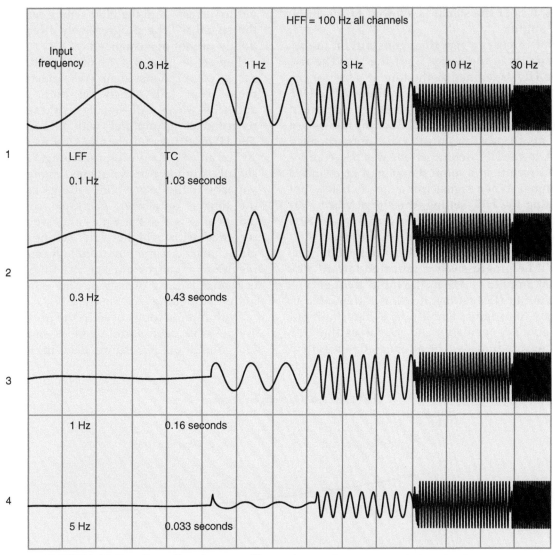

FIGURE 4-16 The effect of low-frequency filter settings on sine wave output at varying frequency.

the signal amplitude, are allowed to pass through the filter as amplifier output.

Setting the HFF too close to 35 Hz can attenuate EEG abnormalities such as sharps and spikes. Muscle twitches from arousals, teeth grinding, and body movements can also be difficult to distinguish from brain activity.[6] In fact, these may be misinterpreted as epileptiform spikes on the recording when the HFF is set too low. For this reason, applying an HFF setting of 60 Hz or 70 Hz should be considered when epileptiform activity is expected or suspected. Furthermore, because many patients only exhibit epileptiform activity during sleep, it is probable that for some undiagnosed patients, the abnormal brain discharges will be first identified during a sleep study. The HFF setting recommended by the AASM for the EEG channel is 35 Hz;[10] however,

this setting should be applied according to attending physician and recording technologist judgment, as it may not be appropriate for all patients.

Spikes are defined as having a 20- to 70-ms duration, which equals 14 to 50 Hz.[7] An HFF setting of 35 Hz will certainly attenuate frequencies within this range below the filter setting, but it will also result in attenuation of the faster frequencies to some degree. The HFF setting of 70 Hz will not have a negative effect on the recording of epileptiform spikes.

Reducing the HFF in response to artifact is not often the best response. The best solution may be reapplication of electrodes or a derivation change to preserve the integrity of the recording. Changes to filter settings should not be the first line of resolution unless used as a temporary solution until better options can be deployed. Input frequencies at the HFF setting are attenuated to 80% of the signal's original amplitude. As a result, as input frequency increases, less of the signal is allowed to reach the recorder output.

The HFF imposes a **rise time constant** on the recording similar to the decay TC of the LFF. The rise TC of the HFF is defined as the time it takes for the signal to attain 63% of its peak amplitude.[8] The HFF rise TC is responsible for the dampened or peaked morphology of data. A higher HFF setting allows fast components to pass and results in a more peaked output. A lower HFF setting attenuates fast components and results in a more dampened or rounded output signal. When signal frequency is below but approaching the HFF setting, the signal will be attenuated to somewhere between greater than 80% and less than 100% of its original amplitude.

As the input frequency gets closer to the filter setting it will be progressively attenuated toward 80% of original amplitude. When the input frequency is identical to the HFF setting, it will be attenuated to exactly 80% of original amplitude. When the input signal frequency increases and surpasses the HFF setting, the amplitude will be attenuated to less than

80% of the original. The remaining signal amplitude will be reduced by half for each doubling of frequency above the cut-off frequency.[11] If input frequency continues to increase and the filter setting remains constant, the signal will be progressively attenuated until it finally cannot be visualized.

Figures 4-17 and 4-18 were produced to allow easier comprehension of HFF effects, by isolating them from LFF effects on both square waves and sine waves. All signals in these figures were recorded using amplifiers with the LFF set at 0.01 Hz. The HFF settings for channels 1-4 were 3 Hz, 10 Hz, 30 Hz, and 60 Hz during recording. On Figure 4-16, slightly rounded or dampened signal morphology appears at the lower HFF settings as the result of the longer, or slower, rise time constant. Signal dampening is also known as undershoot. On signals recorded with a higher HFF setting, progressively more peaked signal morphology emerges as the result of a faster, or quicker, rise time constant. This is referred to as overshoot and is also known as underdampening (see Figure 4-17).

With filter settings used in the previous example, a sine-wave calibration signal is sent through the four amplifiers recording data in Figure 4-18 at

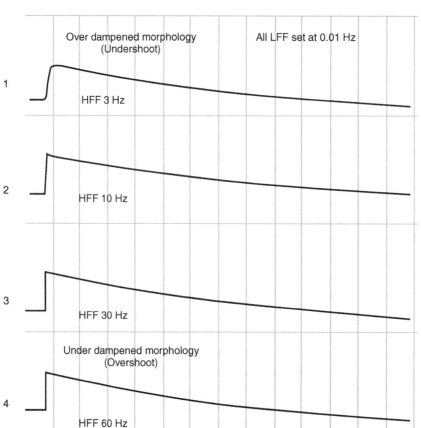

FIGURE 4-17 The effects of various high-frequency filter settings on square wave morphology.

HFF Attenuation of Fast Input Frequencies

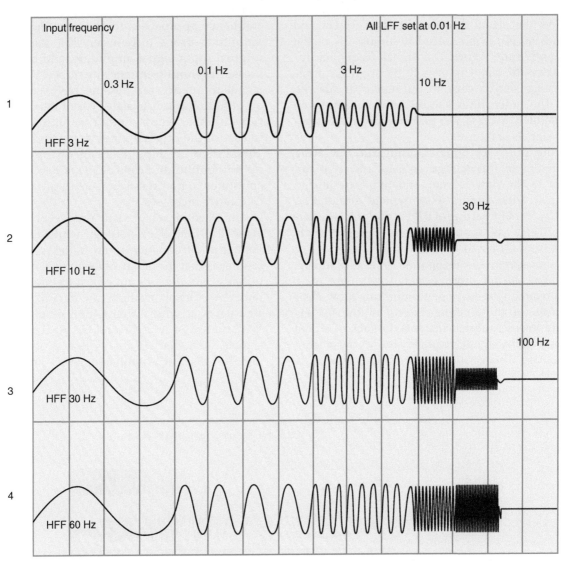

FIGURE 4-18 Attenuation of signal amplitude at various high-frequency filter settings as input frequency increases.

increasing frequency. Note the progressive attenuation of amplitude as input signal frequency increases, particularly at the lower HFF settings. On channel 1 with an HFF setting of 3 Hz, input signals of 0.3 Hz and 0.1 Hz are too slow to be affected by the HFF. However, at 3 Hz the input signal is significantly attenuated. The input signals with a frequency of 10 Hz and 30 Hz are much faster than the 3 Hz HFF set on this channel. The amplitude of these input signals has been attenuated by the 3-Hz filter to the point that they are essentially nonexistent (see Figure 4-18).

THE 60-Hz FILTER

Because the world is powered by electricity, there is constant bombardment by electrical fields emanating from home or office wiring, lighting, and electrical equipment. In the United States, electrical line frequency is 60 Hz, whereas in most other countries line frequency is set to cycle at 50 Hz. Because the human body is a relatively good conductor of electricity, when an electrode is placed on the body, 60 Hz line current can be readily detected.

Although modern laboratories and equipment are well grounded, shielded, and isolated, it is difficult to completely eliminate 60-Hz signals from the PSG. Because EEG, as an example, is typically recorded at a gain setting of 20,000, any artifact, including line noise, is also amplified 20,000 times on the EEG channel. When the slightest hint of 60-Hz noise contaminates the recording, once it is amplified it may obscure the channel.

A device used to reduce power line signals obscuring EEG recordings is the 60-Hz filter or **notch filter**.

This filter attenuates frequencies of 58 to 62 Hz. The attenuation curve is very sharp with a notch in the middle. As the signal frequency passes 58 Hz and approaches 60 Hz, it is reduced to almost 0% of the original amplitude. When the signal frequency increases above 62 Hz, it returns to its original amplitude. Because signals close to the notch can also be reduced, the notch filter should only be employed when absolutely necessary to prevent unwanted attenuation of signals of interest.

If having difficulty understanding the operating characteristics of filters, Figures 4-19 and 4-20 can be useful to the new learner and the experienced technologist alike. Figure 4-19 depicts attenuation imposed by the LFF setting of 0.3 Hz and the HFF setting of 70 Hz as input frequency progressively increases from 0.1 Hz to 100 Hz.

Initial assessment of the top data set makes understanding the second much easier. These data were recorded from a sine-wave generator and allow clear visualization of the filtering effects of the 0.3 Hz LFF at the lowest frequencies and the lack of signal attenuation as the signal frequency moves away from the LFF setting. Throughout the midrange of the wide

amplifier bandwidth created by these filter settings, signal amplitude remains at 100%. As the input frequency approaches the HFF setting of 70 Hz, the amplitude drops to between 80% and 100% of the original input signal amplitude, and continually decreases as input frequency increases. When the input signal frequency reaches the HFF setting of 70 Hz, amplifier output is exactly 80% of the original amplitude. In other words, output amplitude is attenuated to 80% of the original input signal and attenuated by 20%. When the input frequency surpasses the HFF, output amplitude drops below 80% of the input and continues to progressively decline as the input signal frequency increases.

The second set of data was recorded using the same LFF and HFF settings while identical signal voltage and frequencies were being recorded. The difference is that the 60-Hz notch filter is in use. Note the difference in the amount of fast frequencies being attenuated. Closely evaluate the data to determine the frequency at which attenuation of the data begins. With both a 70-Hz HFF and the 60-Hz filter in place, signals with frequencies as low as the high 20s or low 30s become attenuated. With an input signal

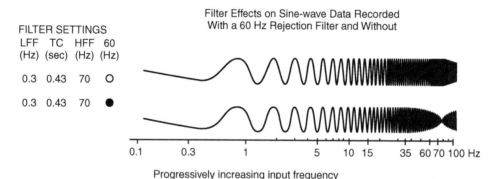

FIGURE 4-19 The effects of filters on sine-wave data with progressively increasing input frequency with and without a 60-Hz filter applied.

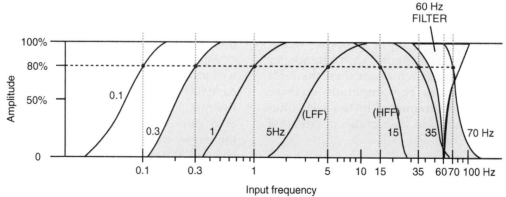

FIGURE 4-20 A frequency response curve from which signal attenuation can be estimated when amplifier settings and input signal amplitude are known.

frequency around 35 Hz, amplitude begins dropping much more rapidly than when the 60-Hz filter is not applied, as in the top channel. This is why the 60-Hz filter should not be used as a first-line remedy for unwanted electrical signals.

The technologist should become proficient at equipment troubleshooting and use his or her skills rather than simply applying a filter that distorts the data being acquired. Artifacts and their resolution are thoroughly covered in a later chapter. Obviously the effects of a 60-Hz filter along with a 70-Hz HFF are profound. When the HFF is set too low, even 35 Hz, distortion of fast-frequency signals becomes even more prominent, making data less reliable. In a worst-case scenario, signals originating from the body can be distorted to the point that they no longer appear to be of physiological origin.

DIGITAL FILTERING

Digital filtering offers the advantage of changing filter settings during the scoring and review of the sleep study. Widening the bandwidth of the bioelectrical signal on the tracing can reveal information not otherwise noticed by the recording technologist. Digital filters produce less peak distortion backward (LFF) and forward (HFF), respectively.

There are three types of digital filters: the finite impulse response (FIR), the infinite impulse response, and the fast Fourier transform. Most PSG systems use the FIR, which averages the amplitude of adjacent digitized signal samples. The FIR creates a wider HFF bandwidth, thereby attenuating signals of lower frequency.

Digital filters use algorithms to perform the work that analog filters did in the past. Digital filtering takes place after the raw data is converted from analog to the digital form. Unfortunately, there are no industry standards for the digital filter types used by the various system manufacturers. Some filters attenuate at 20% of the raw signal and others at 30%-50% of the raw signal. Most modern polysomnographs sample and digitize bioelectrical signals at the bedside, and transmit the signal to the acquisition computer in the control area. The bioelectrical signals can then be visualized and digitally filtered during the study or later during playback.

FREQUENCY RESPONSE

Filters act to attenuate signal components outside of the set cutoff frequency and maintain the signal components inside of the cutoff frequency. All filters have a cutoff frequency, which is by definition the frequency at which the output declines to 80% of the original amplitude.[8] This is also known as the *3 dB point* because a voltage ratio of 80%, expressed in decibels, is −3 dB or 3 dB down in amplitude.

In monitoring bioelectrical data, such as EEG, the convention is that the signal is attenuated to 80% at the cut-off frequency. However, in electrical engineering the signal is attenuated by 30% at the cut-off frequency. That is 10% for each decibel up or down. In reality, the 80% amplitude convention is only followed by certain equipment manufacturers. Depending on the manufacturer, or even the model or revision of a digital acquisition system, amplifier attenuation at the cutoff frequency may be 80%, 70%, or even 50%.

Regardless of the actual signal attenuation that a particular amplifier imposes, the technologist must have a functional understanding that amplifiers do not simply cut off all signals when they reach the frequency of the selected filter. Rather, there is progressive attenuation as a signal increases in frequency toward the HFF setting or decreases in frequency and begins approaching the LFF setting. By evaluating a **frequency response curve**, as depicted in Figure 4-20, an estimation of signal attenuation for a variety of amplifier settings can be determined, when the frequency of the input signal is known or can be measured.

On the y-axis (left) in Figure 4-20, output amplitude is represented as a percentage of the original input signal amplitude. On the x-axis (bottom) the frequency of acquired data is assessed in a range from less than 0.1 Hz up to 100 Hz. Any number of filter options can be displayed on a single frequency response curve graph, but one must only plot one set of amplifier data to begin understanding the dynamics of amplifier filters. On this particular graph, the attenuation characteristics of four LFF settings are displayed as downward slopes to the left. These LFF options include 0.1 Hz, 0.3 Hz, 1 Hz, and 5 Hz. On the right side of the graph, attenuation characteristics of the four HFF options of 15 Hz, 35 Hz, and 70 Hz can be seen as the downward slopes to the right. Any one of the LFF curves can be paired to any one of the HFF curves to form a frequency response curve and assess the amplifier cut off at these settings.

To help simplify this explanation, the frequency response curve for the common amplifier settings of 0.3 Hz for the LFF and 70 Hz for the HFF have been highlighted. Using this information, it can be determined if, and to what degree, an input signal with a specific frequency will be attenuated when data are recorded with these amplifier settings. With the 60-Hz filter turned off, 100% of the input amplitude will exit the amplifier to be recorded for frequencies ranging between approximately 0.5 Hz and approximately 60 Hz at these settings.

Moving from the middle of the graph to the left, the line representing 0.3 Hz eventually begins to descend representing a decrease in signal output amplitude. Moving farther to the left, the line progressively descends until it reaches 80% of the original amplitude on the y-axis of the graph. Notice along the x-axis that the frequencies aligned with this 80% to 100% amplitude range are above the filter setting of

0.3 Hz. Because the assumed convention is attenuation by 20%, or attenuation to 80%, at an input signal frequency of exactly 0.3 Hz, the original signal amplitude will be reduced to exactly 80%. As the input frequency falls below the LFF setting, less than 80% of original amplitude will get through the amplifier to the output.

If the frequency continues to progressively drop, the output amplitude will also progressively drop until it can no longer be visualized. For any HFF or LFF setting, an input frequency equal to it, will be attenuated to 80% of the original amplitude.

To recap, as the input frequency decreases, at some frequency above the LFF setting its amplitude will begin being attenuated for an output that is less than 100% but greater than 80% of the original. When the input frequency equals the LFF setting, exactly 80% of the amplitude will reach the recorder output. As the signal frequency drops below the LFF setting, it is progressively attenuated to less than 80% of original amplitude. Using a straight edge, it is possible to estimate the percent amplitude of any signal as long as the filter settings and the signal frequency are known.

The HFF attenuates data amplitude in exactly the same manner. As input frequency increases and begins approaching the HFF setting, at some frequency the output amplitude is attenuated to less than 100% but greater than 80% of the original input amplitude. When the input frequency equals the HFF setting, exactly 80% of the input amplitude will reach the output. Finally, when the input signal frequency is faster than the HFF setting, less than 80% of the amplitude will be present at the amplifier output. As previously described, the 60-Hz filter notches out frequencies between 58 and 62 Hz when in use and is only effective for reducing artifact from electrical sources. When a 60-Hz filter and HFF are used together, signals with frequencies far outside of the 60-Hz filter's discreet range will be distorted. For this reason, the 60-Hz filter should not be used unless the source of artifact cannot be eliminated.

ADDITIONAL TESTING EQUIPMENT AND CONSIDERATIONS

TRANSDUCED SIGNALS

Signals representing respiratory effort, temperature, pressure, and other mechanical functions are **transduced** into electrical signals capable of interfacing with the polygraph. A polygraph records the electrical difference between two input signals, or in the case of ancillary devices, the voltage of a single input. However, much of what is obtained during a sleep study is not directly related to the rising and falling of electrical potentials recorded directly from the body's surface. Instead, mechanical activity, like that associated with breathing, must be converted into a signal that can be interfaced with the acquisition system.

A **transducer** is a device that converts one form of energy into another. For polysomnography, a transducer converts a mechanical signal into an electrical signal. Thermal sensors used for obtaining an airflow signal actually measure the relative change in temperature that occurs as cool room air is pulled across the sensor and then warm air is exhaled over it.

This relative temperature change results in a difference in voltage that travels through **conductors** to the polygraph for display in a sinusoidal signal used to represent airflow. Likewise, the nasal pressure airflow signal is derived from pressure changes exerted on the opening of a **cannula** that resides at the nares during inspiration and exhalation. The other end of the cannula, or tube, is attached to a pressure transducer that converts the pressure changes into an electrical signal.

Similarly, when a cannula is placed in the esophagus for **esophageal manometry**, the changes in **intrathoracic pressure** exerted on the esophagus and the tube during breathing are converted by a pressure transducer into a usable signal. **Respiratory inductance plethysmography** belts and older sensors using **piezo crystal technology** transduce movement or pressure on a sensor, respectively, into an electrical signal for display on the recording. Conversion of a mechanical to electrical signal can be found in other common sleep-testing devices, including snore sensors and snore microphones, position sensors, and movement sensors.

ANCILLARY EQUIPMENT

Free-standing devices capable of providing diagnostic information when used alone are often interfaced with the sleep study recorder to complement other measures being obtained. When devices are interfaced with the polygraph to supplement diagnostic or therapeutic data, these machines are collectively referred to as **ancillary equipment** or **devices**.[5]

Ancillary devices such as oximeters and capnometers provide the final complement of information recorded during a sleep study. These free-standing machines and signal transducers, along with the electrodes that record bioelectric signals directly from the surface of the body, are connected to polygraph amplifiers for simultaneous recording. A **pulse oximeter** provides **oxyhemoglobin saturation** data and a **capnometer** is often employed to continuously monitor the patient's CO_2.

A **positive airway pressure (PAP) device** is used to deliver **continuous positive airway pressure (CPAP)** or bilevel positive airway pressure (BPAP). A transduced airflow signal is derived from the PAP device during the therapeutic phase of testing. The PAP device is typically capable of sending additional data to the polygraph, including the amount of pressure being delivered to the patient as the technologist continually adjusts it in response to sleep-disordered breathing events and the amount of air leaking from around the patient's PAP interface, such as a nasal mask. Most ancillary devices communicate with the acquisition system using low-voltage signal such as 0-1 V DC.

More details, including how ancillary devices are set up with the recorder, and the need to calibrate before each use to ensure accuracy of data, are covered in subsequent chapters.

THE POLYSOMNOGRAPH

A standard sleep study is segmented into 30-second increments called **epochs**, each of which must be assigned a sleep stage score by either the recording or scoring technologist. The 30-second epoch recorded on paper required a paper speed of 10 mm/s. For clinical EEG, a 10-second epoch is used. When recorded on paper, this requires a paper speed of 30 mm/s. Standard ECG paper speed is 25 mm/s. When comparing data from an ECG reference, PSG data will be compressed by 2.5 times.

In addition to sleep-stage identification the scoring technologist must identify, quantify, and tabulate occurrences such as EEG arousals, sleep-disordered breathing events, and EMG changes that are possible signs of a disorder. The tabulated data are organized into a report to be interpreted by a sleep medicine physician. These data are used alongside clinical evaluation of the patient with a possible sleep disorder to aid in diagnostic decision making and to determine the effectiveness of established therapy. If a therapeutic intervention, like CPAP or supplemental oxygen (O_2) is administered during the sleep study, the technologist must also report whether the intervention was effective.

VIEWING THE STUDY

According to the AASM, the screen resolution for scoring raw data must be a minimum of 1600×1200 pixels. The video data must be synchronized with the PSG data and have an accuracy of at least one video frame per second. A viewing screen of 25 to 30 cm or larger optimizes fine detail and avoids eye strain. Vertical spacing between channels should be 15 mm. The American Clinical Neurological Society recommends a minimum of 2 pixels of resolution for each vertical millimeter.

Earlier paper tracings allowed the technologist the flexibility to change paper speed from 1 to 30 mm/s. A paper speed of 10 mm/s would produce a 30-second epoch. Of course, once the tracing was produced, there was no method to look at the data differently by increasing or decreasing the paper speed. These recordings were WYSIWYG. Once recorded, the data were there.

Digital systems provide the user a time scale range from 1 second to the entire recording time for retrospective evaluation. The mechanical electrode selector on analog recorders allowed the technologist to change derivations by flipping switches or manually changing inputs to create a new montage. On modern digital recorders, these functions are easily accomplished within the software and offer almost unlimited options.

The AASM mandates digital systems must provide montage-changing controls without relying on a common reference electrode. In addition, a 60-Hz filter and an impedance meter for each channel are mandatory. There should be a toggle switch permitting visualization of the 50 µV calibration signal for all channels to demonstrate polarity, amplitude, and TC settings for each parameter studied.[10] Each channel should also have a separate sampling rate selector.

All digital systems must retain and display all sensitivity, filter, montage, and derivation changes. The user must be able to turn off the automatic scoring programs and enter and save manual scoring.[10] Essentially, the digital system must be capable of producing a study equal to a paper tracing. Rapid tabulation and manipulation of data is the salient strength of digital software. Most digital polygraph systems produce an all-night or hourly histogram for sleep stage, respiratory events, oxygen saturation, arousals, and other parameters.

DATA STORAGE

Digital technology's greatest contribution to sleep technology may be related to data storage. Previously, a 17-lb box of Z-folded paper held one 8-hour PSG. Today that same data can be archived to a digital server, a 1-oz DVD, a compressed tape backup system, or a variety of other digital storage devices.

A sleep study is a medical-legal record, which should be archived according to the regulatory guidelines of the specific state or country and the facility's accrediting bodies. The amount of digitized information to be stored depends on the sample rate of the analog-to-digital converter, the number of bits used to store the sample, and the length of study time. There are 8 bits in 1 byte. Using a 12-bit system, each bit is equal to 1.5 bytes. For example, four EEG channels sampled at 200 times per second, for a 1-hour period would total:

$$(4 \times 200 \times 60) \times 60 = 2,880,000 \text{ samples} \times 1.5 \text{ bytes} = 4320000 \text{ bytes}$$

$$1024 \text{ bytes} = 1 \text{ kilobyte so } 432000/1024 = 4219 \text{ kilobytes}$$

$$1 \text{ million bytes} = 1 \text{ Megabyte (Mb)}; 1000 \text{ Mb} = 1 \text{ Gigabyte (Gb)}$$

An 8-hour sleep study can produce 40 to 50 Mb of data. Most CD and DVD storage media can hold between 650 Mb and 5 Gb and can last up to 25 years. Other methods of storage for digital technology exist that have limitless archival space and long-lasting endurance.

RECORDED DATA

When preparing a patient for a sleep study, most technologists start with the head measurements, scalp preparation, and application of cephalic electrodes. Although a particular order is not crucial, eye movement and chin EMG electrodes may be placed on the face next, followed by ECG electrodes on the trunk and leg EMG electrodes. Next, respiratory airflow and effort sensors, a snoring microphone, and a nasal cannula connected to a pressure transducer are applied to the face, neck, and trunk. Finally, an oximeter probe is applied to a finger and a body position sensor is attached.

THE ELECTROENCEPHALOGRAM (EEG)

The EEG represents biopotentials from the brain as recorded at the scalp's surface. They are the result of potential currents generated by networks of cortical cells. When these potential changes are recorded continuously, the frequency, duration, amplitude, and polarity of acquired data combine to create a visual pattern, which is consistent with wakefulness, the stages of sleep, and other findings.

Many of the individual patterns and components of the EEG are assessed on a defined channel derived from electrodes overlying specific cortical areas. Because brain potentials are small, in the range of microvolts, potential fields are sampled to obtain a summation of potentials from many nerve cells underlying an exploring electrode.[7] These signals are directed to the polygraph through a selector panel, which pairs two leads for input to the differential amplifiers. Groups of paired electrodes make up the montage, which determines which data are viewed on the channels of the tracing.

THE ELECTROOCULOGRAM (EOG)

Eye movements can be easily recorded because the retina at the back of the eye is negative with respect to the cornea at the front of the eye. As the eyes move, the potential difference between the EOG electrodes is recorded based on their placement in relation to the cornea and retina. Most commonly, one electrode is affixed 1 cm above the right outer canthus and one electrode is affixed 1 cm below the left outer canthus. Both electrodes are referenced to the M2 electrode for a right and left EOG channel.

This configuration is designed to record vertical and horizontal eye movements. Electrodes placed precisely on the same horizontal plane will collect only horizontal and oblique eye movements. When the eye moves so that the cornea is in closer proximity to the electrode than the retina, a positive potential will be recorded as a downward deflection on the respective channel. When the eye moves so that the retina is closer to the electrode, a negative deflection will be generated.

THE CHIN ELECTROMYOGRAM (EMG)

Biopotentials from chin muscle activation are recorded from the skin's surface as an EMG signal. Muscle tone in the submentalis decreases as the patient falls asleep, and is at its lowest during rapid eye movement sleep. The **submentalis muscle group** consists of the genioglossus, and the hyoglossus and the palatoglossus. These muscles coordinate the control of the tongue and airway space.

Three electrodes are placed to record chin EMG: one midline above the inferior edge of the mandible and two others 2 cm below the inferior edge of the mandible with one 2 cm to the right and one 2 cm to the left. When placed properly, the two lower electrodes lie directly over muscle that is activated by having the patient swallow.

THE LIMB ELECTROMYOGRAM

Bursts of muscle activity recorded from the anterior tibialis of each leg are used to identify periodic limb movements. This neurosensorimotor disorder causes frequent limb jerks, EEG arousals, and a reduction in the quality and quantity of sleep. Electrodes for recording leg EMG activity are placed 2-3 cm apart, longitudinally, along the belly of the anterior tibialis muscle group.

CHAPTER SUMMARY

- The PSG is a recording of many physiologic parameters, including bioelectric signals that are represented on the recording by waveforms.
- Waveform characteristics and the variety of other physiologic parameters obtained during a sleep study must be thoroughly understood by the sleep technologist.
- Bioelectrical signals travel to an input board via electrode wires. Signals from other sensors and equipment are also interfaced with the input board.
- Input signals are routed to amplifiers where the difference between two signals is calculated and amplified.
- Maintaining data quality is one of the most important duties of the technologist. Unless underlying

signals are intact, manipulation of data will be ineffective.

- Full knowledge of instrumentation operating characteristics provides the sleep technologist with the ability to perform an optimal recording.
- Recorded data are eventually routed to a computer where they are further filtered, amplified, digitized, processed, and stored.

References

1. Chokroverty S: *Sleep disorders medicine: basic science, technical considerations and clinical aspects*, ed 2, Woburn, Mass., 2000, Butterworth-Heinemann.
2. Guyton AC: *Structure and function of the nervous system*, ed 2, Philadelphia, 1972, WB Saunders.
3. Ranson SW, Clark SL: *Anatomy of the nervous system*, ed 1, Philadelphia, 1959, WB Saunders.
4. Mattice C, Brooks R, Lee-Chiong T: *Fundamentals of sleep technology*, ed 2, Philadelphia, 2012, Lippincott Williams & Wilkins.
5. Lee-Chiong T, Sateia M, Carskadon M: *Sleep Medicine*, ed 1, Philadelphia, 2002, Hanley & Belfus.
6. Fisch BJ: *Fisch and Spehlmann's EEG primer: basic principles of digital and analog EEG*, ed 3, Philadelphia, 2000, Elsevier.
7. Rowan AJ, Tolunsky E: *Primer of EEG: with a mini atlas*, ed 1, Philadelphia, 2003, Elsevier/Butterworth-Heineman.
8. Tyner F, Knott J, Mayer W: *Fundamentals of EEG technology*, vols 1 and 2, Philadelphia, 1989, Lippincott Williams & Wilkins.
9. Kryger M, Roth T, Dement W: *Principles and practice of sleep medicine*, ed 4, Philadelphia, 2005, Elsevier/Saunders.
10. Berry R, Brooks R, Gamaldo C, et al: *The AASM Manual for the Scoring of Sleep and Associated Events V2.0*, Darien, Ill., 2012, American Academy of Sleep Medicine.

REVIEW QUESTIONS

1. A trough to trough measurement along the x axis is performed to confirm:
   a. Amplitude
   b. Polarity
   c. Duration
   d. Chart speed

2. The measured vertical height of a waveform is known as:
   a. Polarity
   b. Impedance
   c. Duration
   d. Amplitude

3. The shape and characteristics of a waveform define:
   a. Resting potential
   b. Morphology
   c. Action potential
   d. Common mode rejection

4. When the amount of potassium leaving a cell equals the amount of potassium entering a cell, the cell potential is described as:
   a. Action
   b. Resting
   c. Monopolar
   d. Bipolar

5. The rapidly changing cell membrane potential is known as:
   a. Resting
   b. Action
   c. Monopolar
   d. Bipolar

6. A small device constructed of conductive metal for the measurement of bioelectrical signals is known as a (an):
   a. Electrode
   b. Amplifier
   c. Montage
   d. Meter

7. An impedance meter measures:
   a. Polarity
   b. Frequency
   c. Resistance
   d. Duration

8. The minimizing of signals common to input 1 and input 2 is known as:
   a. Frequency
   b. Polarity
   c. Common mode rejection
   d. Sampling rate

9. Which of the following rejects common signals recorded at input 1 and input 2?
   a. A differential amplifier
   b. A common mode amplifier
   c. A referential amplifier
   d. A WYSIWYG amplifier

10. A listing of derivations defines which of the following?
    a. Sampling rate
    b. Montage
    c. GIGO
    d. Channels

Chapter 5

Bioelectric Signals of Interest in Sleep Medicine

Kristine Servidio • Buddy Marshall •
Bonnie Robertson • Margaret-Ann Carno

CHAPTER OUTLINE

LEARNING OBJECTIVES

After reading this chapter, you will be able to:
1. Describe the EEG and its importance to the study of sleep.
2. Explain waveforms of interest to the sleep technologist.
3. Identify correct electrode placement for EOG monitoring.
4. Recognize how eye movements display on the polysomnogram.
5. Differentiate slow eye movements, rapid eye movements, and blinks.
6. Describe characteristics of both the chin EMG and leg EMG
7. Identify key characteristics of each sleep stage presented in the chapter

KEY TERMS

alpha activity	eye movement	stage N2
beta activity	interfaced	stage N3
bioelectrical signals	low-amplitude, mixed frequency	stage R
biopotentials	(LAMF)	stage W
cup electrodes	neuron	summed ionic flux
data acquisition system	P waves	T wave
delta activity	QRS complex	theta activity
electrocardiography	slow eye movements (SEMs)	vertex sharp waves
electromyography	stage N1	wake

Recalling that a nerve cell, or **neuron**, is simply a highly specialized animal cell, at one end, the dendrites receive signals from other cells in the form of chemical mediators. On the opposite end of the neuron are the axon terminals, which release chemical mediators across the synapse if the signal is propagated through the cell body and across the axon. These structures lie between the dendrites and the axon terminals.

Through the normal function of neurons and other cells of the body, **bioelectric signals**, also known as **biopotentials**, are produced. The biopotential measured on the skin surface is actually the collective activity of large groups of cells. This additive change in the extracellular fluid is known as **summed ionic flux**.

The mechanism within neurons creates action potentials through the movement of sodium and potassium ions in and out of the cell, respectively. As a result of the movement of sodium and potassium ions, the extracellular fluid becomes more positively charged and the fluid inside the neuron becomes more negatively charged relative to the outside of the cell. The resulting concentration gradient from this rapid ionic movement is responsible for action potentials.

These basic concepts, related to neurochemical and positive-negative charges that create an action potential, are essential for a basic understanding of the data a sleep technologist acquires. The polysomnogram (PSG) is actually an expression of the many bioelectric signals generated by physiologic function.

PARAMETERS TYPICALLY EVALUATED BY POLYSOMNOGRAPHY

The PSG is a compilation of three basic signal types: bioelectric, transduced, and those incorporated from ancillary equipment. Bioelectric signals directly represent the rising and falling of electrical potentials as obtained at the surface of the body. These include the **electroencephalogram (EEG)**, electromyogram (EMG), electrooculogram (EOG), and electrocardiogram (ECG). The EEG is recorded using small **cup electrodes** constructed of precious metal, often silver or gold-plated silver. The EMG,

ECG, and EOG can be recorded using the same cup electrodes, although it is acceptable to use other types of electrodes to record these noncephalic parameters.

A transduced signal is recorded using a **transducer**, a device that converts one form of energy into another form of energy. For example, a microphone converts sound waves to electricity that can be saved as an audio file or displayed graphically to represent volume.

The third type of signal is derived from monitoring equipment that has been **interfaced** with the **data acquisition system**. The term interfaced means the quality of being connected together. These devices can be used as stand-alone monitors to provide data, typically on a built-in screen, or they can be connected to the sleep study recorder as an additional parameter of the PSG. The most typical ancillary device used with sleep testing is the pulse oximeter. Pulse oximetry measures the oxygen saturation of blood and displays the value as a percentage. Interfaced data can be sent to the sleep study recorder and displayed on the PSG in numerical form, as a tracing on a graph, or both.

The skilled technologist must ensure excellent patient care, provide effective therapeutic interventions, and produce an artifact-free PSG recording. The exceptional technologist provides all of these services, but also possesses a solid understanding of all instrumentation used in PSG technology while making knowledgeable and timely decisions in a linear fashion, to troubleshoot and resolve any issue that might compromise the PSG recording.

ELECTROENCEPHALOGRAPHY

The EEG records the amplitude, morphology, and frequency of encephalographic bioelectric signals for visual display. Over many years of research, the sleeping brain was observed to generate distinctive electrophysiologic changes that were categorized into waveform types and allowed for categorization of sleep into various states.

Behaviors, such as eye movements and muscle activity, help differentiate sleep from wake and provide essential information used to discriminate non–rapid eye movement (NREM) sleep from rapid eye movement

(REM) sleep. Muscle activity can also indicate whether sleep issues may be related to a movement disorder or can help distinguish between parasomnias and potential seizure activity. Automatic or anatomic functions such as heart activity and breathing provide additional information about sleep and can yield valuable diagnostic information, as well as information regarding the efficacy of treatment for a previously identified disorder.

The signals typically recorded during PSG, as described in the following paragraphs, should be recorded with all characteristics intact using filters set above and below the individual parameter's frequencies of interest to produce the most accurate recording of sleep. Example settings for the low-frequency filter, high-frequency filter, and other amplifier controls for each recording parameter are provided by the American Academy of Sleep Medicine (AASM).[1] The AASM-recommended settings, or those determined for use in a specific workplace, should be set at the start of each recording and be appropriately altered to enhance the quality of recorded data. Judicial adjustment of parameters must be employed only when the underlying signals remain intact and other means of correcting an issue have been exhausted.

The following are descriptions of the types of wave activity:

- **Alpha activity:** EEG data in the range of 8-13 Hz, most prominently recorded from the occipital region. Waveform morphology is typically sinusoidal, often appearing in a crescendo-decrescendo pattern
- **Beta activity:** waves with frequency > 14 Hz interspersed throughout the EEG with eyes opened, and alpha activity when eyes are closed
- **Delta activity:** EEG data with frequency of 0.5-2 Hz and peak-to-peak amplitude of >75 μV measured over the frontal region
- **Theta activity:** EEG activity with a frequency of 3-7 Hz predominantly central in origin. Theta is a prominent component of low voltage mixed frequency activity

A list of waveforms and patterns of interest to the sleep technologist as defined by the AASM follow.[1] Examples are presented after the description of key features of some of these waveforms.

LOW-AMPLITUDE, MIXED-FREQUENCY (LAMF) WAVES

Frequency: predominantly 4-7 Hz
Amplitude: relatively low
Features: predominantly consists of theta activity in the 4-7 Hz range during sleep, although other fast frequencies such as alpha and beta can be interspersed throughout the pattern. When the subject is awake with eyes open, more alpha and beta are present.

Alpha Waves

Frequency: 8-13 Hz
Location: prominent in the occipital region

Amplitude: 10-150 microvolts
Features: sinusoidal morphology; seen during wake with eyes closed and attenuated by eyes opening; can be interspersed throughout the **LAMF** pattern. It should be noted that approximately 10% of the population does not generate an alpha rhythm when the eyes are closed.
Example: Figure 5-1

Delta Waves

Frequency: 0.5-2 Hz
Location: measured over the frontal region
Amplitude: >75 μV
Features: stage N3 (slow-wave sleep [SWS]) scored when >20% of an epoch consists of delta activity; chin EMG amplitude is variable, often lower than seen in stage N2 sleep and sometimes as low as seen in stage R sleep, but not used for scoring stage N3
Example: Figure 5-2

Sawtooth Waves

Frequency: 2-6 Hz
Location: central region
Amplitude: variable
Features: sharply contoured or triangular waves can be serrated; often but not always heralds a burst of rapid eye movements; not required for the scoring of stage R
Example: Figure 5-3

Theta Waves

Frequency: 3-7 Hz or 4-7 Hz*
Location: temporal and central regions
Amplitude: variable
Features: Makes up the majority of the predominantly LAMF pattern seen in stage N1, stage R, and the background rhythm of stage N2

Sleep Spindles

Frequency : 11-16 Hz (most commonly 12-14 Hz)
Location: central region
Amplitude: variable
Features: bursts with sinusoidal morphology lasting ≥0.5 seconds, seen in stage N2 sleep
Example: Figure 5-4

K Complex

Duration: ≥0.5 second duration
Location: maximal over the frontal region
Amplitude: variable
Features: biphasic morphology; negative deflection followed by a slower positive component; seen in stage N2 sleep, stands out from the background EEG
Example: Figure 5-5 illustrates stage 2 sleep with K complex.

(Text continued on page 85)

---

*Theta frequency range varies among industry standards

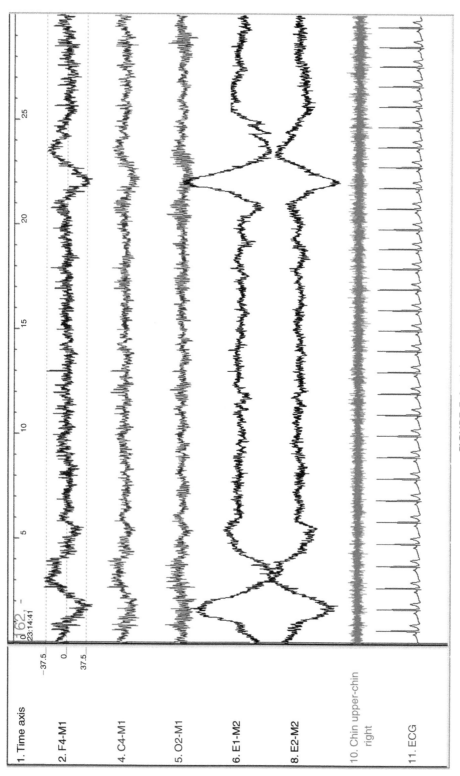

FIGURE 5-1 Alpha waves

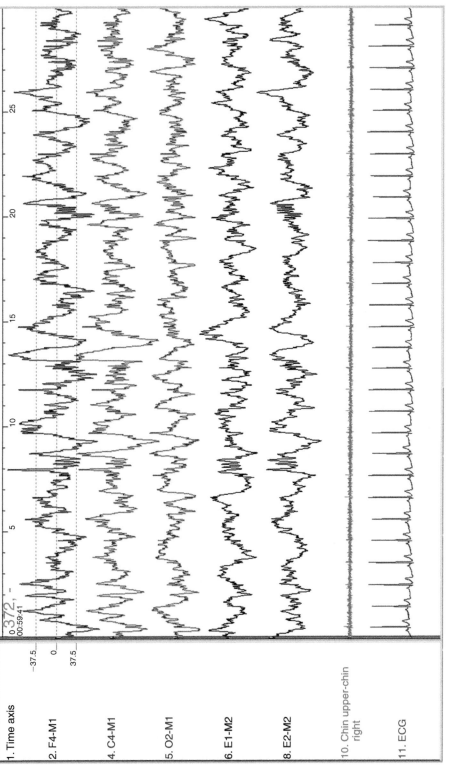

FIGURE 5-2 Delta waves

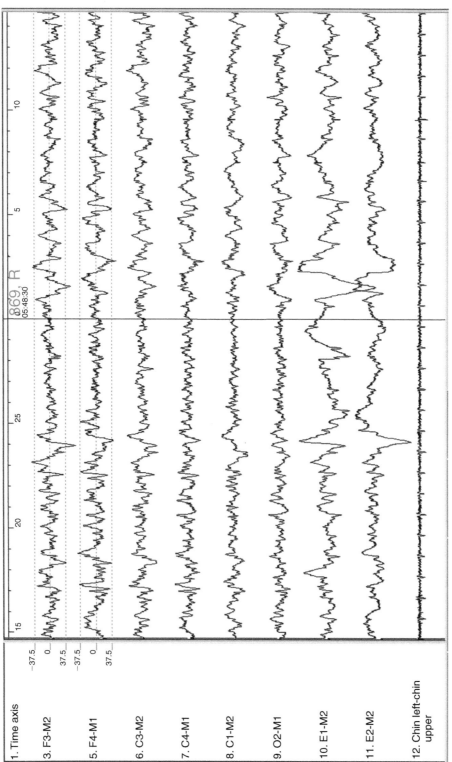

FIGURE 5-3 Sawtooth waves

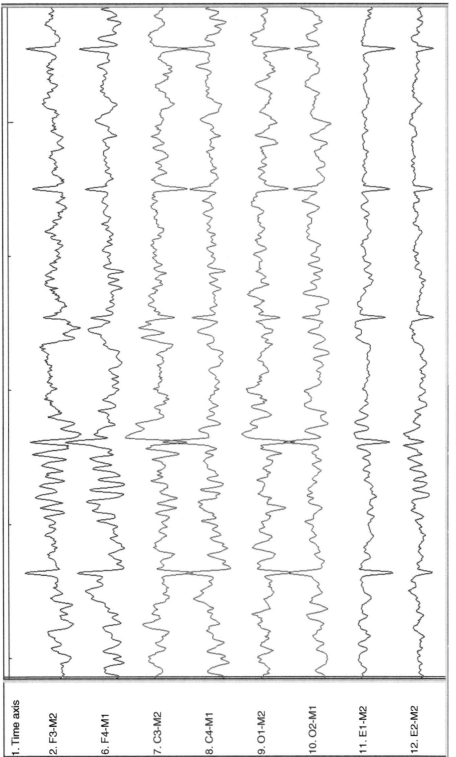

FIGURE 5-4 Sleep spindles

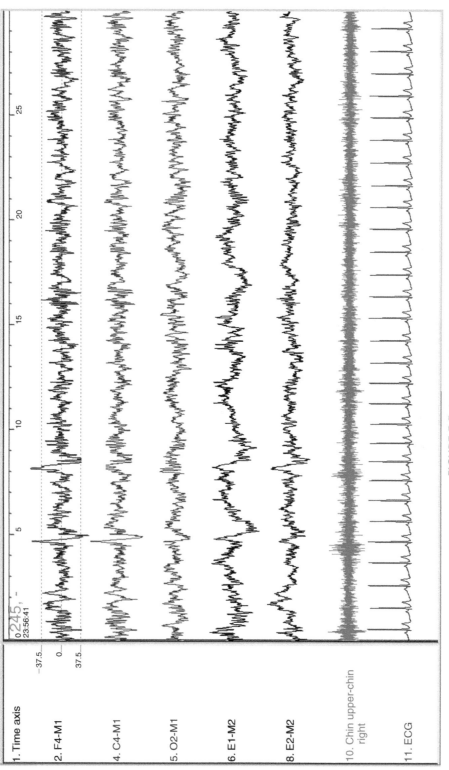

FIGURE 5-5 Stage 2 with K complex

Vertex Sharp Waves

Duration: <0.5 second duration
Location: central region
Amplitude: variable
Features: sharply contoured negative wave, distinguishable from the background activity; may be present, but is not required to score N1 sleep; a normal variant of sleep EEG

ELECTROOCULOGRAM

The EOG records **eye movement** to identify important changes in sleep state. During wakefulness, eye movements may be sharp as the patient watches an object move across the room or while reading in bed. During drowsiness, the eyes may roll slowly.

Slow eye movements (SEMs) often signify drowsiness and the transition into sleep. SEMs are defined as conjugate, reasonably regular sinusoidal eye movements with an initial deflection usually lasting more than 500 ms.[1] In fact, when nonalpha producers begin having SEMs, the start of NREM stage 1 (N1) sleep is scored.

During REM sleep, the eyes dart right and left and up and down. Oblique, or slanted, eye movements also occur during this phase of sleep, although they are not recorded using standard electrode placement. The AASM defines rapid eye movements as conjugate, irregular, sharply peaked eye movements with an initial deflection lasting less than 500 ms. When the patient looks to the right or looks up, the signal on the right EOG channel deflects downward and the signal on the left EOG channel deflects upward. When the patient looks to the left or downward, the signal on the right EOG channel deflects up and the signal on the left EOG channel deflects down. Some sleep testing facilities also place a right inferior EOG and left superior EOG electrode for backup purposes.

Recording Methods and Sleep-Wake Stage Scoring

EOG electrodes are positioned 1 cm below the LOC, or left outer canthus (E1), with another electrode placed 1 cm above the ROC, or right outer canthus (E2).[1] An alternative recording relies on both the right and left EOG electrodes being placed 1 cm lateral and 1 cm inferior to the outer canthus. For these recording channels, the exploring electrodes are connected to a supranasion reference. The supranasion reference is placed midline, above the nasion, at the location referred to as *frontal pole midline (Fpz)*. The main advantage of this configuration is that oblique eye movements are recorded. It can be beneficial to record the EOG with alternative placement when a multiple sleep latency test is anticipated because it is crucial that rapid eye movements be identified during a nap study. Recording from each outer canthus to a right mastoid reference, which are the recommended derivations from the AASM Manual, always yields out-of-phase deflections, as illustrated in Figure 5-6.

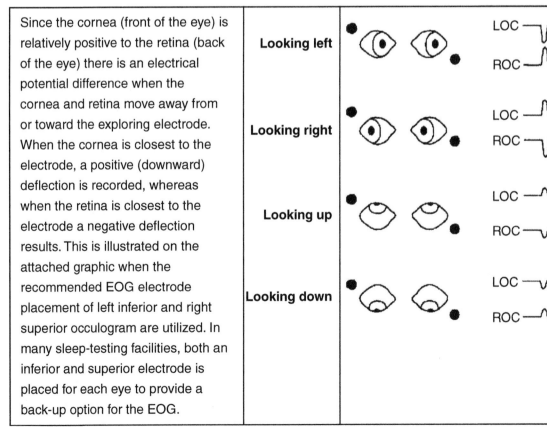

Since the cornea (front of the eye) is relatively positive to the retina (back of the eye) there is an electrical potential difference when the cornea and retina move away from or toward the exploring electrode. When the cornea is closest to the electrode, a positive (downward) deflection is recorded, whereas when the retina is closest to the electrode a negative deflection results. This is illustrated on the attached graphic when the recommended EOG electrode placement of left inferior and right superior occulogram are utilized. In many sleep-testing facilities, both an inferior and superior electrode is placed for each eye to provide a back-up option for the EOG.

Looking left
Looking right
Looking up
Looking down

FIGURE 5-6 Eye movements.

While awake with the eyes closed, the EOG may show little or no movement. Fortunately, most individuals produce alpha-range activity while awake with the eyes closed, making this state easy to identify with certainty. Refer to the *AASM Manual for the Scoring of Sleep and Associated Events* for the rules applied to the sleep-stage scoring of wake and N1 in subjects who do not generate alpha rhythm.[1]

During drowsiness and as sleep ensues, SEMs may commence. The hallmark of N1 sleep onset is an LAMF EEG with elevated chin EMG and most often the presence of SEMs. Unfortunately, it can be difficult to differentiate the wake state, stage N1 sleep, or stage REM sleep with the eyes open because an LAMF background makes up the EEG pattern for these three sleep-wake states with only subtle differences. Chin EMG is essential to help determine REM versus NREM sleep in conjunction with the EOG for correct identification of these states. During wake with eyes closed, the chin EMG will be elevated and the EOG will yield sharp, fast scanning or reading eye movements with blinks. Identification of blinks on the EOG is a skill essential to differentiating this state.

During NREM 1 there will be SEMs, although rapid eye movements often appear when the subject is taking a selective serotonin reuptake inhibitor (SSRI) or selective norepinephrine reuptake inhibitor (SNRI) antidepressant. For this reason, it is imperative for a sleep technologist to know the patient's current and past medical history and medications that have been taken prior to the sleep study. These particular rapid eye movements during NREM sleep are often referred to as *Prozac eyes.*

During REM sleep, as the name suggests, there should be rapid eye movements at some point during the REM period. This is termed "phasic REM" and is the state typically thought of as REM sleep. As long as all other characteristics of stage REM persist, "tonic REM" is said to occur when there are no eye movements following a period of phasic eye movements. REM sleep can be discerned from other sleep-wake stages with a LAMF EEG when rapid eye movements appear without blinks as long as the patient is not taking an SSRI or SNRI medication. To stage-score REM sleep, the chin EMG must be lower than all other stages and at the lowest level of the recording. Chin EMG is primarily useful for differentiating NREM sleep from REM sleep as it has no bearing on scoring the substages of NREM sleep. To ensure a distinct drop in the qualitative chin EMG signal at the onset of REM, the amplifier should be continuously adjusted during NREM sleep to produce a minimal signal deflection of approximately one-half of the channel's peak-to-peak capability. The technologist must also identify and respond to 60-Hz interference. Artifact in the chin EMG should be eliminated to ensure it does not mask a reduction in muscle tone representative of REM sleep.

An alternate method of recording EOG may also be used which allows for the recording of oblique eye movements. Many practitioners find adding these channels enables the identification of REM sleep onset at the earliest possible moment during testing. For this method, EOG electrodes are placed 1 cm lateral and 1 cm inferior to the outer canthus of each eye. Both the left inferior ocular (LIO) and the right inferior ocular electrodes are referenced to a supranasion electrode, which is placed at the Fpz anatomic location. This alternate method of EOG recording yields both in-phase and out-of-phase deflections. The deflections, while looking left and right, will be out-of-phase and identical to those from the recommended method. For up and down eye movements, in-phase deflections moving in the same direction will be recorded. However, looking up will result in a negative (upward) deflection, whereas looking down will produce a positive (downward) deflection. Regardless of which method is employed, expected deflections can be determined by visualizing electrode placement and the direction the eyes move. The correct deflection for the left or right EOG channel can always be determined according to whether the front or the back of the eye is closest to the electrode.

As an example using the recommended EOG derivations, when the patient looks to the left, the left cornea moves toward the LIO electrode. Simultaneously, the left cornea moves away from, and the retina moves closer to, the right superior ocular (RSO) electrode. Because the cornea is relatively positive and the retina relatively negative, when the cornea is closer to the LIO electrode, the deflection is positive (downward) on the left EOG channel. Because the retina is closer to the RSO, the deflection is negative (upward) on the right EOG channel.

ELECTROMYOGRAM

The electromyogram is a measure of the electrical potential difference generated by groups of skeletal muscle cells at rest and during activation. For the purposes of PSG monitoring, the EMG is a qualitative signal, although a voltage threshold must be met for scoring limb EMG events. Overall, the monitoring of EMG is important to the sleep technologist as it provides information on the sleep state of the patient and whether specific body movements cause disruptions in the sleep continuity for the patient.

Chin Electromyogram

During REM sleep, the body is virtually paralyzed, causing chin EMG tone to disappear (atonia) as submentalis muscles become inhibited by the brain. The submentalis muscle, located immediately under the chin, is very useful in identifying wake, sleep, and REM. The AASM recommends a bipolar derivation of the submentalis with two electrodes to record chin muscle tone and one additional back-up electrode.

One electrode is placed 2 cm above the inferior edge of the mandible (jawbone) on the middle of the chin and the other two are placed 2 cm below the inferior edge of the mandible, one 2 cm to the left and the other 2 cm to the right.[1] During acquisition, the anterior midline electrode should be used as input 1 with either of the two electrodes below the inferior edge of the mandible as input 2. The chin EMG amplitude should be high enough that an obvious drop can be seen when the patient goes into REM sleep.[1,3]

Many laboratories expect that during relaxed wakefulness, the minimum chin EMG amplitude should be approximately one half the width of the recording channel. As long as the chin EMG signal is not intruding on adjacent channels, excessive amplitude is never a problem. The primary issue with recording chin EMG exists when the amplitude is insufficient, making it difficult to determine the transition from NREM to REM sleep. This is a particularly troubling issue when reduction in amplitude during this transition uncovers artifact, making the relative change in amplitude nominal. Figure 5-7 provides an example of the chin EMG.

Leg Electromyogram

The leg EMG is important to monitor as it gives information concerning limb movements and any changes in sleep patterns caused by these movements. The anterior tibialis muscle group can be best located by having the patient flex the big toe up and down. During this maneuver the belly of the anterior tibialis can be located for electrode placement by feeling for muscle activation. Electrodes should be placed, one above the other, along the belly of each anterior tibialis 1 to 3 cm apart. If only one channel is available, both legs can be recorded on a single channel by placing an electrode from one leg in the input 1 position and an electrode from the other leg into the input 2 position of a single derivation. This is not recommended, but it will suffice, if necessary. Unfortunately, with this "linked" derivation the long interelectrode distance will almost invariably result in ECG artifact and the likelihood of 60-Hz artifact will be dramatically increased.

Impedance measures of less than 10 K ohms are recommended and typically achievable with good skin preparation.[1,3] However, the technologist must weigh the cost of excessive skin abrasion when impedance measures remain high despite adequate preparation, particularly if the patient is severely diabetic or if other concerns exist regarding the patient's ability to heal and fight infection. The skin should not be breached in this scenario and the technologist's rationale for allowing impedances to remain high should be thoroughly documented. Filters should be set to accommodate a bandwidth of 10 to 100 Hz with a notch filter, if necessary. The sample rate should be set to 200 to 500 Hz.

Figure 5-8 provides examples of both right and left leg EMG with right leg movement shown.

MODIFIED LEAD II ELECTROCARDIOGRAPHY (ECG)

The ECG is a vital parameter for all sleep recordings and is used to document changes in heart rate and ECG signal morphology related to sleep state, abnormal events, and/or underlying pathologic conditions. Nerves in the heart are highly specialized to depolarize and to conduct electrical activity through specific nerve tracts. When stimulated, these nerve tracts cause cardiac muscles to contract in a sequence, which is responsible for the cardiac cycle that sends nutrient-rich, oxygenated blood throughout the body.

Cardiac anatomy is covered in a later chapter; however, for a fundamental understanding, the **P wave** of the ECG complex represents the electrical activity responsible for atrial depolarization and contraction. The **QRS complex** represents the electrical activity responsible for ventricular depolarization and contraction. Finally, the **T wave** represents ventricular repolarization, or relaxation. Contraction of the ventricles results in such a large signal that it obliterates the signal that would otherwise represent atrial repolarization; therefore, the wave form representing atrial repolarization is buried within the QRS complex.

Lead Placement

The lead placement recommended by the AASM is referred to as modified lead II[1]. One lead is placed below the right clavicle, aligned with the nipple and the other on the lower left ribs, aligned with the hip and midaxillary (arm pit). The left lead should be placed over an intercostal space, between the ribs, although this space is sometimes difficult to identify in the patient population served by sleep centers. The right lead is plugged into the negative input and the left into the positive connection on the ECG harness. This lead placement should yield an upright P wave, which is of most importance, at the start of the recording. If not, reverse the inputs so that the P wave is upright. Depending on exact electrode placement, and the patient's cardiac pathologic conditions and body composition, the QRS may either yield an upright or downward deflection. The deflection of the QRS has no bearing on the recorded data.

Many laboratories have historically recorded a modified lead I ECG in which both left and right electrodes have subclavicular placement. Because only one channel of ECG is typically recorded during sleep testing, it is imperative the channel provide the optimal amount of information possible. A modified lead II derivation provides the most detailed cardiac activity as compared with any other single derivation. Although it may be a

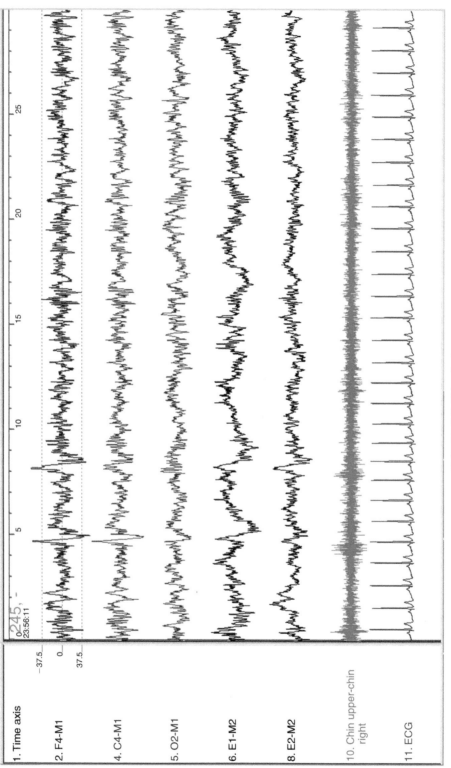

FIGURE 5-7 Chin electromyogram

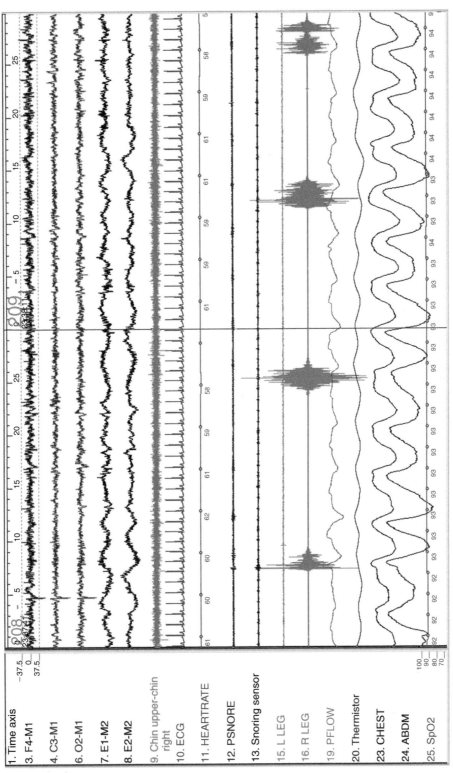

FIGURE 5-8 Right and left leg electromyogram

little more difficult to place the left electrode for a modified lead II configuration, the patient deserves optimized recording during the sleep study, given the frequency of cardiac dysrhythmias identified in the sleep laboratory.

SLEEP/WAKE STATES

Sleep stage is scored in 30-second periods called epochs. Sleep stage scoring of wake, NREM stage 1 (N1), NREM stage 2 (N2), NREM stage 3 (N3), and REM (R) is determined by the waveform information gathered during a sleep recording through the analysis of all recorded bioelectric signals. Although an over-simplification of the process, the sleep-stage characteristics that comprise more than 50% of a 30-second epoch determine the epoch's stage.

AASM GUIDELINES FOR WAKE AND SLEEP STAGES[1]

To establish continuity for the scoring of sleep studies, the AASM publishes guidelines. An overview of the descriptions of the stages of wake/sleep and their properties is listed in Table 5-1.

WAKE

Various differences exist between the appearance of recording parameters during wake with eyes open and wake with eyes closed. Throughout stage wake, however, the chin EMG yields variable muscle tone, typically higher than what is recorded during the various sleep stages. Unfortunately, during stage wake with the eyes open, the EEG can be easily confused with the EEG of stage N1 sleep and stage R sleep, since they are all LAMF patterns; however, a distinct feature of stage wake with eyes open that can resolve this issue is the presence of blinks.

When the subject is relaxed with the eyes open, stage wake is identified by a low-amplitude, mixed-frequency EEG pattern, chiefly made up of alpha waves and beta rhythms. Alpha waves are trains of 8-13 Hz activity that are sinusoidal in nature and primarily seen in the occipital region in most subjects. Alpha amplitude while the eyes are open is much lower as compared to alpha amplitude during wake with eyes closed. Maximum beta amplitude is usually evident in the frontal to central regions and is composed of frequencies greater than 14 Hz. The EOG demonstrates conjugate eye movements consisting of a slow phase followed by a fast phase in the opposite direction when reading, rapid eye movements as the subject scans the environment, and eye blinks with a frequency of 0.5-2 Hz. When the subject closes his or her eyes, there is a proliferation of alpha activity.

During relaxed wakefulness with the eyes closed, more than half of the epoch must contain EEG that consists primarily of alpha activity. Alpha waves are trains of 8-13 Hz activity which are sinusoidal in nature and primarily seen in the occipital region in most subjects. On the EOG, slow eye movements (SEMs) may be present, defined as conjugate, reasonably regular, sinusoidal movements with an initial deflection usually lasting more than 500 ms. Alpha activity is attenuated upon opening of the eyes, giving way to an LAMF EEG pattern, which is primarily seen in the central derivations.[1] Upon transition into sleep, a slowing of background EEG frequencies and attenuation of amplitude are typical.

For individuals who do not produce alpha rhythm, score stage wake if any of the following are present:
1. Eye blinks at a frequency of 0.5-2 Hz.
2. Reading eye movements.
3. Irregular, conjugate, rapid eye movements associated with normal or high EMG tone.

TABLE 5-1
Stages of Sleep

Properties	Stage W	Stage N1	Stage N2	Stage N3	Stage R
EEG	Eyes open: LAMF, little alpha Eyes closed: LAMF with alpha	LAMF, theta, vertex sharp waves	LAMF, K complexes and sleep spindles	> 20% delta waves	LAMF, sawtooth waves
EOG	Eye blinks, under voluntary control, can see SEMs when drowsy	SEM	Occasional SEM	Usually no eye movements	REM—usually phasic
*Chin EMG	Highest, and under voluntary control	High	Lower than N1	Lower than N2	Lowest, with periods of twitching

EEG, Electroencephalogram; *EMG*, electromyogram; *EOG*, electrooculogram; *LAMF*, low-amplitude, mixed-frequency; *REM*, rapid eye movement; *SEM*, slow eye movement.
* Only useful to differentiate REM sleep from NREM sleep

The wake state has two different appearances depending on whether the eyes are open or closed. An example of stage wake can be found in Figure 5-9.

STAGE N1

Stage N1 sleep is scored when greater than half of an epoch contains a LAMF EEG in subjects who generate alpha. The dominant waveform in **stage N1, LAMF activity** is characteristically within the 4 to 7 Hz range. Vertical sharp waves may also be seen in some patients. Slow-rolling sinusoidal eye movements that are conjugate, with an initial deflection usually lasting more than 500 ms are usually seen.[1] This is illustrated in Figure 5-10.

For subjects who do not generate alpha activity, begin scoring stage N1 sleep with the earliest of any of the following:
1. EEG activity in the range of 4-7 Hz with slowing of background frequencies $\geq$ 1 Hz from those of stage W.
2. Vertex sharp waves
3. Slow eye movements

STAGE N2

Stage N2 sleep begins with the presence of either a sleep spindle (12-14 Hz) or K complex each of which must have a duration lasting 0.5 seconds or longer. Spindles are maximal over the central regions but may be seen in the occipital or frontal regions. K complexes are maximal when recorded over the frontal region. A LAMF background EEG continues. Eye movement activity usually disappears. The chin activity can be variable from slightly below wake to as low as seen in REM sleep.[1] Figure 5-11 illustrates stage N2 sleep with both a sleep spindle in the central region and a K complex in the frontal region.

STAGE N3

Often called slow-wave sleep (SWS), **stage N3** sleep often emerges from stage N2 sleep and is characterized by a progressive decline in spindles and an increase in 0.5-2 Hz delta activity with peak-to-peak amplitude of more than 75 μV as measured over the frontal region. When $\geq$20% of the epoch is composed of delta waves, the epoch is scored as stage N3 sleep. On a 30-second epoch, six cumulative seconds of delta activity must be present. Eye activity is typically absent but delta waves may appear as in-phase deflections on the eye channels because of the voltage responsible for their amplitude. The chin tone is typically lower than in stage N2.[1] This is illustrated in Figure 5-12.

STAGE R

During REM sleep (**stage R**), the EEG background is LAMF. Sawtooth waves may be seen. Conjugate rapid eye movements that are sharply peaked and irregular appear in bursts. The initial defection of the eye movements usually last less than 500 ms. The chin EMG drops to its lowest level for the sleep study. The first REM sleep period usually occurs approximately 90 minutes after sleep onset.[1]

Stage R sleep is divided into two types: 1) phasic REM sleep, in which there are rapid eye movements and episodic EMG twitching, known as transient muscle activity; and 2) tonic REM sleep, in which rapid eye movements are absent and chin tone continues to be very low. Tonic REM sleep is only scored following a period of phasic REM sleep when eye movements cease but all other parameters remain consistent with REM sleep. Stage R sleep is illustrated in Figure 5-13 with example of low chin tone, LAMF waveforms, and sharp eye movements.

(Text continued on page 97)

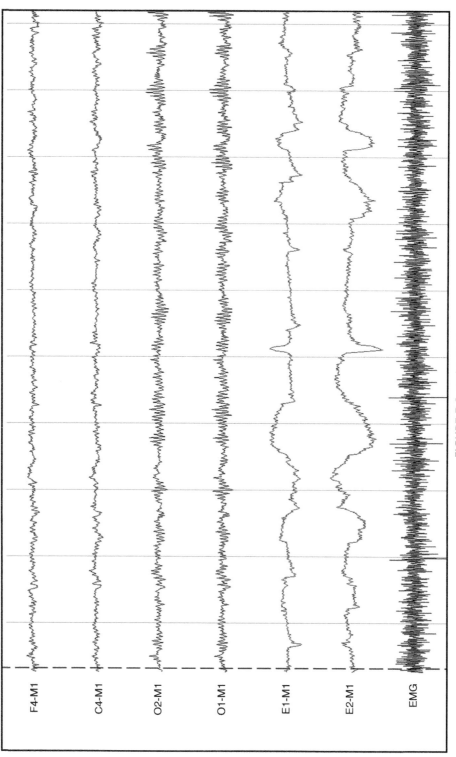

F4-M1

C4-M1

O2-M1

O1-M1

E1-M1

E2-M1

EMG

FIGURE 5-9 Wake stage

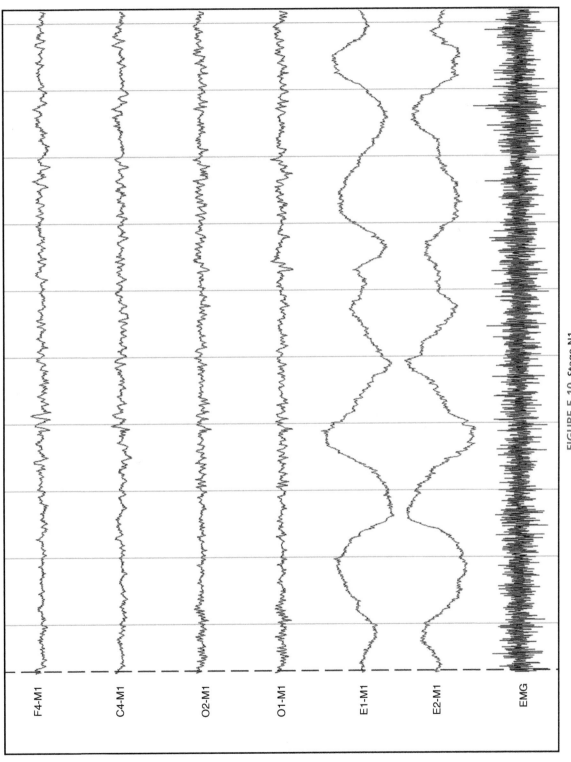

FIGURE 5-10 Stage N1

F4-M1

C4-M1

O2-M1

O1-M1

E1-M1

E2-M1

EMG

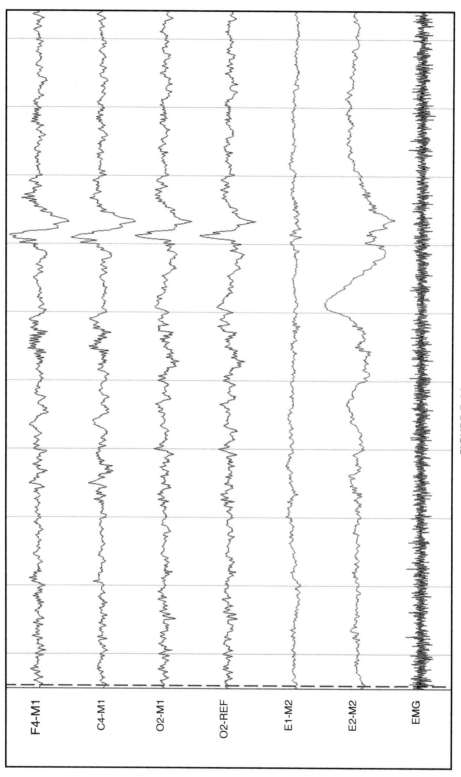

FIGURE 5-11 Stage N2

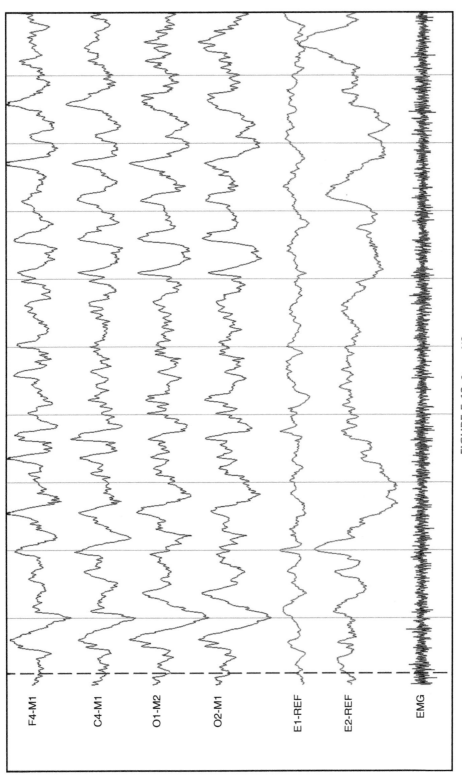

FIGURE 5-12 Stage N3

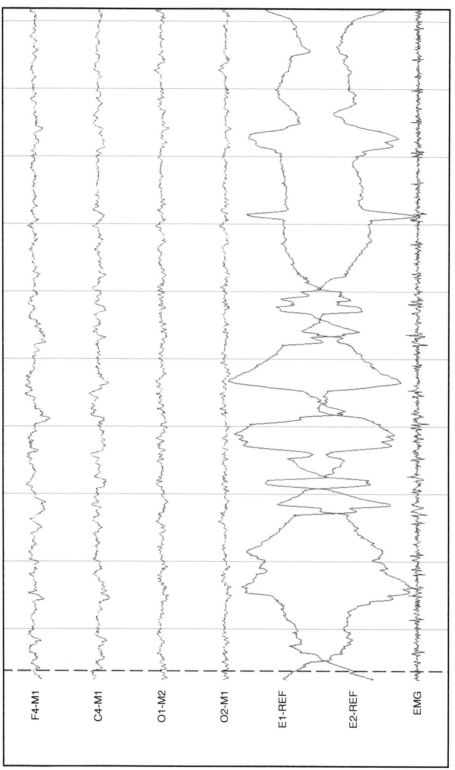

FIGURE 5-13 Stage R

CHAPTER SUMMARY

- The PSG is a compilation of three basic signal types: bioelectric, transduced, and those incorporated from a piece of ancillary equipment.
- Bioelectric signals directly represent the rising and falling of electrical potentials as obtained at the surface of the body. These include the EEG, EMG, EOG, and ECG.
- Through the use of the EEG, each sleep state has been observed to have its own distinctive electrophysiologic, behavioral, and automatic characteristics to allow for specific categorization of each phase of sleep.
- The EOG and the EMG are important to determining stage R versus other sleep stages.
- The AASM has set specific guidelines for the scoring of sleep stages on the polysomnogram.

References

1. Berry R, Brooks R, Gamaldo C, Harding S, Marcus C, Vaughn B: *The AASM manual for the scoring of sleep and associated events V2.0,* Darien, Ill, 2012, American Academy of Sleep Medicine.
2. Scheidt S, Netter F, Heidel W: *Basic electrocardiography,* ed 1, West Caldwell, NJ, 1986, Ciba-Geigy.
3. Mattice C, Brooks R, Lee-Chiong T: *Fundamentals of sleep technology,* ed 2, Philadelphia, 2012, Lippincott Williams & Wilkins.

REVIEW QUESTIONS

1. A device that converts one form of energy to another, such as mechanical energy into electrical energy, is known as a(n):
   a. Oximeter
   b. Transducer
   c. Impedance meter
   d. Capnograph

2. Relaxed wakefulness with eyes closed typically results in:
   a. Alpha activity
   b. Spindle activity
   c. REMs
   d. K complexes

3. A clear pattern of rhythmic alpha activity changing to a relatively low-voltage, mixed-frequency pattern occurs during transition from:
   a. Stage wake to stage N1
   b. Stage N1 to stage N2
   c. Stage N2 to stage N3
   d. Stage N1 to stage R

4. A 0.5-second burst of 12-14 Hz activity describes a:
   a. K-complex
   b. REM
   c. SEM
   d. Spindle

5. A 0.5-second sharp negative deflection immediately followed by a slower positive component describes a:
   a. Delta wave form
   b. K complex
   c. Spindle
   d. REM

6. A 1-second, 75 μV wave form describes a:
   a. Delta wave
   b. Spindle
   c. K complex
   d. SEM

7. Sharply contoured 2-6 Hz waves are typically noted in which stage of sleep?
   a. Stage N1
   b. Stage N2
   c. Stage N3
   d. Stage R

8. Epileptiform activity on the PSG encompasses which of the following?
   a. K complex
   b. Spindle
   c. Spike
   d. Delta

9. An eye movement to the right produces which of the following signals?
   a. Downward deflection on the E2
   b. Downward deflection on the E1
   c. Lateral deflection on the E2
   d. Lateral deflection on the E1

10. An eye movement to the left produces which of the following signals?
    a. Downward deflection on the E1
    b. Downward deflection on the E2
    c. Lateral deflection on the E1
    d. Lateral deflection on the E2

Chapter 6

The Recording of Physiological Parameters and Electrical Safety

Michael Salemi

CHAPTER OUTLINE

LEARNING OBJECTIVES

After reading this chapter, you will be able to:
1. Specify recorded physiologic parameters.
2. Interpret baseline patient data.
3. Classify sleep study calibrations.
4. Distinguish documentation required during sleep studies.
5. Predict factors for optimization of recorded data.
6. Demonstrate the use and limitations of filters.
7. Specify gain and sensitivity adjustments.
8. Describe electrical safety factors for polysomnography.

KEY TERMS

diagnostic polysomnogram
earth ground
electromotive force (EMF)
frequency response curve
ground loop
high-frequency artifact
machine calibrations

macroshock
microshock
montage calibrations
physiologic calibrations
signal polarity
slow-frequency artifact

spectral power
split-night PSG
standing orders
stray capacitance
stray inductance
therapeutic intervention

The recording of a polysomnogram (PSG) requires the sleep technologist to use a comprehensive skill set. Performing a sleep study requires a firm grounding in technical knowledge, from the application of electrodes through electrical safety, electrical signal processing, and display and storage of data in a digital format. A technologist who combines these technical skills with basic sleep science and knowledge of treatment modalities is prepared to effectively provide numerous hours of direct patient care.

In some ways the basics of recording an electroencephalogram (EEG) during sleep from surface electrodes has changed little since 1938 when the first EEG was recorded.[1] EEG remains a significant component of the sleep recording; however, there has been a proliferation in the development of sensors and methodologies used to measure the complex array of physiologic signals. This allows for identification of numerous sleep disorders in a single recording session. This is the "poly" of *polysomnography,* which literally means "many sleep writings."

Of course, much of the "writing" today happens in a digital format. It is the recording process that has changed dramatically during the past 20 years. Analog polygraphs were an impressive collection of circuits, switches, galvanometers, and pens. Computerized sleep recording systems have simplified many aspects of polysomnography. There are no more paper records to store, no ink, and no mechanical parts.

Surprisingly, the amplifier controls that allow manipulation of data have changed very little. The recording technologist must possess full knowledge of these controls in the same way required for effective use of an analog polygraph. Without this skill set, it is not possible to produce a high-quality study representative of physiologic data. Digital systems provide a wide array of clinical tools that have helped advance the role from that of someone who was primarily concerned with acquiring data to the role of technologist, a highly skilled clinician who is trained to make important clinical decisions during a sleep study.

This chapter covers the technical aspects of recording physiologic parameters and electrical safety.

RECORDING PHYSIOLOGICAL PARAMETERS

In simple terms sleep studies can be broken into two primary categories: diagnostic and therapeutic. The **diagnostic PSG** provides a comprehensive analysis of sleep patterns, cardiopulmonary function, and body movements that can confirm or rule out sleep-disordered breathing (SDB), movement disorders, inefficient sleep, and parasomnias. Abnormal cardiac and EEG events may also be identified and recorded. The diagnostic PSG montage is composed, at minimum, of channels for recording the electroencephalogram, electromyogram, electrocardiogram, airflow, respiratory effort, and oxyhemoglobin saturation measured by pulse oximetry (SpO_2).

A diagnostic PSG is also performed to observe and document the efficacy of surgery or pharmacologic treatment of a previously diagnosed sleep disorder. A treatment study is a PSG during which a **therapeutic intervention** is initiated and titrated. Therapeutic intervention is the implementation of the PAP therapy or another treatment such as oral appliance therapy. For a treatment study, the same montage as that for a diagnostic study is typically used, with the addition of a treatment parameter, most often positive airway pressure (PAP) or oral appliance therapy for SDB. A therapeutic study is characterized by active technologist intervention in the therapy being applied. A **split-night PSG** combines a diagnostic portion of study to confirm the presence of SDB along with technologist intervention to apply and adjust the therapeutic modality, which is most commonly PAP or an oral appliance.

Sleep study measurements are derived from electrodes and sensors that are designed to collect data from numerous physiologic systems. Electrical activity from the brain, eyes, heart, and muscles is measured using surface electrodes. The measurement of changes in body position, vocal sounds, and the respiratory system uses more mechanical technologies. Because these signals are so different, it is important to know *what* signal is being recording and *how* that signal is measured to determine what response to expect from each recording sensor during the occurrence of various possible sleep disruptions.

BASELINE PATIENT INFORMATION

Practitioner orders typically stipulate whether a diagnostic, therapeutic, or split-night test is to be performed, and define patient-specific recording parameters. Most laboratories have a predetermined montage for each test type; however, the ordering practitioner may choose to modify these parameters. For instance, additional EEG electrodes may be placed when epileptiform activity or the presence of a parasomnia is suggested by patient history. Prior to recording, the technologist must verify that the practitioner's orders for the test to be performed are consistent with the patient's presentation and medical history. **Standing orders**, or predetermined physician orders, for each of the study types described previously contain information on the montage, from which equipment requirements for the study can be determined. Prior to recording, the filter and gain or **sensitivity** settings, and channel labels should be verified to ensure they match the desired montage.

MACHINE CALIBRATIONS

Once the montage is verified, **machine calibration** signals are recorded and evaluated to confirm amplifier function and amplifier control response for each channel. If the acquisition system is capable of producing an all-channel calibration signal, this should be the first step in the process. The all-channel calibration is performed by simultaneously inputting a known voltage, typically 50 μV, to all amplifiers with each channel gain or sensitivity, low-frequency filter (LFF), and high-frequency filter (HFF) set to identical values. The signals generated are evaluated for consistent amplitude, morphology, and time constant. This provides documentation of overall amplifier response.

If a channel displays signals different from the others, amplifier settings should be confirmed and, if correct, amplifier function should be questioned. If incorrect, set to the proper values and repeat the process. Following the all-channel calibration, or as the first step in the process in the absence of this capability, a **montage calibration** is performed.

The montage calibration serves as visual documentation of initial amplifier settings, and is performed by inputting a calibration signal of known voltage, typically 50 μV, to all amplifiers simultaneously with gain or sensitivity, LFF, and HFF controls set to the values routinely used at the beginning of every study. The primary purpose of the montage calibration is to confirm amplifier function and appropriate channel response to amplifier control changes.

Following the montage calibration, channels with like settings (e.g., EEG channels, EMG channels, respiratory channels) should be assessed for identical output. If a channel output is not as expected, the technologist must first verify correct settings. If incorrect, the calibration should be repeated after correcting the setting.

If settings are correct and output is not as it should be, amplifier function should be questioned. Together, the all-channel and the montage calibration are referred to as *machine calibrations*. Machine calibrations verify the screen order, baseline, labels, and filter settings for each channel. The technologist's role is to visually inspect the amplitude, morphology, and decay time constant of each recording channel.

Amplitude, Morphology, and Decay Time Constant

Signal amplitude is the product of input voltage and the gain or sensitivity setting of the amplifier; morphology is the result of both the HFF and LFF settings; and the decay time constant is determined by the LFF or time constant setting.

The decay time constant, or simply *time constant,* is defined as the time it takes for a square wave to return to 37% of its original amplitude, and can dramatically affect signal morphology. A longer time constant is the result of a lower LFF setting, whereas a shorter time constant is the result of a higher LFF setting. In other words, the time constant has an inverse relationship with the LFF. On some recorders, a time constant setting replaces the LFF setting.

Once the technologist has been trained on the morphology of a square wave signal with specific filter settings, the recording parameters of the PSG can be verified quite quickly. Because all EEG and EOG channels share identical amplifier settings, respiratory channels also most often have identical amplifier settings. Because all EMG channels have the same LFF and HFF settings, visual inspection of montage calibration signals is easily accomplished by ensuring all like channels have consistent morphology and that EEG and EOG channels have identical amplitude.

All-Channel Calibration

The all-channel calibration is performed by simultaneously applying a known voltage to all AC channels with the LFF, HFF, and gain or sensitivity controls set the same for each amplifier. In the example shown in Figure 6-1, the LFF of 1 Hz, HFF of 35 Hz, and sensitivity of 100 μV/division were used. Each channel yields identical signal amplitude, morphology, and decay if functioning properly. The purpose of this procedure is to verify overall amplifier function by assessing these parameters. The all-channel calibration was an important step in preparing an analog polygraph for use, during which mechanical adjustments were made to the instrument. Although it provides a clear overview of function, most digital acquisition systems lack the ability to perform this step because mechanical adjustments are no longer necessary.

Montage Calibration

The montage calibration is similar to the all-channel calibration in that a known voltage is applied to all

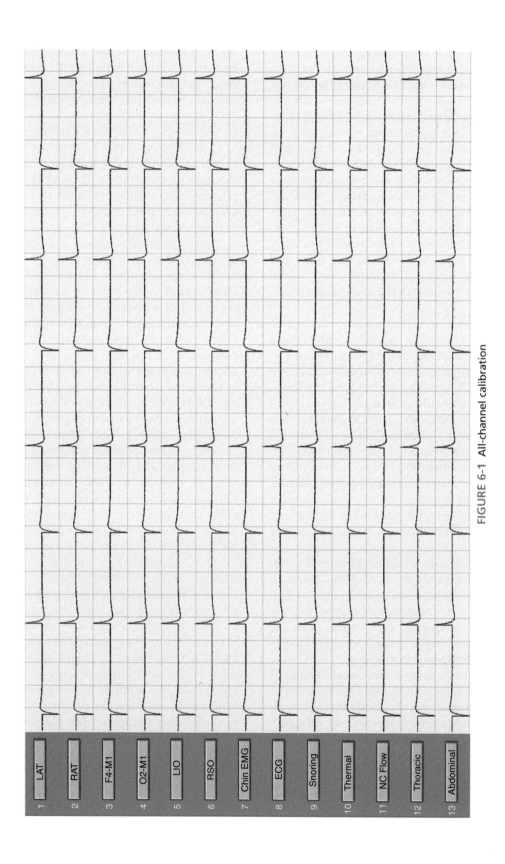

FIGURE 6-1 All-channel calibration

alternating current (AC) channels. The difference is that each channel is set to the recommended values for LFF, HFF, and gain or sensitivity typically used at the beginning of each study. This procedure is also performed to verify amplifier function and more importantly, to verify that individual channels respond appropriately to control setting changes. To evaluate recorder function based on this procedure, the technologist must compare channels with like settings (e.g., respiratory channels, EEG channels, EMG channels, etc.). If a channel displays morphology, amplitude, or decay time different from like channels, the technologist must first ensure that settings are correct. If so, amplifier function must be questioned (Figure 6-2).

SIGNAL CALIBRATIONS

Signal calibrations verify that the direct current (DC) output of ancillary devices such as oximeters, end-tidal carbon dioxide monitors, and pressure transducers are being correctly processed by the PSG recording software. Calibration procedures for these devices are defined by the device manufacturer and PSG software vendor. In general a defined voltage is generated by the ancillary device. For oximeters this is commonly a 1-V DC signal.

From within the software, the technologist types in the physiologic value associated with that signal. In this case 1 V DC equals 100% SpO_2. The software indicates if the voltage range generated by the device is within the acceptable range. Once it is accepted, the device generates a second value. Commonly this is half of the voltage output by the device. Once again this value is entered into the software. The software indicates if the calibration parameters were accepted. If data from ancillary equipment are not as expected during recording, the software file may be corrupted or this may indicate a disruption in the signal from the ancillary device to the recorder. Correction may warrant inspection and/or replacement of the connection between the two devices, or creating a new "calibration file" within the software.

Prior to and following each study, a low-value and a high-value signal should be generated from each piece of ancillary equipment and recorded as part of the pre- and poststudy machine calibrations. This serves as documentation that the recorder is correctly receiving the signal, that the calibration file is intact at the start of the procedure, and that it remained intact throughout the study.

PHYSIOLOGIC CALIBRATIONS

Physiologic calibrations, sometimes called physio-cals, are a series of instructions to the patient that serve as the technologist's first test of signal quality. The primary purpose of physiologic calibrations is to verify that all sensors and ancillary devices are operating correctly while recording patient data.

This assessment of the integrity of recording parameters serves as the time to repair or replace a sensor that is defective, misplaced, or malfunctioning prior to lights out.

Physiologic calibrations also provide a baseline recording of patient data. These baseline patient data are used as an important reference for scoring and interpretation of the study. Because physio-cals are of such critical importance, they are always recorded before each study and at the conclusion of each study.

Physiologic Calibration Commands

Patients should be informed that the sleep study begins with physio-cals. Reading or watching television after the completion of physio-cals is generally not recommended. Ask the patient to complete all bed-time rituals and use the rest room before the test begins. Any patient activity after the physio-cals can result in the need to repeat some or all commands.

Many patients tested in the sleep laboratory are hypersomnolent and will fall asleep during physio-cals. The technologist should strive to complete all calibration commands prior to sleep onset. When severe hypersomnolence exists, or the patient is cognitively impaired or hard of hearing, it may be helpful for a co-worker to remain at the bedside either to keep the patient awake, perform the calibrations along with the patient, or repeat the commands while in view of the patient. All commands should begin with the patient lying still with his or her eyes open. The patient should be encouraged to ask questions regarding the commands and report any discomfort, but casual conversation should end when physiologic calibrations begin.

It is important to understand the purpose of the commands and visually verify that each has been performed correctly and recorded with the highest fidelity. It is also imperative for the technologist to simultaneously document instruction given to the patient as well as any changes made to amplifier settings or sensors for the purpose of obtaining the best possible signal. Because trouble shooting is common during physio-cals, it is critical that once corrective action is taken, the command is repeated until it is recorded cleanly. The following represent the minimum maneuvers performed during physiologic calibrations according to established resources.[2,3]

Eyes Open

The patient should be resting quietly in the bed without talking. Give the command to the patient, "Please lie quietly with your eyes open," and immediately enter "eyes open" into study documentation when there is a visual of the patient's eyes open. Continue recording for at least 30 seconds while ensuring that the eyes remain open. It is preferable to give the command at the very beginning of an epoch so the

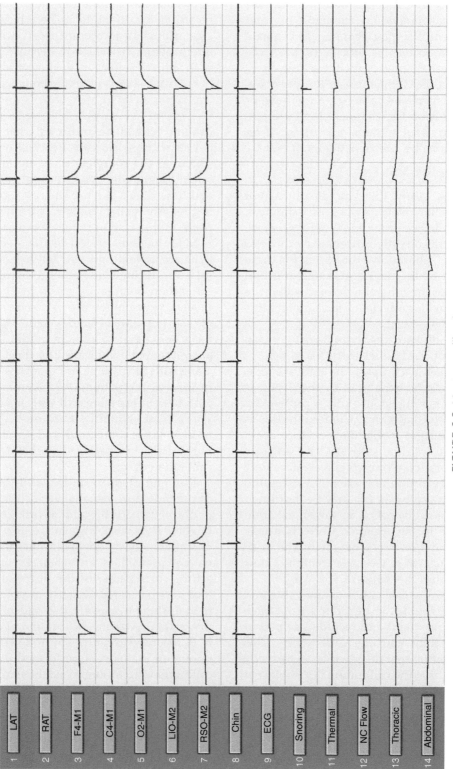

FIGURE 6-2 Montage calibration

30 seconds can be displayed on a single page without manipulating epoch boundaries in playback.

The time with eyes open serves as a baseline to observe waking EEG activity, blinks, and eye movements. This activity is often compared with the patient's EEG activity during rapid eye movement (REM) sleep, which can sometimes mimic wakefulness, and serves as a baseline of his or her alpha attenuation against which questionable epochs can be compared to determine sleep or wake.

Eyes Closed

Give the command to the patient, "Please lie quietly with your eyes closed starting now. I will let you know when to open them again." Immediately enter "Eyes-Closed" into study documentation while visualizing the appropriate deflection on the recording. Again give the command at the beginning of an epoch. It is important that a contiguous 30 seconds of activity is recorded. If the patient does not perform the command correctly, reinstruct and record the activity over. After recording for 30 seconds, ask the patient to reopen the eyes. Make sure the patient has not fallen asleep. If so, gently awaken the patient to complete the activities. Be sure to document any instances where the patient might have fallen asleep.

With eyes closed during wakefulness, alpha activity should be quite visible in the occipital recording channels—and often in other channels as well. The character and amount of alpha activity can vary greatly between patients. Approximately 10% of patients will not display alpha activity and an additional 10% will have reduced alpha activity.[2] The alpha activity at "eyes-closed" serves as a baseline to differentiate sleep from wake. The absence of alpha activity with the eyes closed is the primary indicator of sleep onset.

Alpha will generally be most prominent in the occipital channels during wake with the eyes closed. If alpha activity is not clearly evident, ensure that the patient's eyes are fully closed. If the patient's eyes are open, alpha activity will be attenuated, or minimized, and can be easily differentiated from the eyes-closed recording of a non-alpha producer by the blinks that will be recorded on EOG channels.

If eyes were previously open, repeat the instructions for "eyes-closed" and ensure that the patient's eyes remain closed for the entire 30-second period. If the patient's eyes are closed with an absence of alpha, the patient may have fallen asleep. Enter all instances of sleep into the study documentation. Gently awaken the patient to continue the calibration procedure. If the patient's eyes are closed with an absence of alpha and it is determined that a wake state exists, documentation of the status of a non-alpha producer should be provided to assist in later evaluation of data.

During the eyes-closed command, it is often helpful to begin observing the respiratory channels. Because the command "breathe normally" is nearly impossible to perform once a patient is aware of breathing, it is important to make this observation during the quiet periods of the eyes-open and closed procedures. This is an ideal time to adjust channel **polarity** for an upward deflection as the patient's inspiratory phase of breathing is observed and a downward deflection during exhalation.

It may be helpful to observe and adjust one channel, for instance thermal airflow, to match the patient's breathing followed by adjustment of the phase of all other respiratory channels to match it. This is also a good time to adjust the gain or sensitivity to ensure that respiratory channel deflections are of consistent and sufficient amplitude without intruding on other channels or blocking. Make sure that any modifications to these parameters are noted in the record.

Eye Deflections

Have the patient open his or her eyes and remain lying quietly. Give the command to the patient, "Please keep your eyes open and look straight ahead. Now slowly blink your eyes five times." Enter "blink five times" into the study documentation as you visually verify the deflections on the recording. While the patient's eyes remain open give the command, "Please keep your eyes open and without moving your head look to the right," verify the deflection, and document "eyes right." Once the deflections return to baseline, tell the patient, "Now without moving your head look to the left," verify the deflection, and document "eyes left." Allow the deflections to return to baseline and repeat these commands. Next, tell the patient, "Now without moving your head, look up toward the headboard," verify the deflection, and document "eyes up." When the deflection has returned to baseline, tell the patient, "Now, without moving your head look down toward your feet." Again, verify the deflection and document "eyes down," after which the eyes-up and eyes-down maneuvers are repeated.

During the blink command, large deflections should be observed in both the EOG and EEG channels. During the "look right, left, up, and down" commands, a sharp, out-of-phase deflection should be observed on the EOG channels. If the deflections are in phase, check the polarity settings in the recording montage for proper configuration. If the polarity setting for both eye channels is correct, verify the electrode board pin input as well as the electrode placement to ensure that both are correct. If backup electrodes have been placed, ensure that the left inferior and right superior EOG electrodes are being used. Note any changes and repeat the previous commands.

Grit Command

Give the command to the patient, "Please grit your teeth or clench your jaw," wait 2 seconds and then give the command, "Now relax," wait 2 more seconds, then repeat twice. Enter "grit teeth" into the study documentation each time deflections are visualized on the recording. Three very prominent bursts of EMG activity should be observed in the submental EMG. Muscle bursts should also be expected as a **high-frequency artifact** on the EOG and EEG channels during this procedure. A high-frequency artifact is an unwanted frequency signal recorded in addition to the signals of interest. A muscle burst is similar to what might be seen during an episode of bruxism. Having the patient swallow will yield similar results and may be added as a separate command to simulate what automatically occurs in response to postnasal drip and severe gastroesophageal reflux during sleep.

The "grit" command allows observation of the stark difference between tonic baseline (relaxed) activity and the amplitude increase with muscle activity. The tonic baseline on the chin EMG should ideally be 25 μV ± (50 μV total amplitude variance). It should not be flat. Conversely, the pen deflection during the EMG burst should not be so high that it cannot be fully displayed in the channels' dynamic range. Submental EMG amplitude is qualitative, not quantitative, so the sensitivity or gain may need to be adjusted at sleep onset. Mark any changes in the study documentation. Electrode impedance on the chin EMG should not exceed 10 KΩ. If it does, the baseline activity may in fact be 60 Hz artifact. If the impedance values are questionable, perform an impedance check. If 60 Hz artifact remains, attempt to correct the offending electrode. The 60-Hz notch filter should be used only as a last resort.

Remember that 60 Hz artifact is generally caused by a poor impedance level on one or both electrodes within a derivation, imbalanced impedance levels, or a poor connection anywhere in the patient circuit. Mark any modification to the montage in the study documentation.

Limb Movements

Ideal performance of the activation of the anterior tibialis muscle group is accomplished by having the subject dorsiflex and plantarflex the great toe of each foot individually.[4] This action best isolates the anterior tibialis muscle group from which limb movements are routinely monitored. Patients often have difficulty understanding what is needed for this procedure.

During preparation for testing, the technologist should explain what is needed during physiologic calibrations and have the patient point the great toe up and down to locate ideal placement for the leg EMG electrodes along the belly of the anterior tibialis muscle group. Incorporating this into the electrode application procedure for every patient usually prevents confusion regarding what is expected.

During calibration maneuvers, tell the patient to "point the great toe of the left leg up," wait 2 seconds, "and down," wait 2 seconds, "and now relax." Enter "flex left foot" in the study documentation as the deflections are being recorded. Repeat the process for the right leg. Very prominent bursts of EMG activity should be observed in the anterior tibialis channel recordings.

Take note that the movements are recorded in the correct leg. If not, correct the input selection or reposition inputs in the jack box. Although not recommended, some sleep laboratories combine both legs into a single channel (Figure 6-3). If this is the case, make sure that deflections are observed on the single channel during muscle activation of each leg.

In the leg EMG example shown, the right anterior tibialis (RAT) and left anterior tibialis (LAT) electrodes have been combined for display on a single channel. Although not recommended by the American Academy of Sleep Medicine (AASM), this practice is considered acceptable and is sometimes employed when channel space or amplifier numbers are limited. With the long

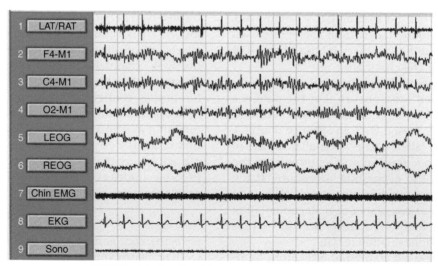

FIGURE 6-3 Combined leg electromyogram channel

interelectrode distance of the RAT-LAT derivation, it is common to record excessive unwanted signals, particularly ECG artifact.

The sample tracing also provides an example of 60-Hz artifact in the chin EMG recording. The transition to REM sleep may be difficult to discern unless this issue is resolved. Attempts should be made to resolve all artifacts prior to lights out. The technologist is also responsible for the correction of artifact as it emerges throughout the study. Since the subject is awake in this example, corrective action should be taken regardless of whether the artifact is occurring at the beginning of the study or sometime after lights out.

The "flex leg" command allows for observation of the amplitude increase during muscle activity. Converse to the chin EMG, the tonic baseline on the limb EMG channels should be flat. Electrode impedance on the limb EMG should not exceed 10 KΩ, although at times this is difficult to achieve on leg channels. When the patient is diabetic, or another medical reason exists to limit skin abrasion, limb impedance must be sacrificed rather than risking harm to the patient. The technologist should document this rationale along with the actual impedance achieved.

Breath Commands

Give the command to the patient, "Please take three deep breaths and hold the last one. I will tell you when to begin breathing again." As the patient begins the first inhalation, enter "three deep breaths" into the study documentation. After the last exhalation, remind the patient to hold for 10 seconds. Observe the deflection slowly return to baseline, thus verifying the setting of the LFF. Once the channel has returned to baseline, instruct the patient to begin breathing normally again. Patients with decreased lung function may have difficulty performing a sustained breath hold or deep breathing. An alternate command in this instance is to instruct the patient to exhale as slowly as the condition allows. If the breath hold is the only issue, a 5-second hold will typically suffice.

In addition to confirming that all sensors are functioning appropriately, this command is performed to verify that the amplifier settings for the airflow and effort channels generate a waveform that allows for the maximum range of adjustment throughout the study. The observations made during the breathing commands will not provide all of the data needed to ensure a high-fidelity signal. Keep the following in mind while recording physiologic calibrations, with regards to respiratory commands.

- Respiratory channels should be observed throughout the physiologic calibration process. "Normal" breathing is best observed during periods of eyes open and eyes closed when the patient is lying quietly in bed and not focused on breathing.
- Ensure that all respiratory signals are in phase with the correct **signal polarity**; an upward (negative) deflection during inhalation and a downward (positive) deflection during exhalation should be observed.
- An incorrect LFF setting will cause the sinusoidal respiratory waveform to be truncated or to deviate from baseline.
- The HFF setting depends on the device used and the signal to be collected.
  - For pressure transducers that are used to observe snoring, an HFF higher than the standard setting of 15 Hz is needed. The HFF setting typically used for a snoring channel (100 Hz) is often employed.
  - Many respiratory measures are obtained through ancillary devices and recorded through analog DC inputs. Each device should be used according to the manufacturers' specifications. Many ancillary devices such as pressure transducers and respiratory inductance plethysmography sensors will have specified filter settings. Gain adjustments should be made only if the device is designed for such modifications.
- The deep breathing command will allow verification that the signal is being recorded within the dynamic range of the channel. The waveform should not block, or intrude on other channels if allowed by the recording system, when the patient inhales or exhales. If it does, an adjustment should be made to the gain or sensitivity setting, depending on the acquisition system.
- The gain or sensitivity of each respiratory channel at lights out should be in the middle of the sleep recording system's available range. This will allow the most flexibility for consistent deflections throughout the study. If any specific gain setting is too close to the top of its range during physio-cals, the technologist should reposition, tighten, or loosen the respiratory belts so that recording begins in the middle of the gain scale.
- Respiratory belts can loosen when the patient is moved from the hook-up chair to the bed. They can also shift during body movements in bed. Respiratory channels are qualitative signals that require vigilance throughout the recording. The technologist may need to loosen, tighten, or reposition the belts to ensure the best possible signal quality is achieved throughout the recording.

Electrocardiogram

Check the ECG signal for the correct amplitude, polarity, and morphology. When recording a single modified lead II derivation of ECG, it is standard practice to adjust polarity at the beginning of the study to ensure an upright P wave (Figure 6-4).

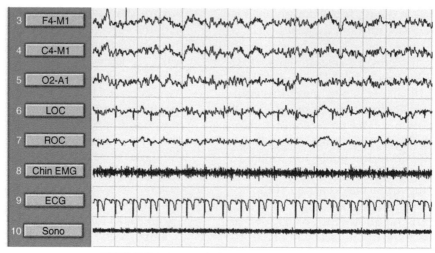

FIGURE 6-4 Reversed electrocardiogram signal

The ECG is inverted as determined by a P wave with a downward deflection. It is common practice to ensure that the P wave is upright at the start of the recording. The direction of the QRS deflection is of little importance, and the P wave and QRS deflections are sometimes opposite one another. In this example, the technologist should change the polarity within the recorder software, reverse the selector panel inputs, or unplug and reverse the inputs when a bipolar jack box is present, depending on the recording system being used. Ideally, all changes made to the recorder settings during data acquisition will remain in place for subsequent study review and scoring.

Final Observations

Review the signal quality on all channels in case any electrodes or sensors became dislodged during the calibration process. Go into the bedroom and check on the patient. Say "good night" and turn off the lights. Box 6-1 outlines the pre- and post-polysomnogram calibration sequence.

Lights Out

Return to the monitoring room immediately after saying good night to the patient and make the notation for Lights out (LT) on the study. The formal beginning of the total recording time (TRT) starts at the LT annotation. Most computerized systems have a specific button or key stroke to mark lights out. Recording time should start at the beginning of an epoch, so LT should be marked within the first seconds of an epoch on a recorder that does not automatically start TRT at the lights out mark. Likewise, lights on (LN) should be documented within the first seconds of an epoch at the end of the study, as this epoch is not counted as part of the TRT.

BOX 6-1
Prepolysomnogram and Postpolysomnogram Calibration Sequence

PRIOR TO LIGHTS OUT
- All-channel calibration (if system is capable)
- Montage calibration on standard settings
- Physiologic calibrations

FOLLOWING LIGHTS ON
- Physiologic calibrations on final test settings
- Montage calibration on final test settings
- All-channel calibration (if system is capable)

DOCUMENTATION DURING THE RECORDING

The standardized recording parameters and adjustments made during physiologic calibrations create a baseline for the PSG recording. One of the most important roles of the data collection technologist is to comment on physiologic changes, and to document any changes to recording parameters. All interactions with the recording are predicated on the baseline data and knowing when changes to the baseline occur throughout the study. For example, an amplitude reduction in the chin EMG is a possible indicator of REM sleep. An amplitude reduction in respiratory effort can be an indicator of hypoventilation, a potentially life-threatening condition.

Sleep technologists and sleep medicine physicians are trained to look for subtle changes that indicate sleep-stage changes and important events such as hypopneas, arousals, and movements. When a technologist fails to recognize signals that need to be

---

BOX 6-2
Recommended Polysomnogram Recording Documentation

- Amplifier changes and the reason for changes
- Attempts to correct a recording problem
- Rationale for allowing artifact to either temporarily or permanently continue
- Interactions with the patient during testing
- Changes made to the testing environment such as temperature adjustment
- The reason expected impedance measures are not achieved
- Any additional equipment issues, including corrective actions

ADDITIONAL OBSERVATIONS THAT MUST BE DOCUMENTED:

- Technologist observations
- Patient response to testing and treatment
- Patient vocalizations or other actions during testing

- Snoring sounds, along with a subjective level of noise
- Breathing sounds and indicators of increased work of breathing
- Abnormal body movements
- Potential epileptiform or seizure activity
- Parasomnia-related behaviors
- Real-time body position changes
- Rationale for therapeutic intervention, as appropriate
- Optimal treatment delivery device, if used
- Anything unexpected or otherwise relevant to the interpretation of data
- Estimated TST and AHI prior to application of treatment
- Any additional technologist interventions
- Patient issues with therapy or delivery device
- Any adverse reactions by the patient
- Patient acceptance/tolerance of therapy
- Technologist-physician communication

AHI, Apnea-hypopnea index; *TST,* total sleep time.

---

adjusted, or makes adjustments without proper documentation, it can result in events being missed. In some cases these failures can lead to misdiagnosis or a need to repeat the procedure. In a worst-case scenario, the patient could either be denied treatment based on data obtained from the study or placed on suboptimal therapy. See Box 6-2 for recommended PSG recording documentation.

Modern digital systems offer numerous ways to document changes. Many systems automatically annotate all changes made to the amplifier settings. The simple computer annotation of "change HFF from 35 Hz to 10 Hz" does not explain why the change was made—and that is often the more important piece of information. Most digital PSG systems are capable of storing a library of common annotations such as the physiologic calibration commands. This allows the technologist to document common occurrences with a single keystroke rather than having to type the entire statement. Most often, calibration commands and some general documentation statements come pre-entered into the acquisition system. However, annotation fields are usually user-definable and can be easily modified for a facility's specific needs. See Box 6-3 for interval PSG recording documentation.

OPTIMIZING THE RECORDED DATA

An important premise to follow during data acquisition is to preserve and record a faithful representation of the patient's actual physiologic state. This simple rule can be a guide in the decision-making process throughout the study.

BOX 6-3
Interval Polysomnogram Recording Documentation

The American Academy of Sleep Medicine recommends that notations on the following parameters be documented every 20 minutes during the recording.[5]
- Sleep stage at the time of notation
- SpO$_2$ nadir during the observation period
- Observed events during the observation period
  - Respiratory
  - Cardiac
  - Movement
- Treatment parameters
  - Treatment modality
  - Treatment level

ARTIFACTS

The first, and seemingly straightforward, approach is to eliminate artifact in the recording. Artifacts are the result of both physiologic and environmental factors. Examples of physiologic artifact include EMG artifact in the EEG and EOG from bruxism and movement artifact from body position changes. An example of an environmental artifact is the intrusion of 60 Hz. Sweat can result in a **slow-frequency artifact** and is a physiologic manifestation of an environmental problem.

Using this premise, it becomes clear that *artifact* is a very broad concept, and each of these examples requires a very different course of action. Artifacts create a series of trade-offs during the recording that require careful thought as opposed to hard rules. The recognition, cause, and prevention or correction of various artifact types is covered in more depth in Chapter 10.

MEDICAL RECORD DOCUMENTATION

Documentation often needs to be made in more than one place. A specific sleep center may have guidelines for what is to be documented in the sleep recorder software, technologist paperwork, paper medical record, or electronic health record. It is always helpful, as a recording technologist, to ask the lead technologist and medical director for information regarding documentation policies and feedback on the appropriateness and thoroughness of documentation. Remember that the purpose of annotation during recording is to allow other clinicians to efficiently review the study so the correct diagnosis and optimal treatment for the patient can be determined.

Technologist notations become medical documentation that may be subjected to legal review. Always use appropriate language that is accurate and stays on point. Never make derogatory statements about the patient. It is beyond the technologist's scope of practice to make inferences about information provided by the patient or otherwise obtained. The technologist should directly report the data as obtained and allow the physician or otherwise qualified practitioner to interpret what it means.

Patient actions such as inappropriate sexual behavior should be reported, but how such information should be communicated is facility-dependent. It is unlikely that the recording software is the appropriate place for such communication.

USE AND LIMITATIONS OF FILTERS

UNDERSTANDING THE WAY FILTERS WORK

For many beginning technologists, the concept of filtering initially seems very straightforward. They imagine a process where two values are set, one high and one low, and only the frequencies between the settings are recorded. This concept can be visualized in Figure 6-5, using a window blind as an analogy. The blind is pulled down to restrict a fixed percentage of the window. But in truth, a filter is much more akin to a venetian blind that from the viewer's perspective appears to gradually filter more light at the top than at the bottom.

A filter gradually attenuates (reduces) the amplitude of signals possessing a frequency that approaches, reaches, and surpasses its setting. The basic process is identical for both LFFs and HFFs, but the learner must imagine the starting point from which frequencies either increase or decrease as a point somewhere between these two settings. The area between the two settings within which data are not affected by the filters should span the range of frequencies of interest being recorded on the particular channel. Overuse of filters occurs when their settings attenuate signals of interest.

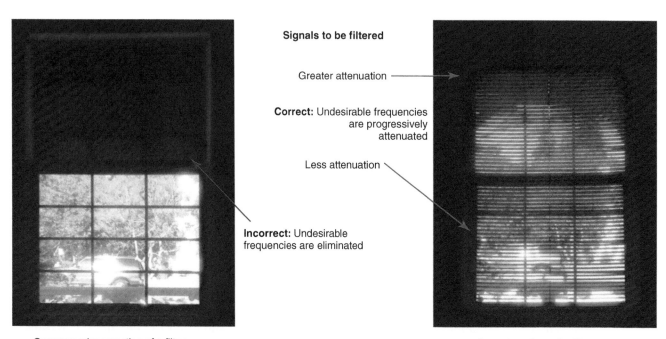

Signals to be filtered

Greater attenuation

Correct: Undesirable frequencies are progressively attenuated

Less attenuation

Incorrect: Undesirable frequencies are eliminated

Common misperception of a filter

Correct analogy of a filter

FIGURE 6-5 Analogy of a filter.

BOX 6-4
Summary of Amplifier Filter Characteristics

- HFFs and LFFs operate in the same manner.
  - Their response can be plotted as a frequency response curve.
- As signal frequency approaches the filter setting, it will begin being attenuated. The amplifier output for these frequencies will be >80% and up to 100% of the original amplitude (attenuation by 0% to <20%):
  - As input frequency decreases toward the LFF setting.
  - As input frequency increases toward the HFF setting.

- When input signal frequency is identical to the filter setting, output amplitude is exactly 80% of the original signal amplitude (attenuation by 20%).
- As input frequency surpasses the filter setting, its amplitude will be attenuated by more than 20%. The output for these signals will be less than 80% of the original amplitude:
  - When input frequency is lower than the LFF setting.
  - When input frequency is higher than the HFF setting.

HFF, High-frequency filter; *LFF*, low-frequency filter.

One example of overuse that is often overlooked occurs when the patient either has known or suspected epileptiform activity. Because the recommended HFF setting for EEG channels as part of a PSG is 35 Hz,[5] consideration should be given to a departmental policy on use of a higher setting either at all times or specifically in this scenario. An HFF less than 70 Hz can both distort or attenuate spikes and render muscle artifact to resemble spikes on the EEG channel.[6] If artifact is present, reducing the HFF to 35 Hz would be well within established guidelines.

It is very important that beginning technologists approach the process of filtering during a recording with a commitment to truly understand what a filter change does to the waveforms being recorded. Although seemingly complex, the way in which amplifier filters work is relatively simple. This is summarized in Box 6-4. Note the significant distortion that can occur when filters are overused.

FREQUENCY RESPONSE

Each amplifier is designed with a given frequency response, or degree of attenuation that is applied to input signals at varying frequencies when an LFF or HFF is set. This can be plotted graphically as a **frequency response curve** from which a prediction can be made regarding the percentage of original signal amplitude that will be present at the amplifier output.

The lower end of a frequency response curve is illustrated in Figure 6-6. This particular curve represents an LFF setting of 5 Hz, as indicated by the attenuation of the input signal to 80% of its original amplitude. On the other end of a frequency response curve, the input frequency that is attenuated to 80% of its original amplitude represents the HFF setting used during recording.

The concept of frequency response is further complicated by the fact that there is no standard amplifier control design between manufacturers; however, the frequencies of interest in a sleep recording are

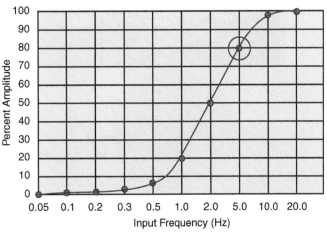

FIGURE 6-6 Attenuation of frequencies

somewhat limited, so the actual influence of these design changes is negligible. Most manufacturers of polysomnography recorders design amplifiers that attenuate signal amplitude for input frequencies identical to the filter setting to 80% of the original, whereas others produce amplifiers that attenuate these signals to 70% of the original amplitude. The sleep technologist should know which degree of attenuation to use and make appropriate changes.

The frequency response curve represents the percentage of attenuation (a reduction in amplitude) for frequencies as they approach, reach, and surpass the frequency cut-off, or filter setting. The set point of the filter is when the signal is attenuated to 80% (attenuated by 20%) of its actual, or original, amplitude. This means that signals with higher frequency than the HFF setting are not completely eliminated from the bandwidth of recorded signals, but rather the signal is progressively attenuated. Likewise, slow signals are not eliminated by an LFF setting. Frequencies approaching the filter setting and those below the setting are progressively attenuated.

PLACEMENT OF ELECTRODES

In the case of EEG, specific brainwave patterns are more prominent in certain regions of the brain. For instance, alpha activity (8-12 Hz) is more prominent in the occipital region; sleep spindles (12-14 Hz) in the central region; and K complexes and delta activity (0.5-2 Hz) in the frontal region.[5,7] Each of these waveforms are a specific marker for sleep-wake staging and arousal identification. It would be incorrect to assume that delta activity *only* happens in the frontal region or that the frontal electrode will *only* record delta activity. Each placement will pick up many frequencies at the same time; what is recorded will be based on the dominant waveforms and the attenuation from the filter settings. Remember that the maximum power of a brainwave in sleep is generally less than 100 microvolts (μV). A microvolt is 1/1,000,000 of 1 volt or 0.000001 V. **Spectral power** is the analysis of dominant waveform frequencies.

A useful analogy for an electrode recording brainwaves is that of a buoy in the ocean (Figure 6-7). The buoy (our electrode) is a stationary object in a medium that is characterized by many waves. As portrayed in the illustration, the water is composed of waves, each of differing heights (amplitude) and widths (wave length). At any given time, the buoy is never being struck by a single wave. Some waves are more dominant because of greater amplitude, but the buoy is also coming into contact with smaller waves and chops, which are still smaller waves.

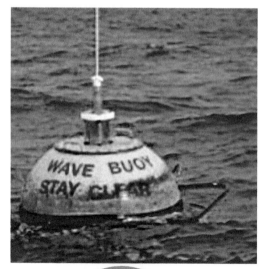

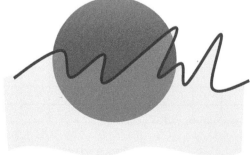

FIGURE 6-7 Analogy of amplitude and wave length.

BOX 6-5

Trouble-shooting Analysis for Root Problem

Who is the patient?	57-year-old man with suspected sleep-disordered breathing—split titration
What is the problem and its root cause?	Low-frequency artifact in the EEG and EOG channels
When is this occurring?	Patient is in stage N2—pretreatment, frequent obstructive apneas
How can this be solved? List:	1. Lower room temperature. 2. Increase LFF. 3. Reapply gel, reattach, or replace electrodes.
Implement appropriate action.	1. Lower room temperature. Yes, temperature of the room should be cooled, but it will take several minutes to have an effect. 2. Reattach, reapply gel, or replace electrode if loosened and moving on skin's surface. Yes, attempt. 3. Increase LFF on the primary EEG and EOG channels. Yes, increase LFF from 0.3 Hz to 1 Hz. Leave backup channels on 0.3 Hz.
Reassess.	Monitor one of the backup EEG channels to observe when sweat artifact has dissipated. When sweat artifact is gone, set LFF back to 0.3 on all channels.
Document.	Make a notation in the record that describes the problem and the exact actions taken to correct the artifact.

EEG, Electroencephalogram; *EOG,* electrooculogram; *LFF,* low-frequency filter.

During a PSG, amplifier settings need to be adjusted to correct artifact. But because each electrode placement records many frequencies simultaneously, the effect that an amplifier modification has on that specific channel, as well as the entire recording, must always be considered. Prior to filter manipulation during the recording it is important to consider the goal and what actions are necessary to accomplish the goal (Box 6-5).

ADJUSTMENT OF SENSITIVITY AND GAIN

Sensitivity and gain are two methods of changing the amplitude of a waveform for display or recording. These terms are often used interchangeably, but it is critical for the sleep technologist to understand that there are important differences between them.

GAIN

Gain refers to the process of basic amplification analogous to the volume control on audio equipment. Gain is often scaled in the percentage of difference from the baseline setting of 1 (i.e., 0.25×, 5×, 10×, 200×, 20,000×). Many digital systems allow the user to input any value for gain.

In a digital recording environment, two more factors affect the size of a signal: **dynamic range** and scale. The *dynamic range* of a channel is defined as the amount of voltage the channel will be able to display in the screen space it is allotted within the software. For EEG this may be 200-250 µv; for SpO2 it may be 0.5 to 1 V. The scaling of a signal is often controlled by the user increasing or decreasing the size of the display window.

Gain is most often used on digital acquisition systems, but some manufacturers continue to use the concept of sensitivity as the way to adjust signal amplitude. Although this is theoretically an outdated concept, the technologist must understand its application to use some modern recorders effectively.

SENSITIVITY

Sensitivity is expressed in µV/mm and represented by the formula $S = V/A$, where S = sensitivity, V = voltage, and A = amplitude. With this simple formula, one can calculate any one of the three variables when the other two are available. Through simple algebra, $S = V/A$ can be rearranged as $A = V/S$ to determine the amplitude to be expected from a known input voltage and $V = S \times A$ to determine the input voltage responsible for a given amplitude. A sensitivity setting of 1 µV/mm literally means that 1 µV of input voltage (from the patient) will yield a 1-mm deflection on the recording. Remember that there is an understood "1" in front of any units that stand alone; therefore, a sensitivity setting of 70 µV/mm means that 70 µV of amplifier input is required to produce a 1 mm deflection on the recorder. At this same setting, an input to the amplifier of 210 µV will produce a 3-mm deflection; however, if the sensitivity setting is changed to 10 µV/mm, the same 210 µV input will now produce a 21-mm deflection. This is because the recorder now produces a 1-mm deflection for every 10 µV of input.

To calculate sensitivity one needs a known input voltage, which is why AC channels in polysomnography are calibrated with a 50-μV square wave. The standard recording sensitivity setting for recording adult EEG is 5 μV/mm, so a 50-μV signal will produce a deflection of 1 cm.

The sensitivity settings for polysomnography were developed during the age of paper recording when 1-cm squares were clearly delineated on the recording paper. On a digital system, the denotation of a centimeter is somewhat meaningless when channels in a flexible display window can be dragged to any size on the screen. The sensitivity formula is still helpful to understand that the scale of the space that represents 1 cm can be increased or decreased at will.

WAVEFORM RULER

In polysomnography, there are two AC channels that have associated scoring rules with specific amplitude criteria. For EEG, delta waves must attain amplitude greater than 75 μV before being included toward scoring stage N3, and limb movement events require an amplitude increase at least 8 μV above the resting baseline. Because the scaling of a channel can vary widely, many digital sleep systems feature a tool that is often referred to as a "waveform ruler." This tool automatically adjusts the sensitivity scale in microvolts to scaling of the channel.

In Figure 6-8, a segment lasting 0.5 seconds was selected from the central EEG channel to determine if the highlighted burst meets the sleep spindle scoring criteria. Frequency can easily be counted as approximately 6.5 cycles from the 0.5-second magnified segment for an average frequency of 13 Hz, as also calculated by the software and listed on Figure 6-8. Because this burst is in a central derivation at the beginning of the epoch, lasts at least 0.5 seconds, and is within the 12-14 (11-16) Hz range, it is scored as a spindle and warrants a stage change to N2 sleep from N1 on the previous epoch.

In Figure 6-9, the distance between vertical gridlines on the PSG data represents 1 second, and the distance between the red horizontal gridlines represents 75 μV. A segment of approximately 6 seconds (5.99) of data was sampled to illustrate the 75-μV and 0.5-second duration criteria being reached during at least 20% of the 30-second epoch. If either criterion is questionable, individual waveforms should be measured for inclusion in the 6 seconds.

In Figure 6-10, the waveform from the frontal EEG channel, highlighted by the purple line, was assessed to determine if it meets the duration criterion for delta activity. The trough-to-trough duration, which must be ≥0.5 seconds is measured as 0.67 seconds.

To measure the voltage responsible for this deflection, only the area between the initial trough and the peak of the waveform should be selected within the

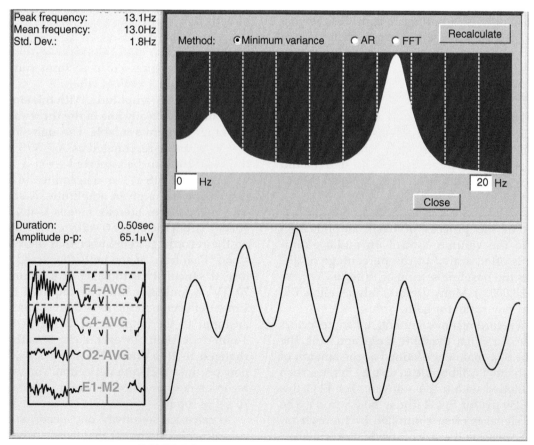

FIGURE 6-8 Waveform ruler, sleep spindle frequency

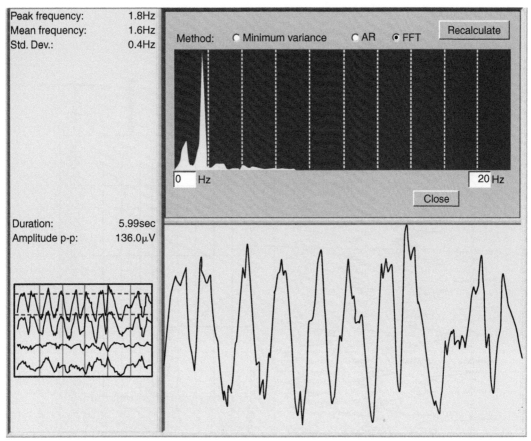

FIGURE 6-9 Waveform ruler, delta wave determination

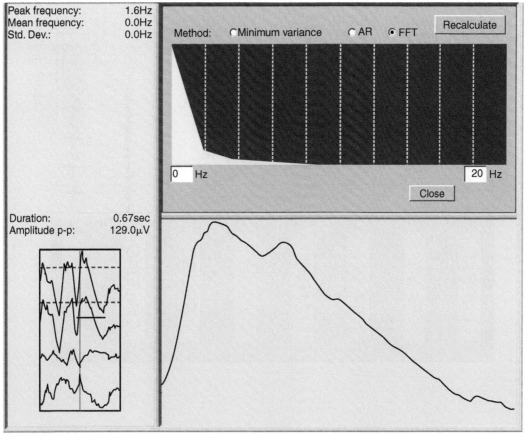

FIGURE 6-10 Waveform ruler, trough-to-trough determination

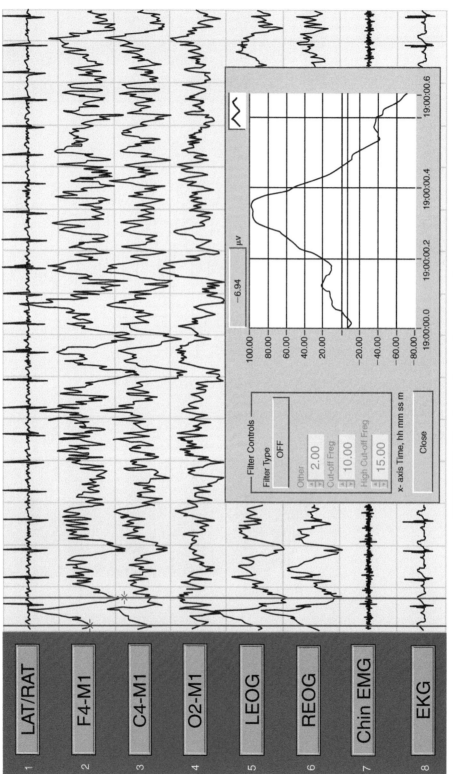

FIGURE 6-11 Waveform ruler, x-axis versus y-axis

waveform ruler function. The peak-to-peak amplitude listed on Figure 6-10, which actually represents the voltage responsible for the deflection, is calculated by the software based on the highest and lowest points selected within the window. The value displayed represents peak-to-trough voltage rather than trough-to-peak voltage, as is correctly measured for polysomnographic monitoring.

On the waveform ruler from this software program, the x-axis represents duration, and the selected waveform is clearly at least 0.6 seconds as measured from trough to trough. The y-axis is calibrated in millionths of volts, or microvolts (Figure 6-11). To assess the voltage responsible for the negative deflection of the selected waveform, the first cursor could be placed at the initial trough and the second at the peak (peak-to-peak in EEG terminology). Because a calibrated voltage scale exists on the y-axis, however, it is easy to see, while evaluating the entire waveform, that the initial, upward deflection was generated by approximately −100 μV. The value of any waveform ruler relies on the user's understanding of how measures are obtained and the careful selection of data points.

ELECTRICAL SAFETY

CURRENT, VOLTAGE, AND RESISTANCE

The movement of charged particles through a circuit is called *current,* which is measured in amperes (amps). Charged particles are always present in a conductive material such as copper wire, but there is no current until a power source is connected to the circuit.[3] Current is produced when electrons begin moving through the circuit. Electrical current is generally classified into two types: alternating current (AC) and direct current (DC).

DC refers to the movement of charged particles in a single direction. A battery is an excellent example of stored DC electricity. Each battery has a negative and positive pole. If a wire is placed between the two poles, a DC circuit is created, and current will flow in a single direction from negative to positive as long as the circuit is patent and the electrochemical reaction responsible for the battery's energy continues.

Commercial electricity is an example of an AC current. In an AC circuit, electrons flow in both directions at a known frequency, which in North America is 60 Hz. In an electrical outlet, current is delivered through the "hot" (black) terminal and returns through the "neutral" (white) terminal. Modern electrical outlets contain a third (green) terminal, which is connected to a building ground that eventually ends at an **earth ground**.

Voltage can be thought of as electrical force, or the electrical "push" within a circuit. It is defined as the difference in electrical potential between two points. Voltage may represent electrical force from a generator, known as **electromotive force (EMF)**, or it may represent stored energy such as that in a battery. Ohm's law defines the relationship between voltage, current, and a third property called **resistance**. Resistance is the property of materials to restrict current, which is measured in Ohms (Ω).

The equation for Ohm's law is $I = V/R$, where I is the current through the conductor in units of amperes, V is the potential difference measured across the conductor in units of volts, and R is the resistance of the conductor in units of ohms. The equation is often expressed as $I = E/R$, where E stands for electromotive force and is used synonymously with *voltage* (Figure 6-12).

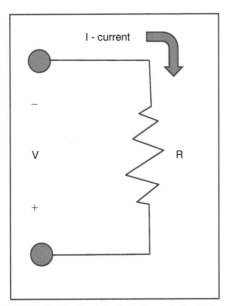

FIGURE 6-12 Graphic depiction of Ohm's law.

A simple analogy for an electric circuit is water flowing through a set of pipes that is driven by a pump. The system of pipes is the water circuit. Voltage is represented by the water pressure that exists between any two points when the pump is turned on. The electrical potential is the water. Even if the pump is not on, the system still contains some water pressure, and this represents the electronic potential. Resistance is created by foreign materials in the water. This analogy will help us throughout the remainder of this chapter. To avoid confusion, keep in mind that the flow of electricity is from negative to positive, which is opposite conventional flow. With conventional flow, like the water in this analogy, movement is from positive to negative or higher pressure to lower pressure.

GROUNDING AND LEAKAGE CURRENT

The electrical ground in a standard three-prong outlet creates an alternate pathway for leakage currents to travel. Leakage currents originate from two primary sources, **stray capacitance** and **stray inductance**. Stray capacitance is a process that results in leakage of stored electrical energy; stray inductance is a process that results in an electrical inductance of energy.

Capacitance is a process that stores electrical energy; the devices that perform this process are called capacitors. Capacitors are constructed by placing two closely spaced conductive plates in parallel and placing an insulator between them, called a dielectric. When current is passed through a capacitor, free electrons flow through the insulator from the plate with the positive charge to the plate with the negative charge. When the circuit is broken, the capacitor remains charged.

Stray capacitance in device power cords and power supplies is the most common source of leakage current.[4] One only needs to look at a diagram of a power cord to recognize that the wires running parallel to each other and separated by insulation in a power cord act as a capacitor (Figure 6-13). Capacitors running in parallel have a cumulative

effect. Device manufacturers must consider the construction materials and length of the power cord, which can both have an effect on the potential leakage current build-up.

Inductance is a term that describes the electromagnetic field that is created around a wire when current is passed through. An inductor is a coil of wire within an electronic circuit that amplifies the magnetic field and is able to store some of the energy.

The green grounding wire in an electric power cable connects to a building's earth ground. An earth ground creates a pathway for the stray electrons in a leakage current. As its name suggests, an earth ground connects the electrical grounding wire to the earth. Because the earth will always have a lower potential than a charged circuit, any electrons leaking from the circuit will be attracted to the lower potential of the earth where they dissipate.

Returning to the water analogy, imagine that the buildup of capacitance in an electrical cord is like condensation building up on the outside of a pipe. As the capacitance (condensation) builds up, electronic potential is stored. The leakage current will be drawn away by the ground because of its conductive properties in much the same way a sponge will absorb condensation (Figure 6-14).

GROUND LOOPS

A **ground loop** is created when leakage current from two different electronic devices flows through a patient. This is an extremely dangerous situation that can cause severe injury and even death. All medical equipment must be approved by the Food and Drug Administration (FDA), which verifies that electrical safety tests on all equipment have been provided by a qualified independent laboratory. The use of safety measures such as isolation transformers prevent patients from exposure to dangerous levels of electrical current from FDA-approved medical equipment. Additionally, with the advent of computerized PSG,

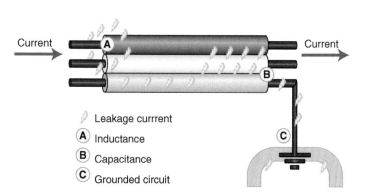

Leakage currrent
(A) Inductance
(B) Capacitance
(C) Grounded circuit

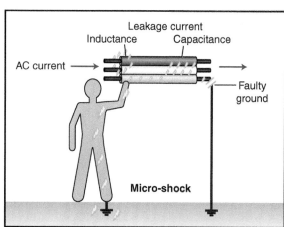

FIGURE 6-13 Leakage currents

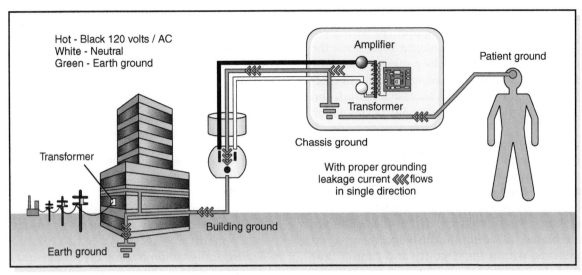

FIGURE 6-14 Proper grounding

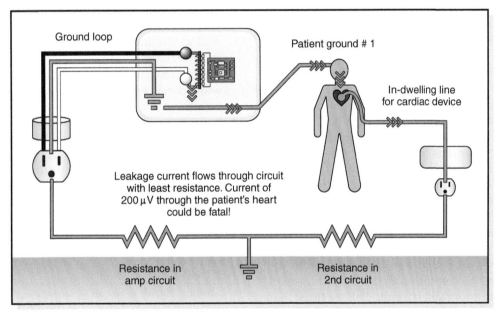

FIGURE 6-15 Ground loop

a greater amount of patient protection has been achieved because the digital signals are transmitted at extremely low voltages.

Patients are generally attached to multiple devices during a sleep study. Most sleep center bedrooms have nonmedical equipment such as lamps, fans, and audiovisual equipment in close proximity to the patient. Because all of these devices have some leakage current, sleep technologists must be vigilant to eliminate and avoid all situations that could create a ground loop. Ground loops can occur when two patient grounds are attached to a patient from two pieces of medical equipment, as illustrated in Figure 6-15.

Another ground loop scenario occurs when a patient comes in contact with an electrical device with improper or faulty grounding. Both situations can be easily avoided by understanding how the ground loop occurs and how it can be avoided.

In the case of patients connected to multiple devices in a clinical setting, first understand what devices are attached to the patient and how those devices are attached. The most dangerous scenario occurs when a patient is connected to a secondary monitor with a ground wire directly attached to the patient, such as an ECG machine or an in-dwelling line (for example, a cardiac catheter). As illustrated in Figure 6-15, this can create a pathway for the stray current to flow through the body instead of being shunted to the building ground. If a secondary piece of equipment with a patient ground is in use, the technologist must leave the polygraph ground electrode off the patient to avoid the possibility of a ground loop. Leaving the ground electrode off the patient will result in excessive artifact, and thorough documentation of the rationale for this action is crucial.

Because sleep studies are performed in environments that are purposely designed to feel less clinical, the use of nonmedical devices creates additional potential for unsafe grounding. It is important to use all equipment according to the manufacturer's recommendations. Many modern electrical devices are double insulated, meaning that leakage current has been contained within the circuitry and cannot flow to a part of the device that can come in contact with the skin. Double-insulated devices are generally labeled as such and have two-prong plugs. Never allow a device with a replacement plug, modified wiring, or an extension cord to come into contact with a patient during a sleep study. If a sleep study is performed in a home or other nonclinical location, any questionable electronic device should be unplugged for the duration of the study.

ELECTRICAL SHOCK

Not all electrical shocks are lethal. The body is partially protected from current because skin has a high resistance. Humans begin to perceive electrical current at approximately 300 microamps (300 μA).[5] The current flowing through the body (following Ohm's law) is determined by the voltage of the source and the resistance of the skin. When the skin is wet, resistance is reduced, allowing more current to flow through the body. The use of electrodes is a purposeful method of decreasing resistance to increase the flow of biopotentials between the skin and the polysomnograph circuit. This means that current can more easily be conducted through the body as well. Refer to Table 6-1 for current levels and their effect on the body.

Macroshock refers to large currents that pass through the body when the body completes a circuit, as with a ground loop. **Microshock** occurs when a smaller voltage passes through the body. A

microshock of 100 μA is not noticeable if the current is diffused through the entire body; however, if that same current flowed directly through the heart, it could cause ventricular fibrillation and possibly death.[6]

CHAPTER SUMMARY

- The laws of electromagnetism provide the foundation for the collection and recording of physiologic signals.
- Sleep technologists must understand these laws to ensure patient safety and the proper usage of PSG equipment.
- During polysomnography, electrodes are used to record electrical energy arising from the body. These tiny voltages, measured in microvolts (μV), are subject to artifact caused by physiologic and environmental phenomena.
- Technologists must be able to recognize both the proper morphology of physiologic waveforms, as well as the many types of artifacts that can affect these signals.
- Digital PSG amplifiers provide tools to collect a wide range of physiologic signals and attenuate unwanted artifacts during a sleep study.
- Improper filtering can mask key physiologic signals.
- A keen understanding of recording principles and electrical safety will allow technologists to record high-fidelity signals and document all filter modifications so that sleep disorder patients may be properly diagnosed and treated.

References

1. Loomis A, Harvey E, Hobart G: Distribution of disturbance patterns in the human electroencephalogram, with special reference to sleep, *J Neurophysiol* 1938;13(suppl):231-256.
2. Butkov N: *Atlas of clinical polysomnography* (Vol. 1), ed 2, Medford, Ore., 2010, Synapse Media.
3. Keenan SA: *Polysomnographic technique: an overview. Sleep Disorders Medicine: basic science, technical considerations, and clinical applications*, ed 3, Sudhansu Chokroverty, Ed. Philadelphia, 2009, Saunders.
4. ASDA Atlas Task Force: Recording and scoring leg movements. The Atlas Task Force. *Sleep* 1993;16(8):748-59.
5. Berry RB, Brooks R, Gamaldo CE, et al., for the American Academy of Sleep Medicine: *The AASM manual for the scoring of sleep and associated events: rules, terminology and technical specifications*, Version 2.0. www.aasmnet.org, Darien, Ill, 2012, American Academy of Sleep Medicine.
6. Deuschl G, Eisen A, Eds: Recommendations for the practice of clinical neurophysiology: guidelines of the International Federation of Clinical Neurophysiology, ed 2, *Electroenceph Clin. Neurophysiol,* 1999, Supplement 52.
7. McCormick L, Nielsen T, Nicolas A, et al: Topographical distribution of spindles and K-complexes in normal subjects. *Sleep* 1997;20:939-41.

TABLE 6-1
Current Levels and Their Bodily Effect

CURRENT LEVEL IN 1 SECOND	BODILY EFFECT
300 μA	Perceptible level
1 mA (1000 μA)	Pain threshold
10-12 mA	Cannot let go
50 mA	Injury threshold

REVIEW QUESTIONS

1. Which of the following literally means "many sleep writings"?
   a. Endoscopy
   b. Oximetry
   c. Polysomnography
   d. Electroencephalography

2. A sleep study performed to establish baseline data leading to recommendations and treatments is known as a:
   a. Diagnostic PSG
   b. Therapeutic PSG
   c. Split-night PSG
   d. Nocturnal oximetry sleep study

3. Which of the following physiologic parameters is *not* verified by command during physiological calibrations?
   a. Breath hold
   b. Heart rate
   c. Eye blink
   d. Snore

4. The movement of charged particles through a circuit is measured by:
   a. Current
   b. Amperes
   c. Watts
   d. Hertz

5. Which of the following terms refers to a form of leakage current?
   a. Stray dielectric
   b. Stray capacitance
   c. Stray resistance
   d. Electromotive force

6. Each amplifier is designed with a given frequency response that is applied to the input signals. This affects the output signal in a process known as:
   a. Attenuation
   b. Amplification
   c. Resistance
   d. Gain

7. Which of the following helps protect a patient from electrical shock?
   a. Earth ground
   b. Amplification
   c. Voltage
   d. Resistance

8. Which of the following is a direct measure of the voltage of an EEG signal within a PSG?
   a. Dynamic range
   b. Gain
   c. Sensitivity
   d. Scale

9. Which of the following describes the underlying theory of how grounding protects a patient from electrical shock?
   a. As the capacitance builds up, electronic potential is stored.
   b. The use of an isolation transformer prevents patients from exposure to dangerous levels of electrical current.
   c. With proper grounding, leakage current flows in a single direction away from the patient.
   d. The FDA verifies that electrical safety tests on all equipment have been provided by a qualified independent laboratory.

10. Large currents that pass through the body when the body completes a circuit are known as:
    a. Macroshock
    b. Microshock
    c. Resistance
    d. Voltage

Chapter 7

Data Acquisition Systems

Michael Salemi

CHAPTER OUTLINE

LEARNING OBJECTIVES

After reading this chapter, you will be able to:
1. Identify the components of digital recording technology.
2. Identify various recording methodologies.
3. Explain available software options for data manipulation.
4. Recognize sleep-wake stages on the polysomnogram.
5. Recognize clinically relevant sleep-related events.
6. Identify advancements in digital polysomnography.

KEY TERMS

aliasing
analog-to-digital (A-to-D)
  converter
caching
differential recording
dynamic recording
jack box (head box)

montage
Moore's law
multiplexing
Nyquist principle
random access memory (RAM)
referential derivation
remote monitoring

respiratory effort–related arousal
  (RERA)
spectral analysis
static recording
system referencing

After the first use of an analog polygraph to record sleep electroencephalograms (EEGs) in the 1930s,[1] 50 years passed before significant changes occurred in the technology. Early digital systems were greatly hampered by the lack of processing power as well as the limited screen size and low resolution of the available monitors. Another significant barrier to early digital polysomnography (PSG) systems was the cost and space restrictions for storage. At that time a personal computer (PC) hard drive might only hold 250-500 megabytes (MB) of data. Full sleep studies were approximately 50-125 MB, meaning the recording would need to be quickly archived to other storage media, which was extremely expensive and often could not be used for record playback.

In 1965, the future cofounder of Intel, Gordon Moore, presciently predicted that the number of transistors incorporated in a chip would double every 24 months.[2] This is often referred to as **Moore's Law**. Although not a formal scientific law, it has proven to accurately characterize the rapid pace of advancement in digital technology. As processing speed and storage volume increased, the economics of digital PSG began to compete head-to-head with analog equipment. The advancements in PC operating systems in the 1990s allowed for improved user interfaces. As digital operating costs continued to drop and the feature content of software increased, analog recording began to wane.

Today's digital systems have rich feature content and capitalize on many "off the shelf" technologies such as universal serial bus (USB) connectors and high-definition liquid crystal display (LCD) monitors. This chapter provides guidance on the proper use of common hardware components and software features by describing the basic components of a digital PSG system and the most common and useful tools provided by the majority of manufacturers.

PRINCIPLES OF DIGITAL RECORDING

The recording of digital PSG is governed by the same principles as recording digital audio or video

data. Digital photography is a useful analogy that closely mirrors the collection of computerized PSG data. The analog technologies for photographic prints or film create smooth palates of color and chromatic tones. A digital photo, whether displayed on a PC monitor or on paper, is a collection of dots, or samples, and the human brain is easily manipulated into believing that these dots create a picture. This phenomenon is quite similar to the way movement is perceived from quickly updating a series of still photos—24 frames per second in traditional movie making. Each data point in PSG recording is like the snapshot of a movie, although modern technology now allows the display of thousands of samples in 1 second.

Although sampling can be done at very high rates, the binary format is almost always a lower resolution than that of an analog signal. As an example, the EEG is an analog waveform that is picked up by an electrode. With an analog PSG system, the EEG signal is directly amplified and written onto paper as a continuous, unbroken line. For a digital recording, the EEG signal travels to an **analog-to-digital (A-to-D) converter** where it is read and converted to binary language.

DIGITIZATION AND MANIPULATION OF DATA

Physiologic signals travel through electrodes and other devices to a common connection point called the **jack box**. Between the jack box and PC, analog signals must be converted to a digital format that can be read by the software. This takes place in the A-to-D converter. The first stage of PSG software organizes the data for display and allows the user to specify the data collection criteria. This concept of organization and collection of properties to be displayed on the LCD monitor is called the **montage** and represents a listing of the type, order, and recorder settings for each channel of data being acquired.

The next stop for the signal is the amplifier, where it passes through the first set of filters that are designed to accept data acquired from either a bipolar or referential derivation which are described later in this chapter. The data then enters the PC through a port, usually the USB or a proprietary board docked in the PC. Data are initially cached into **random access memory (RAM),** which allows the software to quickly read the data and apply the software filters set in the montage. At this stage, the data are displayed on the screen within the window configurations, or montage, the user has chosen. Annotations made by the technologist (technologist notes, sleep stage, event scoring, etc.) are collected, entered into the software, and merged with the signal data. As data stream into RAM, small segments are stored to the hard drive in a process called **caching**.

Data Storage

Until data are cached to the hard drive for permanent storage, there is generally no degradation, or loss, of the digitized signal strength. For the signal to be compressed for storage, it must be modified. Storage compression is controlled in the montage

and expressed as hertz or samples per second. The original rule of thumb for storage was called the **Nyquist principle**, which states that any single waveform must be stored with a minimum of 2 points. In other words, the sampling rate must be at least twice the frequency of the fastest signal of interest to minimize distortion of the digitized data. For example, to store a signal with a high-frequency filter (HFF) setting of 75 Hz, the minimum storage rate would need to be 150 Hz.

A 2:1 ratio was commonly used when digital storage was limited and expensive, but storage capacity has increased exponentially in recent years, making it now possible to store signals at much higher sampling rates. A 3:1 ratio is now the American Academy of Sleep Medicine (AASM) minimum recommended storage rate.[3] Sampling data at a higher rate produces a digital signal that more closely approximates the original analog signal, but requires more storage space on the recording media. A lower sampling rate requires less space for data storage, but results in distortion of the original signal, referred to as **aliasing** (Figure 7-1).

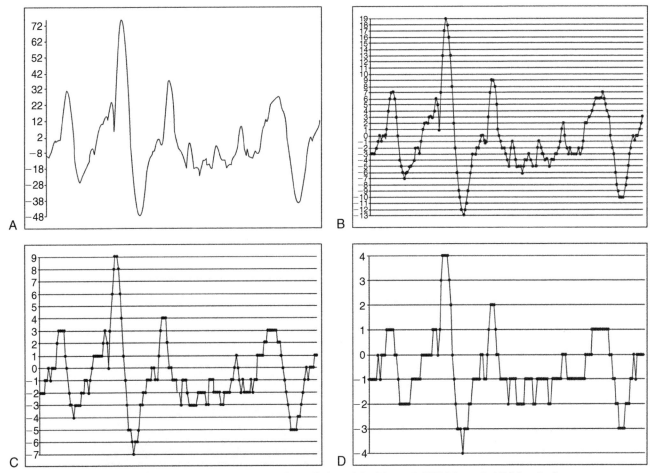

FIGURE 7-1 Signal aliasing. *From Fisch BJ:* Fisch and Spehlmann's EEG Primer, 3rd Edition Basic Principles of Digital and Analog EEG. *Philadelphia, 2000, Elsevier.*

SYSTEM COMPONENTS

Digital PSG systems are composed of software and hardware components. The software can be segmented into three primary functions: data acquisition, data storage, and data review. In an analog world, storage is often thought of as a final destination (e.g., a book is printed and the information is "stored" within the book). In digital PSG, storage is a central determining factor for acquiring and reviewing data. Figure 7-2 illustrates the process of digital PSG starting with the physiologic origin of data through study acquisition and review. For an overview of terminology and processes of digital polysomnography, see Table 7-1.

Hardware Components

Each manufacturer has different hardware design modifications and specifications. The jack box often serves as a useful tool to understand how the system hardware is configured. It is generally broken up into several sections that correspond to the number and types of amplifiers (Figure 7-3). The jack box, or head box, also provides a glimpse into the montage controls for referential bipolar and differential derivations. Derivation describes the type of input signal and reference signal used to create data on a given recorder channel. Some PSG systems include ancillary technologies such as an oximeter, amplifiers, and A-to-D converters inside the jack box, whereas other jack boxes simply provide an interface between sensors and the recorder input cable.

Jack box inputs are designed for repeated use, but great care should be taken to carefully insert and remove connectors. Experience has shown that this is often the first point of failure for this piece of hardware, as well as the sensors being repeatedly

connected. A properly treated jack box can remain in good working condition for several years.

MONTAGES

One of Webster's Dictionary definitions of montage is "a composite picture made by combining several separate pictures." In digital PSG, the term montage describes the use of several different processes of combining signals into derivations and it also describes the master control panel within the software. The term **multiplexing** refers to any process of combining two or more signals into a single channel and can be performed by both analog and digital processes. Because PSG software uses the montage to control multiplexing, the term montage will be used to describe the control interface, whereas multiplexing will be used to describe the process to create channel derivations.

In PSG software, montage is a common term to describe the control panels for data acquisition, recording, and display. Montages can be saved as templates for the many types of recordings: diagnostic PSG; split-night PSG; treatment PSG or positive airway pressure (PAP) titration PSG; multiple sleep latency testing; and so on. Acquisition montages define the number and the storage rate for each channel to be collected. The display montage controls attributes for the display such as channel order and window configuration. It may be helpful to think of a display montage as the user's "eye glasses" through which the data will be viewed.

Although PSG system manufacturers will use many different terms to describe these controls, the concept of separating controls into acquisition and display is common among digital systems. Many sleep centers require montage configurations to follow a specific protocol that outlines the order in

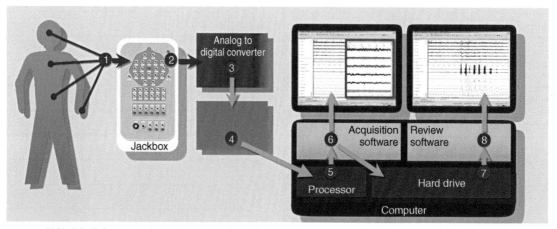

FIGURE 7-2 The data pathway during digital polysomnography from acquisition through review.

TABLE 7-1

Processes and Terminology of Digital Polysomnography

Name	Purpose	Output Signal Type
Sensors and electrodes	• Collect physiologic signals from the body	Analog
Jack box (aka head box or Input Board)	• Receives and organizes numerous signals into referential, differential, and dedicated channels. These channel types create derivations to be sent to the amplifier. • Differential channels may be sent to the amplifier as monopolar (to be referenced in the software) or bipolar (combined physically in the jack box) inputs. • Jack boxes may also contain other imbedded ancillary devices such as pressure transducers and oximetry.	Analog
A-to-D converter	• Converts analog data to digital data. • This is where data are first manipulated. • Can reside in the jack box, the computer, or may be a separate device.	Signals enter as analog and leave in digital format
Amplifier	• Steps up the amplitude of physiologic signals so they can be read in the software. • The number of amplifiers in the device will equal the total number of embedded (nonancillary) channels. • Signals are filtered once again based on their group—referential, differential, and dedicated channels. • Always review the amplifier specifications to determine if sections of the jack box are dedicated to specific signal types such as EEG, EMG, etc. • Outputs are increasingly being formatted into standard PC inputs like USB. • Some amplifier outputs may be directed to a proprietary circuit board docked in the PC.	
Processor	• Controls the speed and processor power of the PC. It works in conjunction with the PC's OS. • The OS may control aspects of the PSG software such as window configurations.	
PSG software	• Provides the user interface to control the collection, display, recording, and review of data. • Separate filters may be applied for data display only versus permanent changes stored with data.	
Data cached to hard drive	• The storage sampling rate is set in the software montage. • Data file size varies but is typically in the hundreds of MB.	
Hard drive—internal	• Stores data for review according to the settings within the PSG software. • Data are rapidly displayed during review. • Data storage capacity is limited and resides on the hard drive only during the time it is needed by the clinical team. • Hard drive capacity increases annually; currently in the hundreds of GB.	
Data review software	• Data are displayed at the storage sampling rate. • Long-term storage media are generally slower than an internal hard drive. They may be used for brief data review but not detailed analysis. • When using long-term storage media, visually confirm that files have been written to the archival media before removing original data.	

A-to-D, Analog-to-digital; *EEG,* electroencephalogram; *EMG,* electromyogram; *GB,* gigabytes; *MB,* megabytes; *OS,* operating system; *PC,* personal computer; *PSG,* polysomnogram; *USB,* universal serial bus.

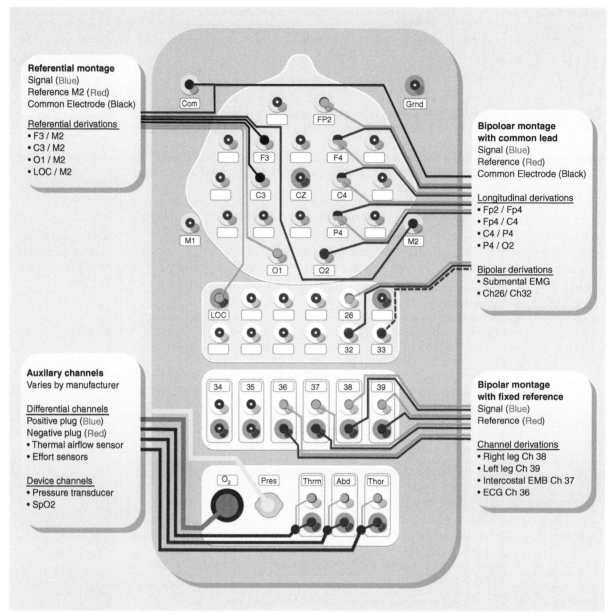

FIGURE 7-3 A jack box with referential inputs, bipolar inputs, and direct current–equipment interface.

which the channel data are displayed visually to the sleep technologist and the interpreting physician.

STATIC AND DYNAMIC RECORDING METHODS

Digital PSG systems provide numerous options for the recording process. Data storage provides the frame of reference for the other montage settings because all aspects of data display are influenced by how the data will be stored. The central concept that influences all aspects of storage is the choice between **static recording** or **dynamic recording**. In a static recording, channel modifications made during

acquisition are permanently written to the disk. In a dynamic recording, data are stored with settings that allow for a broad array of modifications during review. The decision to modify must be made judiciously to minimize degradation of signal integrity. Software systems control these options differently and provide numerous ways to mix and match recording options while providing some options for dynamic recording.

On the surface, dynamic recording appears to be a universally applauded feature until one realizes that this technology makes it possible to review previously recorded sleep data and have no clear idea what the recording technologist actually saw during the test. To address this, many systems have a setting to display data during review as collected even if the data were recorded dynamically. It is the role of the PSG technologist to follow sleep center standards and understand how these policies will affect the review options during data recording, record review, and sleep study scoring.

FILTERING

Each individual amplifier is built with a fixed filtering range that defines its maximal high- and low-frequency limits. A typical amplifier for EEG and electromyography (EMG) has an HFF cut-off of approximately 150 Hz and a low-frequency filter (LFF) cut-off at 0.1 Hz. The software filters are constrained to operate within this range and if the channel is stored statically, filtering options during data review are limited or unavailable. This places an onus on the recording technologist as all artifactual data are permanently recorded and stored.

Dynamic recording allows the sleep technologist to adjust filter options after the recording, a practice known as post-hoc changes. For example, during review a physician or technologist may increase the LFF to minimize sweat artifact that was recorded during acquisition for a more reliable representation of physiologic activity on a channel.

DERIVATIONS

Derivations are a description of the signal inputs that are combined to create a physiologic signal on a PSG recording. For instance, to record central EEG data from the area over which the C4 electrode lies, the physiologic signal of interest is compared with a reference electrode such as M1. Although the signal may often be referred to as C4, it is more accurately described by its derivation of C4-M1. The first position in any derivation is known as input 1 and the electrode connected to input 1 is always the exploring, or recording, electrode. The second position, input 2, is where the reference electrode is connected.

Derivations may be created by selecting the exploring and reference electrode via hardware or software. When derivations are created electronically within the jack box or amplifier, this is known as **system referencing**. Many manufacturers design their systems with a balance of system and software referencing. One of the primary differences between EEG and PSG systems is the degree of system referencing in the product.

Sleep systems streamline the inclusion of respiratory probes and bipolar channels such as EMG by designing jack boxes with specific sections for the different types of derivations and matching sets of amplifiers to those sections. At one end of the spectrum, the PSG systems, which have a highly structured set of system references with a limited degree of flexibility, are designed to focus on sleep-disordered breathing. At the other end of the spectrum, EEG systems have very few system references to allow a maximum degree of referential flexibility. Many contemporary PSG systems use a large number of channels (44-64) to combine the attributes of both ends of the spectrum.

Derivations can be segmented into two primary classifications: referential and bipolar.

Referential

Input 1 overlies an electrically active recording area (e.g., C4) whereas input 2 overlies a site that is relatively inactive (e.g., M1). Using the Input 1–Input 2 (also referred to as G1-G2) convention, the data recorded at M1 will be subtracted from the data at C4, and the remaining data will be displayed.

Bipolar

Both G1 and G2 overlie an electrically active recording site, such as the anterior tibialis. Channel output is equal to G1-G2. The G1-G2 convention is the basis for common mode rejection.

Most bipolar derivations are created via a mechanical connection in the jack box. These signals cannot be re-referenced after they are written to the hard drive and can only be re-referenced during data collection by switching jack box inputs. The most common examples of bipolar derivations are EMG signals. These are ideal bipolar signals because polarity is not a concern and the electrodes can be plugged into either the negative or positive input at the jack box. Electrocardiogram (ECG) is also commonly collected as a bipolar signal: lead 1 (negative)–lead 2 (positive). The polarity of the signal during display will be transposed if lead 1 is connected to the positive jack box receptacle.

RECORDING OPTIONS

Referential Recording

Referential recording refers to a method of data collection in which several signals share a common reference. For instance, to create a dynamic recording in a digital PSG system it is typical to record numerous signals with a common reference. This means that EEG and electrooculography (EOG) signals are recorded with the following derivations: C3 – M2, F1 – M2, O1 – M2, and E1 – M2. Alternatively, signals on both the right and left hemispheres can use CZ as a common reference, creating C3 – CZ, C4 – Cz, M_1 – CZ, M2 – Cz, and so on.

Any signal sharing the common reference can be re-referenced dynamically either during or after data collection. This method of re-referencing is also known as system referencing. Through common mode rejection, the signals C3 – CZ and M2 – CZ are combined via software to create the single derivation

C3 – M2 for display. Using the principles of common mode rejection as described in Chapter 4, the data recorded at CZ is eliminated because it is common to both channels. This allows the derivation C3 – M2 to be displayed on screen. Mathematically this can be described as:

$$C3 - M2 = (C3/CZ - M2/CZ)$$
$$\mathbf{C3\text{-}M2} = \mathbf{C3\text{-}Cz} - \mathbf{(M2\text{-}Cz)}$$
$$= C3\text{-}Cz - M2 + Cz$$
$$= C3\text{-}M2$$

Differential Recording

Differential recording refers to the process of collecting data from devices such as effort belts and thermal airflow sensors that attach to the jack box with separate positive and negative connectors. All digital PSG systems have an input area for differential leads. Some digital PSG systems have proprietary connectors for sensors that are self-manufactured.

GENERAL SOFTWARE OPTIONS FOR DATA DISPLAY

It is important to understand that a digital PSG system displays signals in the data collection window prior to being stored on the hard drive. This means that the sampling rate for data display during collection can be higher than it is during review. Data being written to the hard drive will be subject to the storage sampling rate selected in the software. Depending on the software's design, the sampling rate for data display is only limited by the A-to-D converter and the monitor. Increased storage rates lead to more data points being recorded and stored on the hard drive.

As previously discussed, the sampling process for data storage is an additional manipulation of the physiologic data. A child's "connect-the-dots" drawing is a simplistic but apt analogy. The object in the drawing is recognizable, but there is also significant distortion because each curved line is broken into a series of dots connected by straight lines. The more dots used to complete the picture, the smoother the curved line will be. If looking at a typical EEG signal, the same thing will happen as the signal is sampled at decreasing rates. Remember Figure 7-1 illustrated that, as the sampling rate decreases, higher frequency signals are significantly affected by aliasing.

Although hard drive storage capacity is expanding at a tremendous pace, the advance of technology has also resulted in more things to record, such as time-synchronized audio and video. To prevent a memory storage constraint, the storage sampling rate for physiologic signals must be set by each laboratory. The AASM published recommendations for storage sampling rates most recently in 2012 based on a 3:1 ratio for sampling rate as compared with the maximum HFF for the signal. The 3:1 storage rate minimizes aliasing for data display, but other software functions such as frequency analysis for automated scoring or research applications may require higher sampling rates.

MONTAGE COLLECTION AND REVIEW

The flexibility of software varies greatly between manufacturers, between different versions of the same software, and even between the same versions of software in two different laboratories.

The montage interface is the control panel for data collection and storage. Although the interface varies from system to system, the following attributes are generally controlled from within the montage:
- Channel assignment controls the order of jack box inputs within the display. *Eye 1 (E1) = Ch 1, E2 = Ch 2*
- Channel label allows the user to define the abbreviation for the channel name. *E2 = right eye*
- Signal input and reference, modern PSG systems have a mix of preset inputs on the jack box as well as channels that may be openly assigned.
  - Bipolar signals often have a high degree of flexibility and can be used to collect signals from various locations (e.g., submental EMG, anterior tibialis EMG, intercostal EMG, etc.).
  - Referential signals are recorded as "monopolar" inputs, meaning they are stored on the hard drive along with the common reference (typically Cz) signal. This allows a referential signal to be referenced to any other monopolar channel for display during data collection or review.
- Sensitivity is actually an outdated concept from the days of paper recordings when the voltage of an input signal was determined by measuring the deflection (amplitude) of recording data to calculate a value. Although outdated, some manufacturers continue to employ sensitivity either in the recorder, reviewer, or both. Sensitivity is literally the amount of input voltage recorded from the patient that is required to produce a 1-mm deflection on the recorder. The units of sensitivity are most often microvolts per millimeter ($\mu V/mm$).

Remember, every unit has an understood 1 in front of it in the absence of another value. For any given sensitivity setting in microvolts per millimeter, there is an understood 1 in front of mm. If the sensitivity is set at 10 $\mu V/mm$, it means that 10 μV of input recorded from the patient will result in a 1-mm deflection. It also means that 100 μV of input will result in a 10-mm deflection. Given two of the three variables, the other can easily be calculated using the simple formula: sensitivity (S) = voltage (V)/deflection (D), commonly reffered to as "S=V/D". The *S* represents the sensitivity control setting, the V represents the input voltage in microvolts, and the D represents deflection (amplitude) in millimeters. The three versions that can be employed to determine the missing variable are:

$$S = V/D$$
$$D = V/S$$
$$V = S \times D$$

- Gain is a tool used to increase or decrease the amplitude of a qualitative waveform or change the scaling of a quantitative wave form such as EEG. Each software system has its own set of controls for gain that are displayed during the PSG and the settings for permanent storage.
- Polarity can be adjusted.
- 50/60-Hz notch filter can be turned on and off.
- Storage rate can be adjusted.

VISUAL DISPLAY

There is clear delineation between filter and gain settings for display and storage on the montage control screen of most software programs. Many manufacturers allow each user to save his or her own visual display preferences so they can be immediately accessed during data acquisition or review. It is common for users to save display windows with specific channel groups such as signals used for sleep-stage scoring (EEG, EOG, chin EMG) or respiratory event scoring (flow, pressure, effort, SpO_2). These views should be used judiciously because the cause and effect of events can be masked when a full montage display is not being viewed. For instance, an arousal seen in a sleep-stage scoring window may be caused by any number of events, including leg movements (LMs), respiratory events, noise, and so on. A full montage provides a comprehensive view of all physiologic signals and should be the primary window used during data collection.

Display Position

In a full montage view, it is important to group families of channels together (EEG, EOG, respiratory variables, etc.). The order of the channel group can be left up to the user because it is generally possible for the data collection technologist, scoring technologist, and physician to display these channels according to a user preference. A common example is the user preference to display EEG in the top channels with EOG to follow. Many clinicians prefer to have the EOG in the top position. Software programs have hotkeys that allow a user to focus on respiratory signals only, toggle to sleep-stage scoring channels, and back to a full montage. Hotkeys are often set in the visual display to determine which channels are seen.

Display Color

Display color is an individual preference, although it should be noted that any color other than black must use more than one pixel to display. Black lines can be displayed with a single pixel, which may be more appropriate for viewing EEG signals. Many technologists select colors by the display groups mentioned previously: black for EEG, red for EOG, blue for respiratory variables, and so on.

Window Configuration

Window configuration is an extremely valuable tool for the sleep technologist. The window configuration allows the technologist to save collections of physiologic signals, histogram summaries, and tabular numeric data, and display those groups in specified areas of the display screen.

Look-Back Window

The look-back window allows a technologist to review data recorded earlier in the session. Many look-back windows allow the recording technologist to stage sleep or score events during data acquisition.

Histogram

A histogram is a summary of signals and data displayed in a compressed fashion along a common time axis. The histogram window typically allows the technologist to click on a specific area of data and have the look-back window jump to that epoch.

Tabular Data

Tabular data are numeric data saved for each epoch within the study. Common tabular entries are epoch number; sleep stage; SpO_2 events; technologist notes; and direct current (DC) signal high, mean, and low values.

Respiratory Window

Many technologists like to look at respiratory events on a screen with a compressed time base. This allows some respiratory events like hypopneas and Cheyne-Stokes breathing to be more easily observed. Compressed windows of EEG are generally less valuable, so some manufacturers allow the user to have a window dedicated to respiratory signals that can be permanently available in the display.

Full Display

The full display allows the user to display each PSG data signal in its own window. A full montage may contain 20 or more signals; however, the full display allows the user to view a single derivation of each EEG placement and not display the redundant channels unless, or until, they are needed. The display window is generally displayed in real time. The scrolling style can often be switched between dynamic scroll that emulates paper where waveforms roll across the screen, or a static mode in which the waveforms do not move but are replaced as data are refreshed.

Visual Filters

Visual filters allow the recording technologist to impose a filter setting on a channel during acquisition without affecting the data that are recorded on the hard drive. This is a valuable tool that should be used with caution. On the positive side, visual filters allow a technologist to see how different settings will reduce artifact without changing the recorded data; however, as mentioned before, this tool also allows a technologist to view data in an incorrect fashion, leading to misidentification of, or a failure to score, some events. With visual filters in place, it is possible that recording artifacts emerging during acquisition will be masked from display while being recorded to the hard drive without intervention. During review of the data, it may appear the recording technologist failed to identify or respond to the artifact.

Automated Sleep Staging and Event Scoring

Automated sleep staging and event scoring is now commonplace in digital PSG systems even though its use remains controversial. Each software vendor has proprietary methodology to analyze signals for staging and events.

From a clinical perspective, most PSG technologists who have employed automated analysis can point to sleep studies in which the software performed excellently as well as quite poorly. A pragmatic approach to the use of automation considers the time and cost savings of computerized versus manual scoring. At the time of this publication, there were little or no peer-reviewed data on this comparison. Although the science of automation is compelling, its practicality remains unsubstantiated. It should be noted that the AASM staging guidelines from 2007 and updated in 2012 employ a visual review of frequencies and waveforms.

It is arguable that visual staging standards limit a software program's ability to analyze human sleep in a clinical setting. It can also be argued that software is superior to human sight for quantitative frequency and amplitude analysis. The SIESTA database was formed by Penzel and colleagues to develop new ways of analyzing digital PSG data and create a database of these methodologies.[4]

There are very few studies to date that look at laboratory-based comparisons of automation and human scoring with the AASM scoring rules. A 2007 metaanalysis of digital staging based on Rechtschaffen and Kales's staging rules[5] suggested that "computer scoring and quantitative analysis of

sleep is still in the formative stage of development" and that "the level of agreement cannot be generalized from one system to another."[6] One of the grade 1 papers in the metaanalysis found the percentage of agreement between human scorers and an automated system to be 79.6%.[7] Interestingly, the same paper showed only a 76.9% agreement between the human scorers, but several other papers reported manual interrater reliability for staging to be between 87.5 and 95.1%.[8]

Event scoring guidelines were also included in the AASM's scoring rules from 2007 and updated in 2012. Pittman and colleagues published a comprehensive study of automated staging and event scoring within a single system as compared with human scorers. Their results showed poor agreement for arousals (76%) but far better results for respiratory events based on respiratory disturbance index (89.7%) and limb movements (92.2-93.1%).[9] Human interrater reliability was 83.7%, 94.9%, and 95.6%, respectively.

THE RECOGNITION OF SLEEP-WAKE STAGES AND EVENTS

AASM RECOMMENDATIONS

In 2012, the AASM updated the scoring standards for sleep staging, arousals, movements, and respiratory events.[3] The original 2007 publication used a large metaanalysis of clinical and technical publications to ensure that the new rules were set on a strong foundation. These manuals and the published set of support materials are the basis for much of the next section. Figure 7-4 provides recommendations for polysomnography recording parameters.

As the field of sleep medicine has expanded, the sleep technologist's role has evolved from a recording technician tasked to collect data to that of a clinician with various patient care responsibilities, including the application of treatment modalities. This expansion of responsibility has meant that recording technologists are gaining highly valued clinical skills, the foundation of which is event recognition and sleep-stage scoring. This section focuses on waveform recognition and the identification of the hallmarks for sleep stages and respiratory events. The detailed rules for scoring and staging are contained in the AASM *Manual for the Scoring of Sleep and Associated Events*.[3]

RESPIRATORY EVENTS DETECTION

Historically, there was little agreement on sensors and scoring rules related to these technologies prior to the 2007 recommendations of the AASM task force. The task force set recommendations for the primary

Recommended Recording Parameters							
Physiologic parameter	Signal	Reference	High freq filter	Low freq filter	Sensitivity	Recommended storage rate	Acceptable storage rate
EEG	C_4	M_1	35 Hz	0.3 Hz	5 μV/mm	500 Hz	200 Hz
EEG	C_3	M_2	35 Hz	0.3 Hz	5 μV/mm	500 Hz	200 Hz
EEG	O_2	M_1	35 Hz	0.3 Hz	5 μV/mm	500 Hz	200 Hz
EEG	O_1	M_2	35 Hz	0.3 Hz	5 μV/mm	500 Hz	200 Hz
EEG	F_4	M_1	35 Hz	0.3 Hz	5 μV/mm	500 Hz	200 Hz
EEG	F_3	M_2	35 Hz	0.3 Hz	5 μV/mm	500 Hz	200 Hz
EOG	ROC (E_2)	M_1	35 Hz	0.3 Hz	5 μV/mm	500 Hz	200 Hz
EOG	LOC (E1)	M_2	35 Hz	0.3 Hz	5 μV/mm	500 Hz	200 Hz
ECG	Modified lead 2	Bi-polar	70Hz	0.3 Hz	Gain	500 Hz	200 Hz
EMG	Anterior tibialis	Bi-polar	100 Hz	10 Hz	Gain	500 Hz	200 Hz
EMG	Sub-mental chin	Bi-polar	100 Hz	10 Hz	Gain	500 Hz	200 Hz
EMG	Intercostal	Bi-polar	100 Hz	10 Hz	Gain	100 Hz	25 Hz
Airflow	Thermal sensor	Bi-polar	15 Hz	0.1 Hz	Gain	100 Hz	25 Hz
Airflow	Nasal pressure	DC	100 Hz	—	Gain	100 Hz	25 Hz
Snoring	Microphone or sensor	DC	100 Hz	10 Hz	Gain	500 Hz	200 Hz
Effort	Esophageal pressure	DC	100 Hz	25 Hz	Gain	100 Hz	25 Hz
Effort	Thoricic RIP	Bi-polar	15 Hz	0.1 Hz	Gain	100 Hz	25 Hz
Effort	Abdominal RIP	Bi-polar	15 Hz	0.1 Hz	Gain	100 Hz	25 Hz
Position	Position sensor	Bi-polar	See mfg spec	—	Gain	1 Hz	1 Hz
Oximetry	SpO2	DC	15	—	Gain	25 Hz	10 Hz

FIGURE 7-4 Recommended recording parameters. Data from American Academy of Sleep Medicine.

and alternate technologies for airflow and effort, as well as recommended and optional scoring criteria for respiratory events. For details of these technologies and alternate rules, readers should refer to the latest version of the AASM manual. The focus of this chapter is recognition of events, not formal scoring rules. Refer to the manual's recommendations and definitions as they relate to the examples presented here.

Measurement Technologies

- Oronasal thermal sensor: Device used to detect absence of airflow (apnea)
- Nasal pressure transducer: Device used for the detection of reduced airflow (hypopnea and airflow limitation)
- Esophageal manometry or either calibrated or un-calibrated respiratory inductive plethysmography (RIP): Devices used to detect respiratory effort (central versus obstructive events).

STAGING EXAMPLES

Stage W: Wake

Score in accordance with the following definitions:

Alpha rhythm: Characterized by trains of sinusoidal 8-13 Hz activity recorded over the occipital region with eye closure, attenuating with eye opening.

Eye blinks: Characterized by conjugate vertical eye movements at a frequency of 0.5-2 Hz present in wakefulness with the eyes open.

Reading eye movements: Characterized by trains of conjugate eye movements consisting of a slow phase followed by a rapid phase in the opposite direction as the subject reads.

Rapid eye movements (REMs): Characterized by con-jugate, irregular, sharply peaked eye movements with an initial deflection usually lasting less than 500 msec. Although REMs are characteristic of stage R sleep, they may also be seen in wakefulness with eyes open when subjects scan the environment.

Slow eye movements (SEMs): Characterized by conjugate, reasonably regular, sinusoidal eye movements with an initial deflection usually lasting more than 500 msec.

Score epochs as stage W when more than 50% of the epoch has alpha rhythm over the occipital region.

During stage W with the eyes open, a low voltage mixed frequency pattern EEG will be present.

Score epochs without visually discernible alpha rhythm as stage W if *any* of the following are present:

a. Eye blinks at a frequency of 0.5-2 Hz
b. Reading eye movements
c. Irregular, conjugate rapid eye movements associated with normal or high chin muscle tone
   Refer to Figure 7-5.

Stage N1

Score in accordance with the following definitions:

SEMs: Characterized by conjugate, reasonably regular, sinusoidal eye movements with an initial deflection usually lasting > 500 msec.

Low-amplitude, mixed-frequency EEG activity: Low-amplitude, predominantly 4-7 Hz activity.

Vertex sharp waves (V waves): Sharply contoured waves with duration < 0.5 seconds maximal over the central region and distinguishable from the background activity.

Sleep onset: the start of the first epoch scored as any stage other than stage W.

In subjects who generate alpha rhythm, score stage N1 if the alpha rhythm is attenuated and replaced by low-amplitude, mixed-frequency activity for more than 50% of the epoch.

In subjects who do not generate alpha rhythm, score stage N1 commencing with the earliest of *any* of the following phenomena:

a. EEG activity in range of 4-7 Hz with slowing of background frequencies by ≥1 Hz from those of stage W
b. vertex sharp waves
c. slow eye movements
   Refer to Figure 7-6.

Stage N2

Score in accordance with the following definitions:

K complex: A well-delineated, negative, sharp wave immediately followed by a positive component standing out from the background EEG, with total duration of 0.5 seconds, usually maximal in ampli-tude when recorded using frontal derivations. For an arousal to be associated with a K complex, the arousal must either be concurrent with the K com-plex or commence no more than 1 second after termination of the K complex.

Sleep spindle: A train of distinct waves with fre-quency 11-16 Hz (most commonly 12-14 Hz) with a duration ≥ 0.5 seconds, usually maximal in ampli-tude in the central derivations.

Begin scoring stage N2 (in absence of criteria for N3) if *either* or *both* of the following occur during the first half of that epoch or the last half of the previous epoch:

a. One or more K complexes unassociated with arousals
b. One or more trains of sleep spindles

Continue to score epochs with low-amplitude, mixed-frequency EEG activity without K complexes or sleep spindles as stage N2 if they are preceded by epochs containing *either* of the following:

a. K complexes unassociated with arousals
b. Sleep spindles

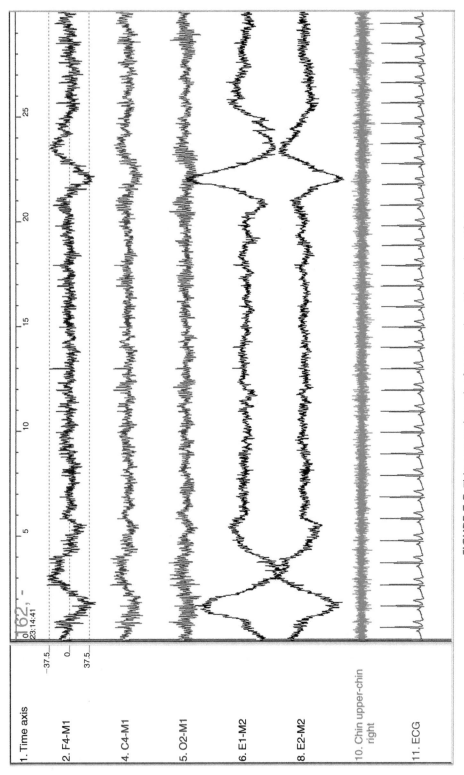

FIGURE 7-5 Thirty-second epoch of stage wake with muscle artifact.

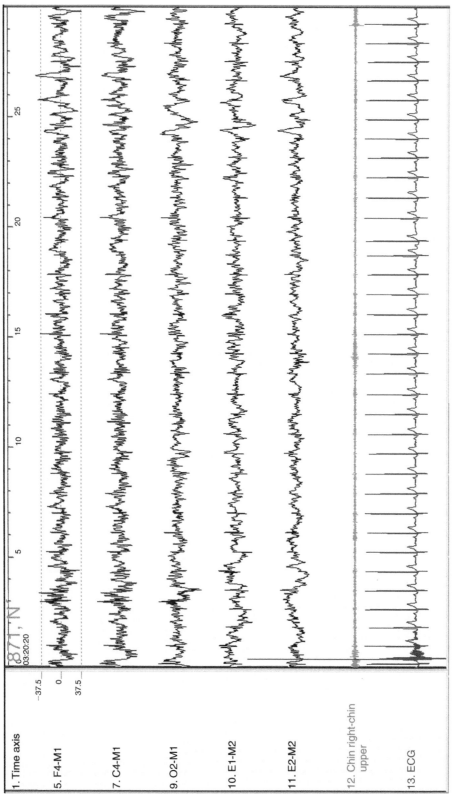

FIGURE 7-6 Thirty-second epoch of N1 sleep.

End stage N2 sleep when *one* of the following events occurs:
a. Transition to stage W
b. An arousal
c. A major body movement followed by SEMs and low-amplitude, mixed-frequency EEG without non–arousal associated K complexes or sleep spindles
d. Transition to stage N3
e. Transition to stage R
Refer to Figure 7-7.

Stage N3

Score in accordance with the following definition:
Slow wave activity: Waves of frequency 0.5-2 Hz and peak-to-peak amplitude > 75 μV, measured over the frontal regions.
Score stage N3 when ≥ 20% of an epoch consists of slow wave activity, irrespective of age.
Refer to Figure 7-8.

Stage R

Score in accordance with the following definitions:
Rapid eye movements: Characterized by conjugate, irregular, sharply peaked eye movements with an initial deflection usually lasting < 500 msec.
Low chin EMG tone: Baseline EMG activity in the chin derivation no higher than in any other sleep stage and usually at the lowest level of the entire recording.
Sawtooth waves: Trains of sharply contoured or triangular, often serrated, 2-6 Hz waves maximal in amplitude over the central head regions and often, but not always, preceding a burst of rapid eye movements
Transient muscle activity: Short irregular bursts of EMG activity usually with duration < 0.25 seconds superimposed on low EMG tone. The activity may be seen in the chin or anterior tibialis EMG derivations, as well as in EEG or EOG deviations, the latter indicating activity of cranial nerve innervated muscles (facial muscles and scalp). The activity is maximal in association with rapid eye movements.
Score stage R sleep in epochs with *all* of the following phenomena:
a. Low-amplitude, mixed-frequency EEG
b. Low chin EMG tone
c. Rapid eye movements
Continue to score stage R sleep, even in the absence of rapid eye movements, for epochs following one or more epochs of stage R (containing a, b, and c, above) , *if* the EEG continues to show low-amplitude, mixed-frequency activity without K complexes or sleep spindles *and* the chin EMG tone remains low for the majority of the epoch (refer to Figure 7-9).

RESPIRATORY EXAMPLES

Respiratory Effort Related Arousal

A **respiratory effort–related arousal (RERA)** is an arousal from sleep caused by increased work of breathing from a partial obstruction of the upper airway (refer to Figure 7-10).
If electing to score RERAs, score a respiratory event as an RERA if there is a sequence of breaths lasting ≥10 seconds. It is characterized by increasing respiratory effort or by flattening of the inspiratory portion of the nasal pressure (diagnostic study) or PAP device flow (titration study) waveform leading to arousal from sleep when the sequence of breaths does not meet criteria for an apnea or hypopnea.

Hypopnea

A respiratory event is scored as a hypopnea if *all* of the following criteria are met:
a. The peak signal excursions drop by ≥30% of pre-event baseline using nasal pressure (diagnostic study), PAP device flow (titration study), or an alternative hypopnea sensor (diagnostic study).
b. The duration of the ≥30 in signal excursion is ≥10 seconds.
c. There is a ≥3% oxygen desaturation from pre-event baseline or the event is associated with an arousal.
If electing to score obstructive hypopneas, score a hypopnea as obstructive if *any* of the following criteria are met (refer to Figure 7-11):
a. Snoring during the event
b. Increased inspiratory flattening of the nasal pressure or PAP device flow signal compared to baseline breathing
c. Associated thoracoabdominal paradox occurs during the event but not during preevent breathing
If electing to score central hypopneas, score a hypopnea as central if *none* of the following criteria are met:
a. Snoring during the event
b. Increased inspiratory flattening of the nasal pressure or PAP device flow signal compared to baseline breathing
c. Associated thoracic-abdominal paradox occurs during the event but not during pre-event breathing

Apnea

Score a respiratory event as an apnea when *both* of the following criteria are met:
a. There is a drop in the peak signal excursion by ≥90% of pre-event baseline using an oronasal thermal sensor (diagnostic study), PAP device flow (titration study), or an alternative apnea sensor (diagnostic study).
b. The duration of the ≥90% drop in sensor signal is ≥10 seconds

(Text continued on page 143)

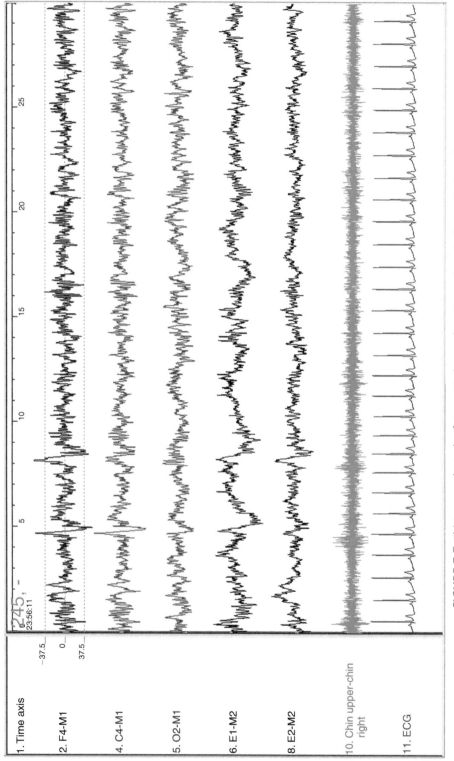

FIGURE 7-7 Thirty-second epoch of stage N2 sleep—clear K complexes in first half of epoch.

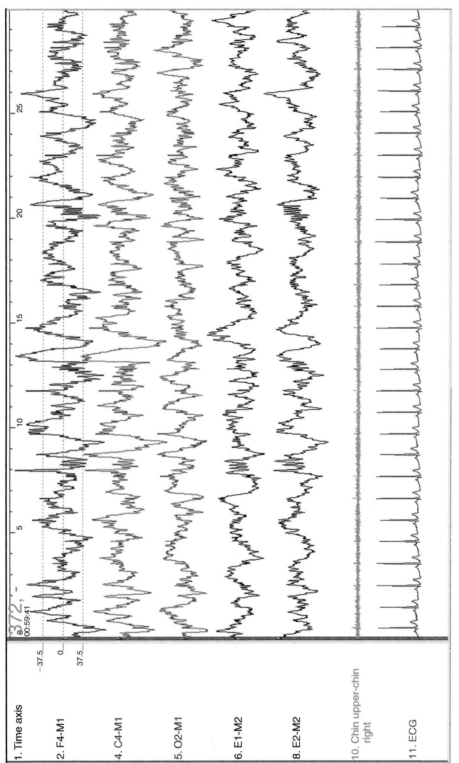

FIGURE 7-8 Thirty-second epoch of stage N3 sleep.

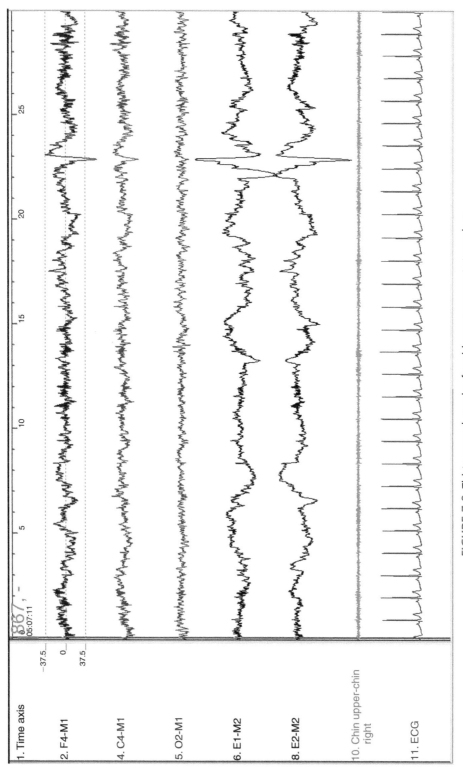

FIGURE 7-9 Thirty-second epoch of rapid eye movement stage sleep.

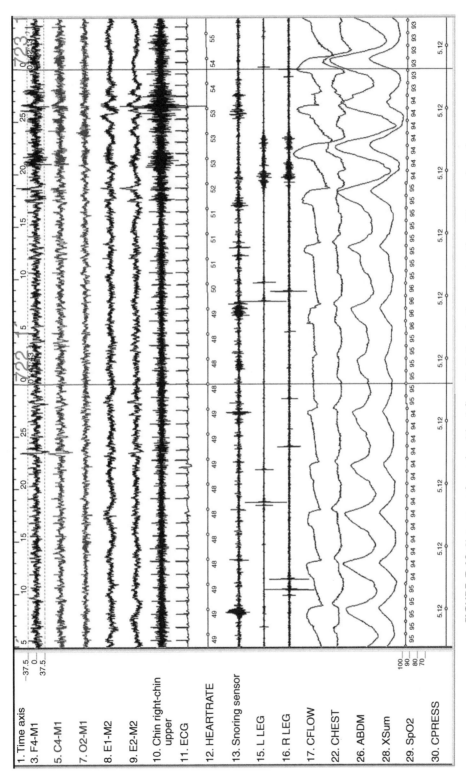

FIGURE 7-10 Sixty-second epoch with airflow limitation lasting greater than 10 seconds and terminating with an arousal—a respiratory event–related arousal.

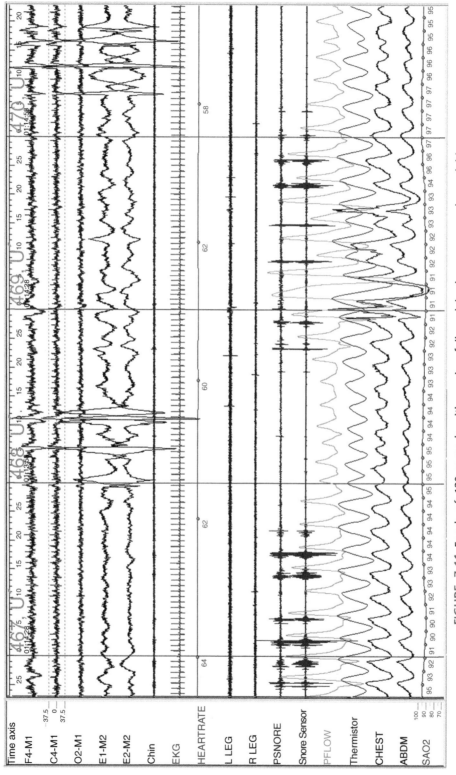

FIGURE 7-11 Epoch of 120 seconds with snoring followed by hypopnea—oxyhemoglobin desaturations follow events.

Score an apnea as obstructive if it meets apnea criteria and is associated with continued or increased inspiratory effort throughout the entire period of absent airflow (Figure 7-12).

Score an apnea as central if it meets apnea criteria and is associated with absent inspiratory effort throughout the entire period of absent airflow (Figure 7-13).

Score an apnea as mixed if it meets apnea criteria and is associated with absent inspiratory effort in the initial portion of the event, followed by resumption of inspiratory effort in the second portion of the event (Figure 7-14).

Cheyne-Stokes Breathing

Cheyne-Stokes breathing is characterized by repeating pattern of crescendo-decrescendo respiratory effort, most commonly seen in patients with heart disease or cerebral vascular injury (refer to Figure 7-15).

Score as Cheyne-Stokes breathing if both a and b apply:

a. There are episodes of ≥3 consecutive central apneas and/or central hypopneas separated by a crescendo and decrescendo change in breathing amplitude with a cycle length of ≥40 seconds.

b. There are ≥5 central apneas and/or central hypopneas per hour of sleep associated with the crescendo/decrescendo breathing pattern recorded over ≥ 2 hours of monitoring.

SLEEP-RELATED MOVEMENT EVENTS

Periodic Limb Movements in Sleep (PLMS)

The following define a significant leg movement (LM) event:

a. The minimum duration of a LM event is 0.5 seconds.

b. The maximum duration of a LM event is 10 seconds.

c. The minimum amplitude of a LM event is an 8-µV increase in EMG voltage above resting EMG.

d. The timing of the onset of a LM event is defined as the point at which there is an 8-µV increase in EMG voltage above resting EMG.

e. The timing of the ending of a LM event is defined as the start of a period lasting at least 0.5 seconds, during which the EMG does not exceed 2 µV above resting EMG.

The following define a PLM series:

a. The minimum number of consecutive LM events needed to define a PLM series is 4 LMs.

b. The minimum period length between LMs (defined as the time between onsets of consecutive LMs) to include them as part of a PLM series is 5 seconds.

c. The maximum period length between LMs (defined as the time between onsets of consecutive LMs) to include them as part of a PLM series is 90 seconds.

d. Leg movements on 2 different legs separated by less than 5 seconds between movement onsets are counted as a single leg movement.

Refer to Figure 7-16.

Rhythmic Movement Disorder

The following define the polysomnographic characteristics of rhythmic movement disorder (refer to Figure 7-17):

a. The minimum frequency for scoring rhythmic movements is 0.5 Hz.

b. The maximum frequency for scoring rhythmic movements is 2.0 Hz.

c. The minimum number of individual movements required to make a cluster of rhythmic movements is 4 movements.

d. The minimum amplitude of an individual rhythmic burst is 2 times the background EMG activity.

REM Sleep Behavior Disorder

REM sleep behavior disorder (RBD) is characterized by the body's failure to suppress muscle activity during REM sleep. RBD is a syndrome and not an event; however, there are several polysomnographic characteristics that can be identified on the recording that should be highlighted for interpretation by the treating physician (refer to Figure 7-18).

Score in accordance with the following definitions:

Sustained muscle activity (tonic activity) in REM sleep: An epoch of REM sleep with at least 50% of the duration of the epoch having a chin EMG amplitude greater than the minimum amplitude demonstrated in non–rapid eye movement sleep.

Excessive transient muscle activity (phasic activity) in REM sleep: In a 30-second epoch of REM sleep divided into 10 sequential, 3-second miniepochs, at least 5 (50%) of the miniepochs contain bursts of transient muscle activity. In RBD, excessive transient muscle activity bursts are 0.1-5.0 seconds in duration and at least 4 times as high in amplitude as the background EMG activity.

The polysomnographic characteristics of RBD are characterized by *either* or *both* of the following features:

a. Sustained muscle activity in REM sleep in the chin EMG

b. Excessive transient muscle activity during REM in the chin EMG or limb EMG

(Text continued on page 151)

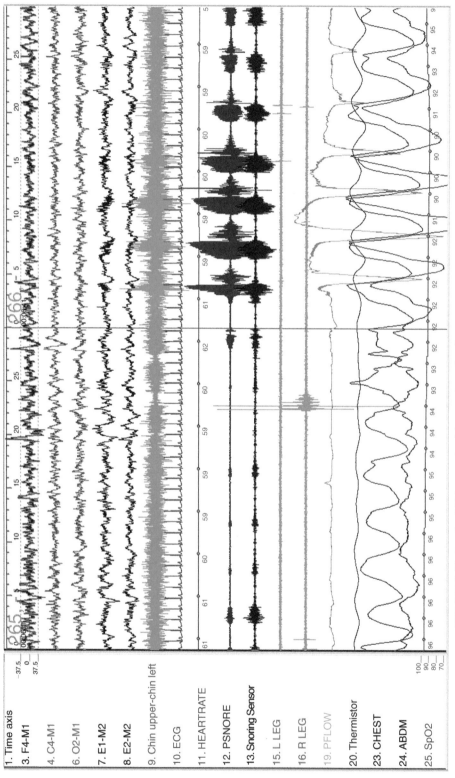

FIGURE 7-12 Epoch of 120 seconds with cessation of airflow and continuing effort—obstructive apnea.

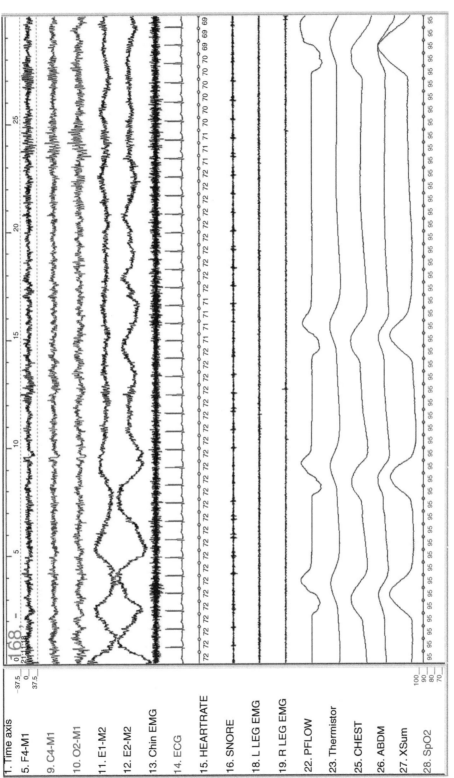

FIGURE 7-13 Thirty-second epoch with central apnea—no effort, no airflow.

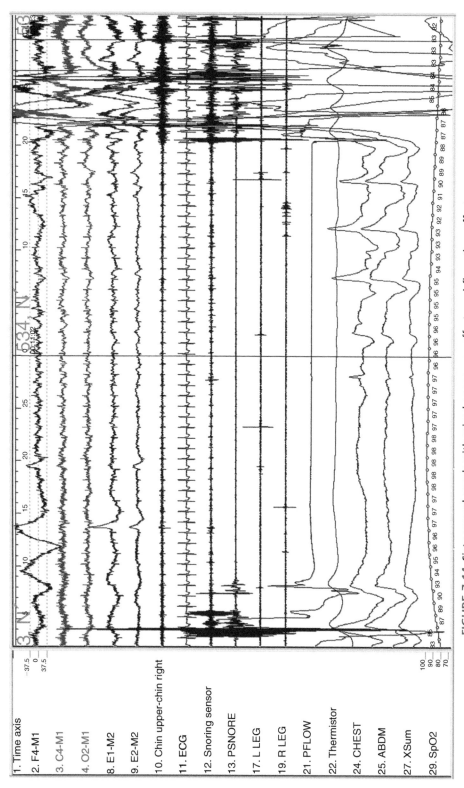

1. Time axis
2. F4-M1
3. C4-M1
4. O2-M1
8. E1-M2
9. E2-M2
10. Chin upper-chin right
11. ECG
12. Snoring sensor
13. PSNORE
17. L LEG
19. R LEG
21. PFLOW
22. Thermistor
24. CHEST
25. ABDM
27. XSum
29. SpO2

FIGURE 7-14 Sixty-second epoch with mixed apnea—no effort or airflow, then effort resumes with no airflow.

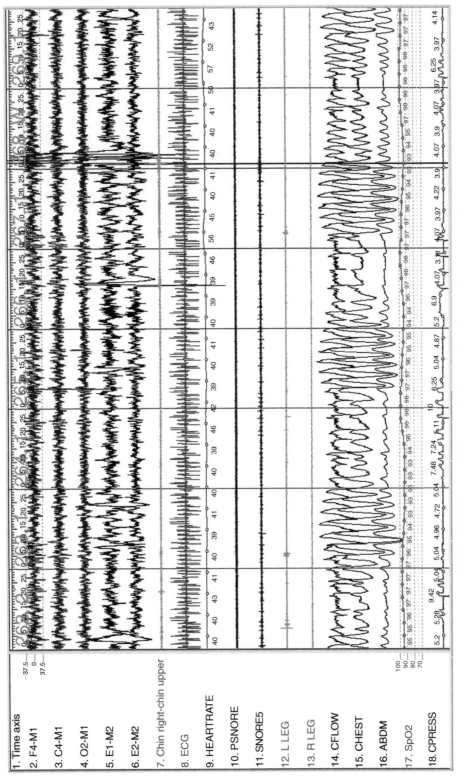

FIGURE 7-15 Epoch of 240 seconds of repetitive Cheyne-Stokes respiration.

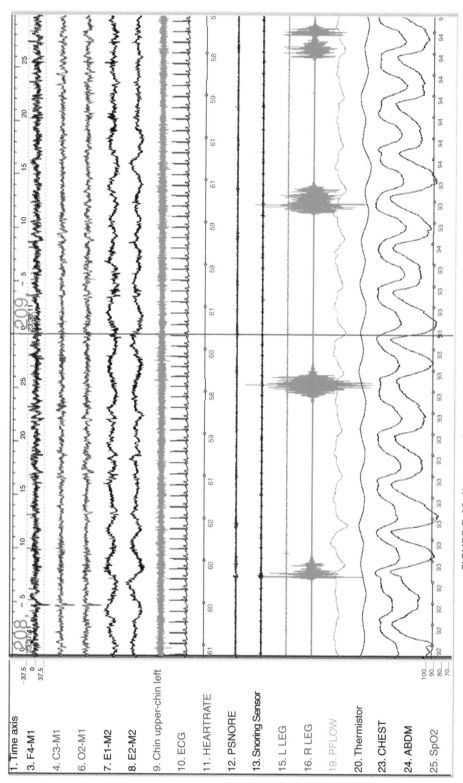

FIGURE 7-16 Sixty-second epoch with four periodic limb movements.

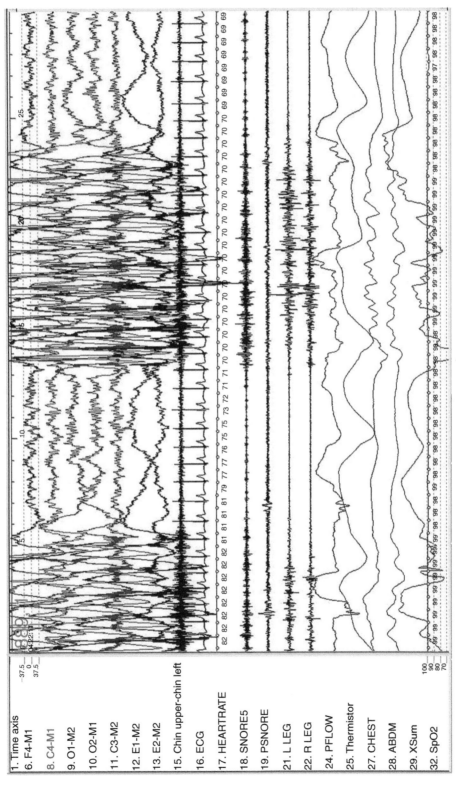

FIGURE 7-17 Thirty-second epoch with body rocking episodes.

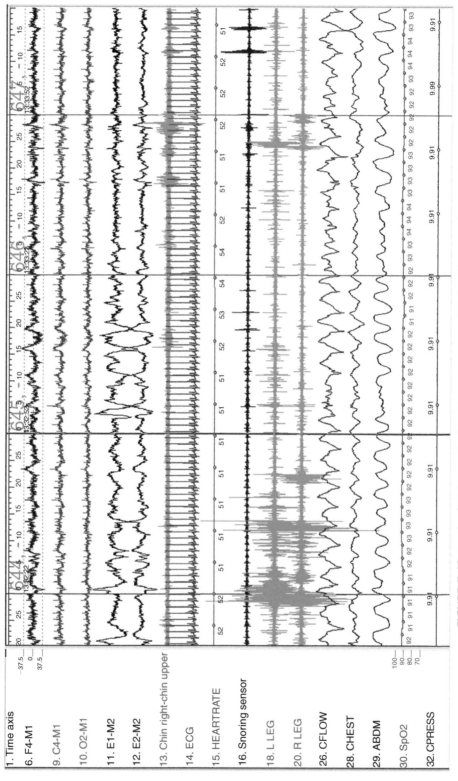

FIGURE 7-18 Epoch of 120 seconds of rapid eye movement (REM) without atonia—REM sleep behavior disorder.

RECENT ADVANCEMENTS IN DIGITAL POLYSOMNOGRAPHY

WIRELESS TECHNOLOGIES

The use of wireless technologies in PSG systems has been primarily applied to transmission between the jack box and amplifiers. This has allowed for greater freedom of movement for patients and elimination of "unhooking" the patient for nocturia. It also allows for the amplifier to be positioned further away from the patient, allowing for a less clinical look to the bedside. A buyer's guide compiled by *Sleep Review Magazine* in September 2011 listed 11 PSG system manufacturers; of these, three listed the availability of wireless technologies.

SPECTRAL ANALYSIS OF ELECTROENCEPHALOGRAM DATA

Numerous technologies such as fast Fourier transform, high-order **spectral analysis**, and "fuzzy logic" have been used to analyze the density and power of EEG frequencies during sleep. There are many advocates for the increased use of digital analysis in the clinical realm beyond automated sleep staging. Spectral analysis has been used to identify central nervous system arousals using the cyclic alternating pattern, as well as autonomic nervous system arousals using ECG signals.[11] Other work has focused on quantifying slow-wave activity to measure the therapeutic response to PAP.[12] These data, although promising, have not been rigorously validated and remain the subject of investigational studies.

PORTABLE POLYSOMNOGRAPHY DEVICES

Although portable systems have been used for many years, the increasing miniaturization of digital technologies and updated reimbursement policies have allowed for rapid advancement of these devices. Portable sleep testing devices range from cardiorespiratory systems focused on sleep-disordered breathing to full PSG systems that are not much larger than a mobile phone. Large-scale, multisite studies, such as the Sleep Heart Health project, have successfully used portable PSG devices to perform thousands of in-home sleep tests. In many clinical settings, both domestically and abroad, the use of in-home cardiorespiratory devices has become the first line of diagnostic testing.

REMOTE MONITORING

The widening reach of broadband internet access and mobile computing have allowed manufacturers to offer the ability to observe PSG data in real time from remote locations. Although at the time of this publication, insurance reimbursement policies do not recognize **remote monitoring** as a form of "attended testing," the technology is being used by a number of clinical facilities throughout the United States.

CHAPTER SUMMARY

- Data acquisition systems allow PSG to be performed with specific individualized montages and protocols.
- Each component of a recording system is intricate and detailed.
- The technologist must understand each component of the signal pathway beginning at the patient and ending with data output visualized on a computer monitor.
- The components and sensors selected to record a sleep study determine the accuracy and viability of acquired data.
- Failure to choose optimum equipment results in poor-quality or erroneous data that may affect diagnostic and treatment decisions.
- Sleep technologists must be proficient when scoring sleep stages and associated events.

References

1. Loomis AL, Harvey EN, Hobart GA: Potential rhythms of the cerebral cortex during sleep, *Science* 82:198-200, 1935.
2. Moore GE: Cramming more components onto integrated circuits, *Electronics Magazine* 4, 1965.
3. Berry RB, Brooks R, Gamaldo CE, et al., for the American Academy of Sleep Medicine: *The AASM manual for the scoring of sleep and associated events: rules, terminology and technical specifications,* Version 2.0. Darien, Ill, 2012, American Academy of Sleep Medicine. www.aasmnet.org.
4. Penzel T, Glos M, Garcia C, et al: The SIESTA database and the SIESTA sleep analyzer, *Conf Proc IEEE Eng Med Biol Soc* 8323-8326, 2011.
5. Rechtschaffen A, Kales A: *A manual of standardized terminology, techniques, and scoring system for sleep stages of human subjects,* Los Angeles, 1968, Brain Information Service.
6. Penzel T, Hirshkowitz M, Harsh J, et al: Digital analysis and technical specifications, *J Clin Sleep Med* 3(2):109-120, 2007.
7. Anderer P, Gruber G, Parapatics S, et al: An E-health solution for automatic sleep classification according to Rechtschaffen and Kales: validation study of the Somnolyzer 24 × 7 utilizing the Siesta database, *Neuropsychobiol* 51:115-133, 2005.
8. Danker-Hopfe H, Kunz D, Gruber G, et al: Interrater reliability between scorers from eight European sleep laboratories in subjects with different sleep disorders, *J Sleep Res* 13:63-69, 2004.
9. Pittman SD, MacDonald MM, Fogel RB, et al: Assessment of automated scoring of polysomnographic recordings in a population with suspected sleep-disordered breathing, *Sleep* 27(7): 1394-1403, 2004.
10. Ferri R, Bruni O, Miano S, et al: Inter-rater reliability of sleep cyclic alternating pattern (CAP) scoring and validation of a new computer-assisted CAP scoring method, *Clin Neurophysiol* 116: 696-707, 2005.
11. Blasi A, Jo J, Valladares E, et al: Cardiovascular variability after arousal from sleep: time varying spectral analysis, *J Appl Physiol* 95:1394-1404, 2003.
12. Bennett LS, Langford BA, Stradling JR, et al: Sleep fragmentation indices as predictors of daytime sleepiness and nCPAP response in obstructive sleep apnea, *Am J Respir Crit Care Med* 158:778-786, 1998.

REVIEW QUESTIONS

1. The waning of analog recording methodology in PSG was a result of:
   a. Increased expense of analog recordings
   b. Decreased expense of digital recordings
   c. Improved storage of analog recordings
   d. Inflexibility of digital recordings

2. The process of transforming a physiologic signal into a format that is digitized is known as:
   a. A-to-D conversion
   b. Multiplexing
   c. System referencing
   d. Data caching

3. The listing of the type, order, and recorder settings for each channel of data being acquired is known as:
   a. Derivation
   b. Montage
   c. Multiplexing
   d. System referencing

4. A recording in which both G1 and G2 overlie an electrically active recording site is known as:
   a. Referential
   b. Multiplexing
   c. System reference
   d. Bipolar

5. A recording in which input 1 overlies an electrically active recording area and input 2 overlies a site that is relatively inactive is known as:
   a. Bipolar
   b. Referential
   c. Caching
   d. Multiplexing

6. The storage of small segments of data to the hard drive is a process known as:
   a. Referencing
   b. Multiplexing
   c. Caching
   d. Signal splitting

7. A distortion of a signal caused by a sampling rate lower than required is known as:
   a. Caching
   b. Multiplexing
   c. Aliasing
   d. Referencing

8. A systematic outline of the description of the inputs used to create a channel of data is known as a:
   a. Derivation
   b. Reference
   c. Cache
   d. Alias

9. Which type of recording describes the process of collecting data directly from devices such as effort belts and thermal airflow sensors in which both inputs receive active data?
   a. Differential
   b. Bipolar
   c. Referential
   d. Common mode

10. The tool used to increase the amplitude of a qualitative waveform or change the scaling of a quantitative signal is:
    a. Gain control
    b. Time constant
    c. HFF
    d. Sampling rate

Chapter 8

Sensors, Transducers, and Ancillary Equipment

Mike Longman

CHAPTER OUTLINE

LEARNING OBJECTIVES

After reading this chapter, you will be able to:
  1. Explain the theory of operation for equipment used for sleep recordings.
  2. Discuss the application, limitation, cleaning, and care of sensors and electrodes.
  3. Identify appropriate sampling rates and voltage requirements.
  4. Identify equipment interface requirements and appropriate amplifier connectivity.
  5. Define nationally recognized recommendations for equipment used for sleep recordings.

KEY TERMS

amplifier
analog-to-digital (A-to-D) conversion
ancillary equipment
cyclic alternating pattern (CAP)

diaphragmatic and intercostal electromyogram
end tidal carbon dioxide ($EtCO_2$)
esophageal pressure (P_{es})
interface

jumper cable
sensor
transducer

SURFACE ELECTRODES

The importance of surface electrode selection and care cannot be overemphasized. Electrodes are the first and most important item in the patient-recorder **interface**. Because bioelectrical signals are very small, extensive amplification is necessary prior to human interpretation of these data. As a point of reference, the **electroencephalogram (EEG)** is typically amplified 20,000 times for visual display. In addition to the biopotentials of interest, any noise or recording artifacts generated at the site of electrode contact with the skin are amplified. Poor electrode selection or application produces a suboptimal recording of the data being collected. This section focuses on electrodes, electrode care, interface options, cables, and connectors for recording parameters of the typical polysomnogram.

ELECTRODE TYPES

The type of surface electrodes used to record physiologic signals is critical to producing a clear, artifact-free recording. The technologist must have basic knowledge of electrode types, artifact potential, and the appropriate method of affixing electrodes to the patient to produce a clean, artifact-free record.

EEG electrodes can be made from a variety of materials. Any two or more diverse metals used in the same recording will result in artifacts being introduced, so the rule is to never mix electrodes made from different materials.

Commonly Used Metals for Electrodes

The most commonly used metals are gold-plated silver, silver, and silver–silver chloride. These three materials are very good conductors of electrical potentials. Historically, the metal type was more important than it is currently because of older **amplifier** technology. An amplifier is an electronic device with controls for manipulating the amplitude and morphology of data, and also to attenuate signals with frequencies above and below user-defined filter settings. Today, with the advances in modern amplifiers, the type of metal used to construct electrodes is less important than the application technique.

For standard polysomnography (PSG) recordings, gold-plated electrodes are the most common choice.

In the past, the silver–silver chloride electrodes needed to have an adequate coating of chloride to obtain the benefits of less low-frequency "noise" than either nonchlorided silver or gold sensors. Sensors are devices used to collect physiological data, including electrodes and transducers such as those used to monitor breathing and oxygenation.

The chloriding process deposits chloride ions on the silver surface and changes the shiny silver appearance of the electrode to a dark gray color. Over time these electrodes oxidize, requiring that they be rechlorided on a regular basis. Modern silver–silver chloride electrodes are sintered, a process whereby chloride particles are baked into the silver. As a result, they do not need regular chloride bathing to keep them coated. Gold electrodes are actually silver with gold plate over their surface. The benefit of this type of electrode is that they do not oxidize like silver–silver chloride electrodes and require less care.

If the plating on the electrode is chipped, cracked, or scratched, the electrode should not be used, as the direct current (DC) offset potential created by the contact of two dissimilar metals will create artifact in the recording. This artifact can be seen as a baseline drift of the signal.

Electrode Cups

Electrode cups can be manufactured in a variety of styles, two of which are stamped and casted. The stamped electrode cups typically are thinner in design and have a slightly bigger cup to hold conductive material (gel or paste). The casted-style cup electrode has thicker walls and a smaller capacity to hold conductive material. These cup electrodes tend to be more durable than the stamped type because they don't bend as easily. Both are equally reliable for recording bioelectrical signals and are typically selected according to technologist preference. The EEG cup electrodes used for adults are 10 mm in diameter and those for pediatric patients are 6 mm in diameter.

Electrode Wires

Electrode wires, also known as leads or lead wires, are attached to cup electrodes and are also manufactured with some differences. Most of these differences are small, and technologist preference is usually the deciding factor. The material used to insulate electrode wires is sometimes a factor in this decision, although durability and recording quality are likely the most important criteria for selection of reusable electrodes. Lead wires insulated with a thin polytetrafluoroethylene coating are durable but tend to tangle more easily than other options. Lead wires coated with a thicker insulation material tend to tangle less readily, but may not be as sturdy as the former.

Specific Use for Electrodes

Although EEG electrodes can be used to record all bioelectric parameters, they are most typically used to record the EEG and electrooculogram (EOG). Many laboratories prefer to use disposable stick-on patch electrodes for recording the EOG, electromyogram (EMG), and electrocardiogram (ECG) because of ease of use and quick application and removal; however, this is also a facility preference.

When deciding whether to use disposable or reusable electrodes, signal quality, recording maintenance, patient comfort, and cost should all be considered. Stick-on disposable electrode patches are not appropriate for recording EEG data. Disposable cup electrodes, similar to the reusable cup electrodes mentioned previously, are available for situations in which it is either impractical to employ the reusable type, or it poses an infection control risk. Some facilities have begun adopting disposable cup electrodes for routine testing as the cost of disposables continues to decline. Silver–silver chloride impregnated plastic disposable cup electrodes are available from many manufacturers of bioelectric sensors.

ELECTRODE CABLES, CONNECTORS, AND JUMPERS

In addition to EEG electrodes, the technologist may use several other electrode types, depending on the parameter being recorded. Each cable may have a different connector depending on the digital polysomnographic recording system being used. Most vendors of bioelectric sensors and **transducers** supply cables that can be ordered with the correct connector to fit a specific recording system. A transducer is any device that converts one form of energy to another.

For EMG and ECG recording, many technologists prefer to use the button snap patches, typically referred to as ECG electrodes, and lead wires with button snap connectors. These come in varying lengths to suit the parameter being recorded, and are quick and easy to use. When selecting lead wires, the patient's girth and height should be considered as well as bed location in relation to the head box location. When using patch electrodes, site preparation is identical to that for cup electrodes and is the most critical step toward obtaining an optimal recording. To lower electrode impedance, site preparation is done by cleansing and rubbing the skin to remove surface oil and superficial layers of the epidermis.

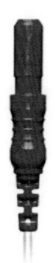

FIGURE 8-1 1.5-mm touchproof. *Used with permission from MVAP Medical Supplies Inc. Newbery Park, California.*

Connectors

Connectors for lead wires vary depending on the type of PSG system being used. When purchasing electrodes and sensors, it is important to consult the PSG hardware technical manual to ensure safety features and the correct selection of electrodes and sensors.

For electrodes and sensors, the 1.5-mm touchproof connectors are most commonly employed (Figure 8-1). An important feature of these connectors, also known as recessed-female connectors, is that they cannot be incorrectly mated. Beginning in 1998, they were required by the Food and Drug Administration (FDA)[1] to avoid accidental electrical shocks. These protected female pin connectors have recessed metal parts; they replaced the single exposed male pin plugs previously used.

There are many other connector types, which are primarily either manufacturer specific or parameter specific. Some of the most common connector types are keyhole (Figure 8-2), phone (Figure 8-3), RCA (Figure 8-4), RJ11 (Figure 8-5), and DIN (Figure 8-6).

FIGURE 8-2 2-pin 1-mm keyhole. *Used with permission from MVAP Medical Supplies Inc. Newbery Park, California.*

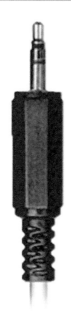

FIGURE 8-3 ⅛-inch (3.5-mm) male phone. *Used with permission from MVAP Medical Supplies Inc. Newbery Park, California.*

The keyhole is a 2-pin, 1-mm connector that is typically used on sensors for specific PSG recording system manufacturers.

The phone connector is a ⅛-inch (3.5 mm) male (or female) plug and is typically used to interface DC signals. The RCA connector is most often used with audio and video equipment, and is sometimes used as an input or output connector on **ancillary equipment**. The RJ11 connectors are often used to transmit signals from a DC device to the amplifier. A DIN connector was originally standardized by the *Deutsches Institut für Normung* (DIN), the German National Standards Organization. There are a variety of DIN connectors; therefore the term DIN connector alone does not identify any particular type of connector unless the relevant DIN standard is added (e.g., DIN 41524 connector).

Jumpers

Jumper cables (Figure 8-7) are typically used for "linked" ear reference or common reference when

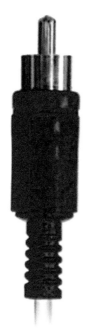

FIGURE 8-4 RCA connector. *Used with permission from MVAP Medical Supplies Inc. Newbery Park, California.*

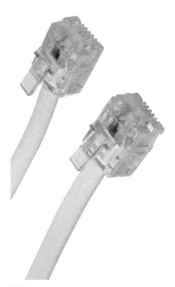

FIGURE 8-5 RJ11 connector. *Used with permission from MVAP Medical Supplies Inc. Newbery Park, California.*

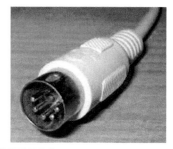

FIGURE 8-6 DIN connector. *Used with permission from MVAP Medical Supplies Inc. Newbery Park, California.*

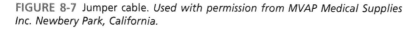

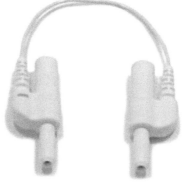

FIGURE 8-7 Jumper cable. *Used with permission from MVAP Medical Supplies Inc. Newbery Park, California.*

the recording system does not offer the capability of accomplishing this by either manual or digital input selection. A jumper cable allows the signals to be referenced together to eliminate common artifact on both references. This is especially helpful when trying to remove ECG artifact from the EEG recording. Jumpers may also be required when a recorder has limited electrode input selection capabilities and the signal from a single electrode must be used in multiple derivations.

As an example, according to the American Academy of Sleep Medicine (AASM), the three recommended EEG channels of a PSG recording use M1 as input 2 of the derivation. When derivations are determined by placement of electrode connectors into the input 1 and input 2 of the jack box for each channel because of hardware or software limitations of the recording system, the M1 signal must be "jumped" across the input 2 connections for each of these channels. Each time an additional connector is introduced to the signal pathway, the potential for recording artifact increases. Additionally, when a signal is distributed by using jumpers, artifact isolation can become extremely difficult because the artifact from a single input will spread across all "jumped" channels.

USE AND CARE OF REUSABLE RECORDING ELECTRODES

Both disposable and reusable electrodes are available in various shapes and sizes. Disposable electrodes are for single patient use. They typically are available with a silver–silver chloride interface and do not require cleaning because they are discarded after one use. Reusable electrodes are for multiple patient use and are typically constructed of silver–silver chloride or gold-plated silver. Because these are intended for multiple uses, they require cleaning and disinfection between applications.

Most facilities use reusable electrodes because of cost, and many technologists believe they produce higher recording quality as compared with their disposable counterparts. Reusable electrodes have historically been a better choice because of superior manufacturing processes and various metal choices. These electrodes can have a varying life span, depending on their use and care. Electrodes must be cleaned according to the manufacturer's instructions as well as the infection control practices at each individual facility. The technologist must have an understanding of infection control definitions so that all electrodes and **sensors** are processed correctly. Principles of infection control will be discussed more in-depth in Chapter 14.

Cleaning

Cleaning[2] refers to the removal of foreign material from the electrode cup. This is accomplished by using water, detergents, and a mild scrubbing action. Cleaning the electrode is the first step before disinfection or sterilization. When cleaning electrodes, care must be taken when scrubbing the electrode cup. A light scrubbing action with water and detergent is all that is required to remove foreign material. Scrubbing too hard can compromise the plating on the electrode, which will cause it to be unusable.

Disinfection

Disinfection[2] refers to the elimination of most pathogenic microorganisms (except bacterial spores) on the electrode surface or rendering them inert. This is typically accomplished by the use of liquid chemicals such as glutaraldehyde, sodium hypochlorite (household bleach), or pasteurization that uses hot water to accomplish high-level disinfection to the surface of articles.

Sterilization

Sterilization[2] refers to the complete elimination of all forms of microbial life, including spores. It is accomplished by physical or chemical processes such as steam under pressure, ethylene oxide, or liquid chemicals. Both disinfection and sterilization can be rendered ineffective if all organic material is not cleansed from the electrode surface or if soap and organic residue are not thoroughly rinsed prior to processing the item.

Semicritical v. Noncritical Items

In the schema of infection control, all electrodes and sensors used in the sleep center can be categorized as noncritical or semicritical items. Noncritical items are electrodes and sensors that come in contact with intact skin, but not mucous membranes, and require only low-level disinfection. Semicritical items are electrodes and sensors that come in contact with nonintact skin or mucous membranes, and require high-level disinfection.

Because the skin, is abraded prior to application of electrodes for sleep testing, the potential for nonintact skin always exists. For this reason, electrodes used for testing patients in the sleep laboratory should be processed using a form of high-level disinfection. A solution of household bleach and water is often used because it has the potential to inactivate prions; however, electrodes used on a patient with known prion disease should be incinerated to eliminate the potential of spreading this debilitating and deadly group of diseases.

INTERFACING ELECTRODES WITH THE INPUT BOARD

Before connecting electrodes or sensors to the input board, commonly called a head box, electrode board, or jack box, it is critical to verify that the type of connector on the sensor matches the input type. Some manufacturers use proprietary connectors, whereas others use standard 1.5-mm touchproof connectors. In addition, many head boxes are designed for a combination of proprietary and standard connectors. For this reason, it is never safe to assume that a particular connector will fit into an electrode board input simply because another sensor uses the same style.

Derivations

No single method of signal derivation is uniquely ideal for displaying all types of activity recorded during PSG; therefore, it is necessary to use various derivation types to obtain the many activities of interest. The electrode inputs on head boxes designed for PSG are used to form at least two types of derivations, referential and bipolar. There may be additional head box inputs for body temperature sensors, SpO_2 sensors, nasal pressure devices, and other transducers. Electrode inputs may be fixed, whereas the sensors that represent input 1 and input 2 of a particular channel must be plugged into designated positions in the jackbox; in addition, inputs may be mechanically switched, or the ability to change derivation inputs may be under software control.

Bipolar derivations measure the difference in potential between two active electrodes. An active electrode overlies an electrically active recording site. An example of this is an EMG recording of chin or limb muscle activity.

Referential derivations measure the difference in potential between one active electrode and one inactive electrode. The inactive electrode is connected to the input 2 or reference position of the derivation, and is usually placed on the mastoid process. A referential derivation, such as C4-M1 or E1-M2, is used for recording EEG and EOG data, respectively.

ECG artifact can be present in the EEG and other channels recording bioelectric signals when contaminated by the relatively high-voltage electrical activity from the heart. To minimize this artifact, it is possible to use a jumper cable between the reference M1 and M2, combine M1 and M2 electrically within the recorder software, or physically make this connection when an electrode selector panel is in use. Regardless of the method available on a particular recording system, this process is known as "double referencing" or "linking the mastoids."

Double referencing works because the ECG components of the two selected signals tend to cancel each other. The closer the impedance values between the two electrodes in the derivation, the more effective the link will work to attenuate ECG artifact. When linking the mastoids, it is important to remember that if either M1 or M2 is contaminated by artifact, all derivations using these reference sources will be contaminated with the artifact. For this reason, attempts should be made to prevent or minimize ECG artifact prior to linking the mastoids. When these channels must be combined, constant attention to the signal quality is necessary. The link may need to be removed if artifact emerges, to allow identification of its origin.

RECORDING EEG, EMG, EOG, AND ECG WITH SURFACE ELECTRODES

Electrodes are placed on the skin to transfer surface potentials to the recorder interface. These potentials are bioelectrical activity arising from the body, commonly referred to as biopotentials. Biopotentials are extremely small and require amplification to be viewed by the human eye.

Site preparation and electrode application techniques are essential for high-quality, low-noise recordings. Poor signal quality is most often caused by poor conduction between the electrode and the skin or electrode movement on the surface of the skin. Excessively high impedance measures caused by inadequate site preparation result in artifact on the recording.

Skin contains oils, sweat, and dead cells, which can form an electrical barrier between its surface and the electrode. If not cleaned and abraded properly prior to electrode application, the impedance will be excessive and will affect the quality of the recording. The skin must be cleaned of all oils, sweat, and dead cells to allow the passage of electrical signals.

Impedance is defined as the combination of resistance and capacitance. Resistance is the electrical barrier created by oil, sweat, and dead skin cells. Capacitance is the ability of a material to store an electrical charge. It is important that impedance between a pair of electrodes is balanced or the difference between them is less than $2 K\Omega$ to provide an artifact-free, quality recording.[3]

The electrode site should initially be cleaned with alcohol to remove oils. An abrading compound such as Nu-prep or Lemon-prep is used to remove dead skin cells. Skin should never be cleansed with alcohol following abrasion, as this can be very painful if the skin is broken. Conductive gel or paste is applied to the electrode either before or after it is affixed to the desired site.

The EEG is a recording of the summed ionic flux that results from the brain's neural activity. This activity changes during the recording, and corresponds to sleep stages. The electrodes used to record EEG are used in a referential derivation.

The EOG is a record of electrical changes that occur during eye movements as the result of the corneoretinal potential difference. The cornea is relatively positive compared with the retina. As the cornea or retina moves more toward the exploring electrode, a positive or negative deflection, respectively, is generated. A referential derivation is used for recording the EOG.

The EMG is a recording of the electrical impulses of muscle groups at rest and during contraction. The electrodes used to record the EMG are used in a bipolar derivation.

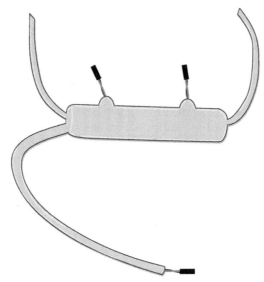

FIGURE 8-8 Thermistor. *Used with permission from MVAP Medical Supplies Inc. Newbery Park, California.*

The ECG represents electrical conduction through the heart. A bipolar derivation is used to record the ECG.

AIRFLOW AND BREATHING EFFORT TRANSDUCERS AND RECORDING SYSTEMS

Respiratory and airflow monitoring is very important and in some cases the main reason patients are referred to a sleep center for testing. There are many options when recording these parameters and these are discussed in detail.

Monitoring Airflow

Thermal sensors, including thermistors (Figure 8-8) and thermocouples, and nasal pressure monitoring are the two most common methods used to record airflow. The thermistor and thermocouple detect airflow based on temperature changes. These temperature changes occur during breathing because inhaled air is cooler than exhaled air. Apneas are detected very well using these devices because of the lack of temperature variation. Hypopneas and other incomplete airway obstructions are not well detected using these devices because the temperature change and flow are not proportional; therefore, the amplitude of the signal may not be reduced or may be only nominally reduced.

Historically, measurement of respiratory airflow was done in research using masks and pneumotachographs. The data that was accumulated during this time showed that resistance in the upper airway could be detected as a plateau or flattening of the inspiratory waveform. Although historically valuable the application of full-facial pneumotachography was not suited to clinical PSG. A more noninvasive alternative was developed for clinical use. This consists of a nasal cannula connected to a pressure transducer.

The pressure transducer detects fluctuations in pressure caused by inspiration and expiration. These fluctuations are proportional to flow and reproduce the pressure signal obtained from full facial pneumotachography in most cases.[4] Airflow monitoring using a nasal cannula pressure transducer is used to identify hypopneas and the flow limitation responsible for respiratory effort–related arousals (RERAs).

Monitoring Respiratory Effort

Respiratory inductive plethysmography (RIP), piezo technology, and **diaphragmatic and intercostal EMG** are the most common methods used to monitor respiratory effort. Other previously used methods to measure respiratory effort included mercury-filled strain gauges and impedance pneumography.

In the past the strain gauges that were used in sleep centers were either fluid-filled elastic tubes or resistive foil mounted on backing material. The strain gauge was mounted to a belt that was placed around the chest and abdomen. Strain gauges operate on the principle of stress. For fluid-filled gauges, the fluid exerts a pressure force on a thin flexible metal diaphragm at the tip of the sensor when the patient inhales or exhales. The strain gauge then converts the pressure stresses to a low-level, millivolt-range signal. For resistive foil, tension during inhalation and compression during exhalation cause an increase in resistance that results in a signal output. The use of the strain gauge only provided information about chest wall movement with no relationship to the volume of air. Other limitations included over-stretching of the strain gauge, causing failure and signal degradation with changes in body position.

Piezo Technology

Piezo electric crystal technology was developed and quickly replaced strain-gauge technology for monitoring respiratory effort. Piezo-electric crystals are artificial or naturally occurring crystals that produce a charge output when they are compressed, flexed, or subjected to sheer forces. When the stress is removed, the electrical output stops. The repeated stress and release caused by the rise and fall of a patient's chest creates the familiar sine wave respiratory effort pattern. The output of the piezo sensor is not linear, which means the waveform is only an approximation of the movement of the chest and abdomen; thus, if a 1-inch stretch of the band creates a 1-V output, then a 2-inch stretch would not create a 2-V output. This lack of a linear response makes it difficult to assess hypopneas.

The piezo-based effort belts measure the tension where the crystal is located, a single point, where the band pulls during breathing. The limitations to this technology include problems with accuracy and readings that can occur when the patient moves and tension is lost. Piezo belts also can produce a phenomenon known as false paradoxing, particularly when the tension on the belt is altered by patient movement or body positioning.

Diaphragmatic and Intercostal EMG

Diaphragmatic and/or intercostal EMG can be recorded to monitor respiratory effort by applying electrodes over intercostal spaces and the upper abdomen. This technique is primarily used to differentiate between central and noncentral respiratory events. Muscle movement is recorded when respiratory effort is present because activity is recorded if any muscle activity occurs, but nothing is recorded in the absence of activity. EMG monitoring of respiratory effort is an accurate way of assessing central versus obstructive events when other data may be questionable. Reliability of these measures is limited by proper electrode placement. It can be difficult to place electrodes in the appropriate area, particularly on the obese patients who make up much of the sleep-disorders testing population.

Respiratory Inductive Plethysmography (RIP)

RIP senses changes in the cross-sectional area of the rib cage and abdominal areas during the breathing cycle. The RIP sensor consists of a belt with a wire woven or sewn in a pattern that is usually sine wave or zigzag along the entire length (Figure 8-9). It contains a module with a circuit board, oscillator, and battery that passes a weak current through the wire, creating a magnetic field. As the patient breathes, the band is stretched and relaxed, causing slight changes in the cross-sectional area. These changes modify the magnetic field, which results in a change in the frequency of the current. This can be measured and converted to a voltage output that creates the waveform that is seen on the polysomnogram. The signal that is produced is linear, which means it changes in proportion to the stretch and relaxation of the belt. Thus, if a 1-inch stretch of the band creates a 1-V output, then a 2-inch stretch will create a 2-V output; the signal amplitude will double on the polysomnogram channel. No electrical current passes through the patient; only a weak magnetic field is created.

Compared with other technologies, RIP is more comfortable for the patient because excessive tension on the band is not required. It only needs to be tight enough to stay in place; over-tightening of the RIP belt can deteriorate signal quality.

Some RIP systems also include a sum channel, useful for detecting paradoxical breathing, which can be displayed on a polysomnogram channel. The sum channel displays the phase relationship between the chest and abdominal bands. When the chest and abdomen signals are out of phase, they will cancel each other out for a flat or diminished sum channel (Figure 8-10). RIP technology does not produce false paradoxical breathing signals like that encountered when using piezo sensors (Figure 8-11).

The RIP signal can be either calibrated or uncalibrated. Calibrated RIP signals represent the actual volume of airflow, and can be used to create a flow-volume loop. Calibrated systems have not achieved widespread use because of expense, frequent calibration requirements, and the technologist time necessary to maintain the calibration, among other reasons. Recent advances in noncalibrated RIP technology, however, have led to widespread adoption of these devices. The AASM includes RIP as one of the recommended sensors for use in accredited facilities. This is likely another reason for the increase in use of this technology in recent years.

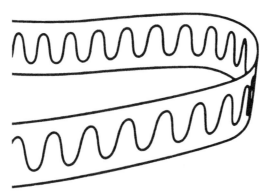

FIGURE 8-9 Sine wave pattern configuration in RIP sensor belt. *Courtesy Mike Longman.*

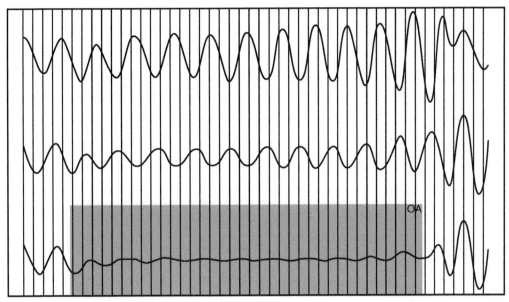

FIGURE 8-10 Thoracic, abdominal, and sum effort channels recorded using respiratory inductive plethysmography technology. When chest and abdomen are paradoxing, the sum channel will be flat or markedly diminished. *Courtesy Mike Longman.*

The technologist should note that RIP systems dedicate a module for the abdomen and one for the chest. The reason these are dedicated is because each module operates on a different frequency in order to prevent interference between channels. If the technologist tries to use two chest modules or two abdomen modules on the same patient, a degraded signal will likely result because they are operating on the same frequency.

SNORE MICROPHONES AND SENSORS

Snore microphones and snore sensors are the most widely used method of recording snoring in the sleep center. The snore devices used in sleep centers record the vibrations or sound associated with snoring, as there is no practical technique to quantitatively measure the intensity of snoring.

A snore microphone is a transducer that converts sound into a small analog voltage. The signal can be interfaced with the recorder and displayed on an output channel. There are several different types of microphones available for use in sleep centers, but the most common types are electret, piezoelectric, and dynamic.

The dynamic types operate with a moveable diaphragm that is displaced by the sound wave and this movement of the diaphragm creates a voltage change that is proportional to the power of the sound wave. The size of the deflection is relative to the power of the sound. These tend to offer a wide frequency range and are sensitive to other sounds in addition to snoring. These are usually encapsulated microphones, which make them durable and moisture resistant.

An electret microphone is a dielectric material that is permanently electrically charged or polarized. The electret forms the diaphragm and its distance from the plate causes a voltage to be induced. These also tend to offer a wide frequency range.

The piezoelectric types operate by responding to vibrations on the skin near the upper airway. They are attached to the patient adjacent to the upper airway, which vibrates when snoring occurs. They respond rapidly to movement associated with snoring. Typically, the piezo sensors are designed with a raised center for increased vibration sensitivity.

Piezo and dynamic snore sensors don't require a power source, whereas the electret type does. The power source is in the form of a battery, usually in line with the sensor cable.

RECORDING PATIENT BODY POSITION

Body position monitoring is important during sleep because of the positional nature of respiratory events in patients who have sleep-disordered breathing (SDB). It is an important parameter that is usually included on the sleep study report. It can be monitored using video and manually documented, or automatically recorded, using a body position sensor. The method used depends on the acquisition system and facility preference. The advantage of using a body position sensor is the ability to capture subtle body position changes that the monitoring or scoring technologist may miss when manually tracking body position changes.

Body position sensors provide data on their position in relation to the direction of gravity. These devices are actually reporting the position of the sensor and not the human body, so it is very important to make sure that they are oriented correctly on the patient. To achieve the correct position output, the band must be firmly secured around the centerline of the chest or

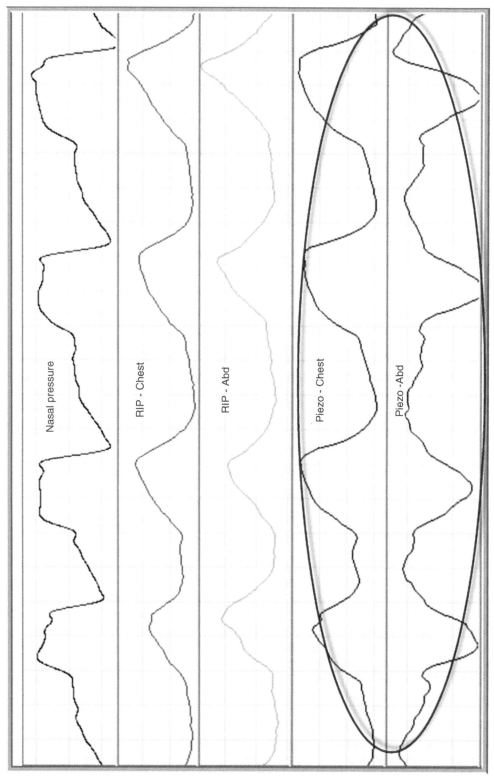

FIGURE 8-11 Nasal pressure airflow along with effort recorded using respiratory inductive plethysmography and piezo technology. Note the false paradoxing in the channels derived from piezo belts. *Courtesy Mike Longman.*

abdomen. These sensors usually report four or five body positions, depending on the particular brand of sensor.

For its power source, a body position sensor relies either on an external battery in line with the sensor cable, or the PSG recorder it is interfaced with.

Body positions may also be reported through video review with manual tracking of body position changes. It is up to each sleep center to decide who has the primary responsibility for ensuring that all body position changes have been recorded or documented accurately. In some centers, the recording technologist is required to document each body position change during data acquisition. The scoring technologist will then verify the accuracy of that documentation. A sleep center may also decide that the scoring technologist is responsible for documenting each body position change using the video as the verifying source.

AUDIOVISUAL MONITORING AND RECORDING

Video and audio recording should be treated as an essential component of the sleep study. It provides the physician and scorer with additional information that may be needed for the correct documentation of respiratory events and body position changes. It will also be of tremendous benefit in the assessment of abnormal movements and behaviors that occur during sleep, and in differentiating sleep disorders, such as parasomnias, from seizure activity. It can also provide objective documentation of both patient and technologist actions in the testing room if legal issues arise.

There is a large variety of audio and video monitoring equipment on the market. Most PSG equipment manufacturers either sell or recommend the equipment that works best with their acquisition system. In general, the video cameras used are either fixed focus or pan-tilt-zoom modules. Regardless of the camera type, an infrared light source is needed so the patient can be monitored in a dark room.

A fixed-focus system uses a lens system in which the distances between lenses are constant, and thus the image will not vary. A pan-tilt-zoom camera is capable of remote directional and zoom control. The newer digital systems allow these functions during monitoring and during scoring or review. This is a tremendous advancement in the technology, as an unnoticed unusual activity can be further assessed if noted during the scoring or review process.

Most sleep centers have two audio monitoring systems. One system records the patient room audio and is only a one-way communication from the microphone to the computer. This system remains on at all times so the recording technologist will hear any speech or other sounds coming from the patient room. The other is an audio intercom system between the control room and the patient room. This allows the technologist and patient to communicate bidirectionally. The microphone in the control room should have a switch that allows the technologist to be heard by the patient only on an as-needed basis.

RECORDING BIOELECTRIC AND TRANSDUCED SIGNALS

The polysomnogram is a recording of electrical and mechanical activity that is amplified and filtered for visual display as channels within a montage. Three basic types of signals are recorded: bioelectric, transduced, and those originating from ancillary equipment.

Differentiating Signal Types

Bioelectric signals represent the summed ionic flux generated by groups of cells or the polarity of one anatomic location relative to another on an organ. These electrical changes can be measured by applying surface electrodes to the skin using conductive material as an interface. Examples of bioelectrical signals include the EEG, EOG, ECG, and EMG.

Transduced signals are derived from a transducer that converts one type of energy to another. Although the term transducer commonly implies use of a sensor or detector, any device that converts energy is a transducer. Transducers used in PSG typically convert mechanical energy to electrical energy; for example, the nasal pressure sensor detects pressure and converts it to an electrical output, which is displayed on the polygraph as an airflow waveform. Examples of transduced signals include body position, nasal pressure airflow, snoring, respiratory effort, and movement.

Ancillary equipment provides the third type of signal typically recorded on a PSG. Ancillary equipment refers to any device that can process data on its own and is simply interfaced with the sleep recording system. Two examples of ancillary devices are the end tidal carbon dioxide monitor and the pulse oximeter. Interfacing an ancillary device to the acquisition system is discussed later in this chapter.

SELECTING AN AC OR DC AMPLIFIER

Sleep recording systems use both AC and DC inputs and devices. To properly record parameters, it is necessary to select the correct method of amplification.

Rapidly fluctuating signals such as EEG, EOG, EMG, and ECG are recorded using an AC amplifier. The designation of AC when referring to an amplifier has nothing to do with the current that powers it. This designation was chosen because the types of signals that are appropriately recorded on an AC amplifier are fast-moving variables with frequencies and morphology similar to that of alternating current. AC amplifiers are easily differentiated from DC amplifiers as they have both a high-frequency filter control and a low-frequency filter control.

Slow-moving or constant variables are recorded using a DC amplifier. The designation DC simply means that this type of amplifier is appropriate for recording signals similar to the constant output of DC electricity. Appropriate signals for a DC amplifier are constant, or relatively constant, signals such as positive airway pressure readings and **end tidal carbon dioxide (EtCO$_2$)** values. The DC amplifier has a high-frequency filter but does not have a low-frequency filter. The lack of a low-frequency filter eliminates the fall time constant, so the signal will not decay.

Because of the decay time constant of the low-frequency filter found on an AC amplifier, signals that are at a constant or near constant voltage are significantly attenuated. A characteristic of an AC amplifier is to force any constant value back to baseline. A DC amplifier will readily accept an input that is at a constant voltage and will produce a constant output amplitude.

Because many sensors can be used with either an AC or DC amplifier, this decision is made by user and facility preference, as well as amplifier availability. As an example, the signal produced by a body position sensor can be recorded using either an AC or DC amplifier.

SAMPLE RATE REQUIREMENTS

A digital sleep acquisition system converts the analog waveforms arising from the patient, transducers, and ancillary devices into a series of numerical values for recording and display. This is known as **analog-to-digital (A-to-D) conversion**. The signals are not stored continuously, but are sampled at a predetermined frequency.

The sampling rate is often referred to as sampling frequency and is expressed in hertz (Hz). Sampling rate is actually expressed in the units of samples per second and not cycles per second, so the former trend can be misleading. Ideally, the samples per second is the number of values per second stored to accurately represent the original analog signal. For example, a sample rate of 5 Hz means that the value of the signal being recorded will be measured and stored in five equally spaced samples in each second. This is then displayed as a continuous tracing by having the computer connect the points to construct a waveform. A higher sample rate provides a better representation of the actual signal (Figure 8-12).

In the past, sampling data at a higher rate was challenging. Although a higher sampling rate increases data resolution, it also increases file size. Even today, a balance must sometimes be found between resolution and data storage in order to avoid unnecessary use of hard drive, DVD, file server, or other archival media space.

EEG Signals

EEG signals are very complex and vary rapidly in both frequency and morphology. They require a much higher sample frequency than slow-moving signals like airflow or respiratory effort. When a signal is recorded, distortion of the data occurs if the sampling rate is too low relative to the frequencies that naturally occur within the signal. For this reason, it is important to understand sampling rates and the effect they can have on recorded data. The rule of thumb states that a signal can theoretically be digitized and later restored to its analog value if the signal is sampled at a frequency greater than twice the highest frequency contained in the signal. This is known as the *Nyquist-Shannon sampling theorem.*

In reality, digitized data are never more than a close approximation of the original analog signal. The AASM has published specifications on minimal and desirable sample rates for signals typically recorded by PSG.[5] The effect of various sample rates on EEG data is evident in the examples in Figures 8-13 through 8-15. A C3-M2 derivation containing some muscle artifact was recorded at a sample rate of 256 samples per second (Figure 8-13). The same segment of data was simultaneously recorded at 8 samples per second (Figure 8-14) and 4 samples per second (Figure 8-15).

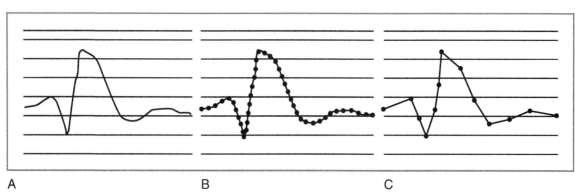

A   B   C

FIGURE 8-12 Signal aliasing. **A,** Original analog waveform. **B,** Sampled at 240. **C,** Sampled at 50.
Courtesy Mike Longman.

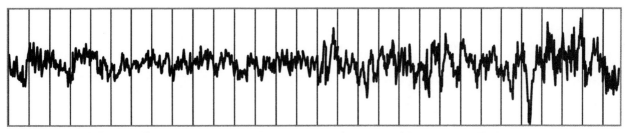

FIGURE 8-13 Original C3-M2 sampled at 256 Hz with 60-Hz artifact. *Courtesy Mike Longman.*

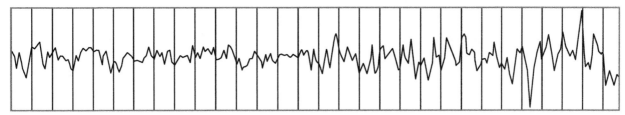

FIGURE 8-14 Same signal sampled at 8 Hz. *Courtesy Mike Longman.*

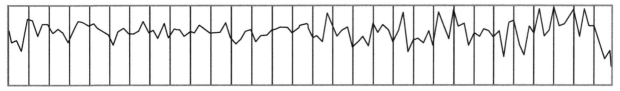

FIGURE 8-15 Same signal sampled at 4 Hz. *Courtesy Mike Longman.*

ANCILLARY RECORDER SIGNALS, EQUIPMENT AND METHODOLOGY

Esophageal pressure (P_{es}) monitoring during PSG, also known as esophageal manometry, is the gold standard for assessing change in respiratory effort. Because the esophagus is a hollow tube lying within the thoracic cavity, pressure changes within the thorax are directly exerted on the esophagus. When monitoring P_{es}, intrathoracic pressure changes are actually being assessed and can be quantified. These changes can provide objective evidence of either airway obstruction or absence of respiratory effort.

In the absence of respiratory effort during a central apnea, there is no change in intrathoracic pressure. During an obstructive apnea, progressively more and more negative intrathoracic pressure is generated until the airway finally opens. Although the gold standard for monitoring respiratory effort, P_{es} it is not widely used in the clinical setting. As an invasive procedure, it may not be well tolerated by the patient. Most clinicians use a nasal pressure sensor attached to a cannula to assess the subtle changes in breathing otherwise only apparent using P_{es}.

During esophageal manometry, inspiratory flow limitation is displayed as progressively more negative pressure with each breath as the individual works harder and harder to maintain a consistent amount of airflow. When a flow limitation event lasts at least 10 seconds and results in an EEG arousal, it is scored as an RERA. These events support the diagnosis of upper airway resistance syndrome (UARS). Although a nasal pressure signal cannot replace P_{es} for differentiating central from obstructive events, it can be used as a surrogate measure for recording RERAs. In fact, researchers found that while simultaneously assessing P_{es} and nasal pressure during UARS, a plateau or flattening of the inspiratory pressure curve consistently appeared on the nasal pressure signal.

RECORDING AND UNDERSTANDING THE CYCLIC ALTERNATING PATTERN

SDB can produce repetitive arousals in sleep. This can result in impaired daytime cognition, reduced sleep quality, excessive daytime sleepiness, and overall decreased quality of life. A feature of SDB is the cyclical nature of the disorder. **Cyclic alternating pattern (CAP)** (Figure 8-16) is a long-lasting periodic activity of two alternate EEG patterns consisting of transient

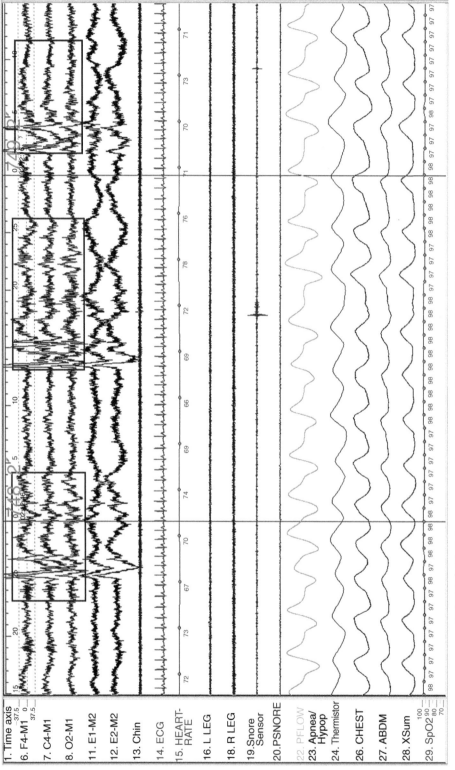

FIGURE 8-16 Polysomnogram showing cyclic alternating pattern (CAP) phase A (*red*) alternating between CAP phase B.

arousals. CAP is divided into two phases, phase A and the following phase B, which make up each cycle of CAP. When CAP appears, arousal fluctuates constantly between two distinct sleep levels. Functionally, CAP is a condition of sustained sleep and arousal instability oscillating between a greater (phase A) and lesser (phase B) arousal level, whereas non-CAP is a prolonged stationary condition of sleep and arousal stability. If a patient demonstrates CAP, the waveforms can be easily identified using standardized recording montages used in the sleep center.[6]

AN OVERVIEW OF PULSE OXIMETRY AND OXIMETER SENSORS

Pulse oximetry is a noninvasive and indirect method to monitor the saturation of the patient's hemoglobin, expressed as SpO_2. The oximeter sensor can be placed on a fingertip, earlobe, toe, or even the forehead using a reflectance sensor. Typically, most sleep centers use the fingertip sensor.

A pulse oximeter shines light from the probe at two wavelengths—red and infrared—through a part of the body that is relatively translucent and has good arterial pulsed blood flow (e.g., finger, toe, or earlobe). The light is partially absorbed by the hemoglobin in varying amounts depending on the degree of saturation, presumably with oxygen.

Pulse oximetry technology cannot differentiate between hemoglobin saturation with oxygen and saturation with another compound. Although it is assumed that saturation represents oxygen saturation, the technologist must be aware that values can be erroneous. As an extreme example, if hemoglobin is 100% saturated with carbon monoxide, the oximeter will read 100% while the patient dies from lack of oxygen. For this reason, it is imperative that the patient's history be reviewed. A heavy smoker may have enough residual carbon monoxide in his or her system to provide a falsely elevated SpO_2 throughout the night, even though severe hypoxemia is present.

By calculating the absorption at the two wavelengths, the oximeter can calculate the portion of hemoglobin that is saturated. Saturation values are typically averaged out over a varying period depending on the manufacturer of the oximeter. The pulse rate is also calculated from the pulsatile signals and averaged out over a similar period.

There are limitations to pulse oximetry that may provide inaccurate measurements such as poor perfusion, anemia, carbon monoxide poisoning, movement, nail polish, and dark-pigmented skin.[7] This will be thoroughly covered in another chapter of this textbook.

INTERFACING AN ANCILLARY DEVICE WITH THE DATA ACQUISITION SYSTEM

Input and output connections vary based on the manufacturer of the acquisition system; however, the concepts are the same for interfacing devices. An external device such as a continuous positive airway pressure (CPAP) machine has an output connection. This output is usually connected to an isolated DC box that is connected to the acquisition system. The external device sends an analog signal, which is converted to a digital signal that the acquisition software reads.

Each external device has output connections on the back of the device. The type of connection varies from device to device. Examples of some output connections are RJ11, ⅛-inch (3.5-mm) male phone connector, and DIN connectors.

An ancillary device may be capable of directly sending data to the PSG recorder in a digital format, or the device may communicate via an analog interface. The majority of devices that can be interfaced with the recorder, however, provide an analog output. Input connections on data acquisition systems also vary based on the manufacturer of the system. All external analog devices need to be calibrated to ensure the data are correctly interpreted by the computer.

When an analog output is interfaced with the polygraph, it is usually in the form of a 0- to 1-V DC signal. Other conventions exist for a low- and high-point calibration, but the 0- to 1-V range is fairly standard. To display the information correctly, the PSG recorder must be calibrated to accept the analog output, and what is represented by 0 V and 1 V, respectively, must be known. This information is usually found in the ancillary device's user's manual, the acquisition system user's manual, or a combination of these documents.

Each device has a high value and a low value that it can output. For example, a CPAP machine may have a low output of 4 cm H_2O and a high output of 20 cm H_2O. The low output value will be associated with 0 V. The high output value will be associated with 1 V. When the calibration is initiated, the acquisition software uses a formula to calculate the difference between 0 V and 1 V and the low-high calibration points. This enables the software to accurately read the output values of the external device. To display the output of an oximeter on the PSG, the range of the analog output of the oximeter, the numerical values each voltage represents, and how to interface this with the recorder must be known.

Consider the following example: After consulting the manual, it is clear that an analog signal at 0 V represents 0% and 1 V represents 100%. Next, the recorder is set to accept these ranges and a 0-V and 1-V calibration signal is sent from the oximeter and captured by the acquisition system. The recorder should now recognize a 0- to 1-V DC range as 0% to 100% and all increments in between. To test the system, known values at 0 V, 1 V, 0.5 V, and 0.1 V are introduced to the recorder. The oximetry channel displays 0%,

100%, 50%, and 10% in unison with the voltage changes. The PSG system software is recognizing the analog signal to represent the corresponding numerical percent in a linear manner. When the oximeter sensor is applied to the patient, the SpO_2 value of 96% is displayed on the recorder. This means that the pulse oximeter reads the patient's saturation as 96% and has converted this to a 0.96-V DC signal, which is being sent to the analog output. The signal travels to the PSG recorder, which interprets it as 96% oxyhemoglobin saturation for display and storage.

CHAPTER SUMMARY

- The theory related to operation, use, cleaning, and limitations of recording electrodes and sensors is extremely important to the sleep technologist if a clean, artifact-free record of physiologic data is to be obtained during a sleep study.
- Accurate data interpretation and subsequent treatment of sleep disorders patients rely heavily on data quality.
- Applying the correct sensor, interfacing the sensor to the recording system, and selecting appropriate recording parameters for the desired result are paramount for effective diagnostic testing and therapeutic intervention during sleep-related procedures.

- Interfacing ancillary equipment to the data acquisition system requires operational knowledge of the device itself, as well as knowledge related to the operation of the recording system.
- Correctly interfaced and calibrated ancillary equipment provides additional physiologic data measures necessary for the most effective diagnostic procedures and therapeutic interventions. This translates directly to the best possible care of the patient population served by sleep-testing facilities.

References

1. *Performance standard for electrode lead wires and patient cables, code of federal regulations,* Chapter 21, Part 898, as published in the Federal Register on May 9, 1997 [62 FR 25497].
2. Rutala WA, Weber DJ, Healthcare Infection Control Practices Advisory Committee (HICPAC)3: *Guideline for disinfection and sterilization in healthcare facilities,* Atlanta, 2008, Centers for Disease Control and Prevention.
3. Khandpur RS: *Handbook of biomedical instrumentation,* ed 2, New Delhi, 2003, Tata McGraw-Hill.
4. Rapoport D, Norman R, Nielson M: *Nasal pressure airflow measurement: an introduction,* 2001, Pro-Tech Services, Mukilteo, WA.
5. Berry R, Brooks R, Gamaldo C, et al., for the American Academy of Sleep Medicine: *The AASM manual for the scoring of sleep and associated events: rules, terminology and technical specifications,* ed 2, Westchester, Ill., 2012, American Academy of Sleep Medicine.
6. Terzano MG, Mancia D, Salati MR, et al: The cyclic alternating pattern as a physiologic component of normal NREM sleep, *Sleep* 8:137-145, 1985.
7. Neuman MR: Pulse oximetry: physical principles, technical realization and present limitations, *Adv Exp Med Biol* 220:135-144, 1987.

REVIEW QUESTIONS

1. Which if the following are recorded using the AC amplifier?
   a. EEG, EOG, EMG and ECG
   b. EEG, EtCO$_2$, EMG and ECG
   c. EtCO$_2$, Therm, Nasal Pressure, Oximeter
   d. EOG, EMG, ECG, Oximeter

2. Which of the following can be calibrated to provide flow- volume loops?
   a. Respiratory inductive plethysmography
   b. Piezo technology
   c. Diaphragmatic/intercostal EMG
   d. Esophageal probe

3. Which of the following can demonstrate false paradoxical movement?
   a. Respiratory inductive plethysmography
   b. Piezo technology
   c. Diaphragmatic/intercostal EMG
   d. Esophageal probe

4. The theory which states that a signal can theoretically be digitized and later restored to its analog value if the signal is sampled at twice the highest frequency contained in the signal is
   a. Analog-Digital Sampling theorem
   b. Digital-Analog Sampling theorem
   c. DC-AC Sampling theorem
   d. Nyquist-Shannon sampling theorem

5. What is the MOST important factor to optimize the physiological signal when using surface electrodes?
   a. Placement
   b. Electrode cleaning between patients
   c. Cleaning of the application site
   d. Metal selection

6. What is the benefit of using gold electrodes?
   a. They do well with the chloride process
   b. They do not oxidize
   c. They mix well with other metals
   d. They are easily plated with silver

7. What is the benefit of the recessed-female connector?
   a. They produce good impedance levels
   b. They cannot be incorrectly mated
   c. They are inexpensive
   d. They cannot be used with analog systems

8. Please identify the BEST description for the disinfection of electrodes.
   a. Removal of foreign material
   b. The use of water and detergent
   c. The elimination of pathogens
   d. The use of high pressure steam

9. An assessment of the audio/visual recording during polysomnography can be MOST beneficial for which of the following?
   a. Abnormal behaviors during sleep
   b. Confirmation of respiratory events
   c. Documentation of spike wave frequency
   d. Containment of future liability problems

10. The airflow transducer records a breathing waveform due to the detection of:
    a. Temperature gradients
    b. Pressure fluctuations
    c. Diaphragmatic muscle firing
    d. Gauge movement stress

The Polysomnogram: Prestudy Procedures, Monitoring Activities, and Poststudy Scoring and Interpretation

Robyn Woidtke • Bonnie Robertson

OUTLINE

OBJECTIVES

After reading this chapter, you will be able to:
1. Define documentation requirements needed prior to the study.
2. Explain the role of the technologist-patient interaction in conducting a sleep study and state components of patient-centered care.
3. Identify patient assessment methods used to obtain a sleep diagnosis.
4. Identify the tools and purpose for recording physiologic data including the montage and equipment selection, and mechanical and physiologic calibrations.
5. Define physiologic aspects of the polysomnogram that require intervention.
6. Define artifactual findings of the polysomnogram that require intervention.
7. Describe poststudy activities required for sleep study scoring and interpretation.
8. Specify patient-related follow-up activities that are outcome based.
9. Describe quality measurements to enhance the patient care experience.

KEY TERMS

10-20 system	patient assessment	scoring
medical record	patient-centered care	sleep efficiency
PAP therapy adherence	quality health care	
patient acuity	recording montage	

"There is a patient at the end of the electrodes."[1] This is a good place to begin a chapter on the preparation of the patient and the recorder. Although not a new concept, **patient-centered care** is coming to the forefront as a way to provide an integrated and holistic approach to caring for patients. The model provides for several constructs: dignity and respect, collaboration, participation, and information sharing.[2] Technologists should be cognizant of these areas and strive to include them in their interactions with patients.[3]

The Institute of Medicine (IOM) defines **quality health care** as "the degree to which health services for individuals and populations increase the likelihood of desired health outcomes and are consistent with current professional knowledge."[4] Furthermore, the IOM cites six quality parameters: care should be "safe, effective, patient-centered, timely, efficient and equitable." Combining these philosophies with facility-based requirements provides an excellent foundation for the technologist to build on in his or her practice. This chapter focuses on the nuances of assessing the patient, the importance of applying standards to the conduct of the polysomnogram and patient care, and the importance of patient-centered care.

The role of the sleep technologist is vital to the practice of sleep medicine. In addition to the technological savvy the practitioner must possess, the technologist is a patient advocate and care orchestrator. The role requires critical thinking skills. Critical thinking skills help the technologist to make sound clinical judgments. Critical thinking skills include analysis, evaluation, inference, and inductive and deductive reasoning, all of which are needed to adequately perform the role.[5] The technologist can use these processes during each patient encounter.

One example of analysis includes the viewing of respiratory data and determining that an increase in positive airway pressure (PAP) is warranted. The technologist must possess knowledge and skills related to sleep physiology, patient preparation for testing, data acquisition, application of electrical concepts, general patient care, sleep disorder–related comorbidities, identifying and correcting artifact, and ensuring that proper documentation occurs throughout the testing procedure. Patient-centered communication should be integrated as a part of standard care.

PATIENT COMMUNICATION

An important aspect of the role of the sleep technologist is to understand the reason the patient has come for testing and to establish rapport with the patient.[6] This is especially true for the recording technologist. These processes include reading and understanding testing orders, effective communication with the patient, applying standard operating procedures for the laboratory, and advocating for the patient. Advocacy is ensuring that the patients' rights and welfare are maintained.[7] Communication should be centered on the patient and based on the principles of mutual respect, harmonized goals, supportive environment, appropriate decision partners, the right information, transparency, and full disclosure and continuous learning.[6]

The technologist has a unique role. Trust is of utmost importance, as patients are at their most vulnerable. Individuals feel vulnerable when they lose control of their person and may exhibit signs of anxiety.[8] If the patient is receptive, touch and active listening provide a connection between the technologist and the patient.

Communication between the technologist and the patient is imperative. The technologist should ask the patient the reason for the sleep study, not necessarily the reason he or she is at the sleep laboratory. In all likelihood, the patient would answer "to have a sleep study" to the latter. It is important for the patient to understand the reason for the sleep study. Early understanding of diagnostic tests can help the patient adjust to a clinical diagnosis; thus, the technologist plays a role in ensuring that the patient has this knowledge.[9] The testing room should present a calming, quiet atmosphere conducive to sleep. The technologist should spend time helping the patient acclimate to the testing bedroom as part of the initial interaction.

Communication with family members or accompanying friends is an excellent way to gauge the patient's support system in the home environment. Educating the family on sleep disorders and treatments can help them provide continued support in the event treatment is recommended. This is especially true for patients with disabilities and for pediatric patients.

REVIEWING PATIENT DOCUMENTS

MEDICAL RECORD REVIEW

The health care provider uses the **medical record** and specific testing orders to communicate vital information to the technologist. The sleep study requires a written order from a health care provider who is licensed to order this type of testing; the order must be documented in the patient's medical record, which provides a complete accounting of the patient's history and physical status.

Review and comprehension of the practitioner's testing orders and the patient's medical record also play a role in advocacy.[7] In some instances, the health care provider writing the orders has limited or no interaction with the patient. Other times, there are few orders accompanying the patient. In addition to querying the patient, the astute technologist seeks out other avenues of information such as diaries and questionnaires to aid in the assessment, understanding of the patient's condition, and reason for the sleep study. Bedtime questionnaires can be a wonderful source of patient information.[10]

Good standards of practice dictate that, at a minimum, a thorough history and physical be available within the sleep center; however, this practice may not always be followed. As **patient acuity**, defined as clinical intensity or severity of a patient's condition, increases and a wide variety of patient populations access the laboratory, availability of these documents is imperative for providing quality of care. The technologist must, therefore, be proactive in obtaining the information required to provide care for the patient if not already present.

The sleep technologist must also be a good documentarian and capture clinical data. The patient should be thoroughly questioned to ascertain whether the written orders are in alignment with the patient's expectation for testing. For many people, having a sleep study is the first step in the realization that they have a chronic, long-term illness. It can be a time of great apprehension.[11] The technologist can play a significant role in educating, comforting, and being a resource for the patient. Using patient-centered communication can reduce the anxiety and apprehension of the patient.

HEALTH CARE PROVIDER ORDERS

The practical aspects of reviewing an order for a sleep test should be addressed. Orders may be preprinted, electronic, and configured in a standardized format. Orders may also be hand written on hard copy. With the emergence of electronic medical records (EMRs), the technologist may access the order electronically; however, all orders should be dated and signed by the ordering physician, whether by hand or electronically. Ensure that the order includes all the requisite information and is not just a request for a sleep study.

The order form should have pertinent patient information, which at a minimum should include the patient's name, date of birth, age, diagnosis, procedure code, and contact information. Information that helps the technologist understand the rationale for the study should also be included. Examples of such information include status of pre- and postsurgical procedures, continuous positive airway pressure (CPAP) titration and use, nocturnal seizure disorder, and necessity of a split-night study. In addition, order forms should include ICD-9 codes. This nationally accepted medical disorder coding system will be upgraded to ICD-10 in 2014.

The technologist is responsible for identifying discrepancies. The ordering practitioner may have never met with the patient, so the technologist must confirm that ordered testing is indicated based on the patient's communications, physical presentation, and available medical records. Any special needs of the patient should be noted and testing may need to be adjusted to accommodate those needs. An example of noted discrepancy is the patient who presents using supplemental oxygen. When the available history does not indicate oxygen use, the technologist must obtain further direction on the testing procedure from an on-call practitioner. The practitioner may make a decision to proceed with testing without the supplemental oxygen to establish a baseline status. The technologist must receive orders to move forward with testing.

MEDICATIONS

A complete list of all medications the patient is taking must be available. Prior to lights out, the technologist should review the medication list with the patient and document any medications that have been taken or will be taken during the sleep study. Some medications may be contraindicated for specific testing procedures. If this is the case, the on-call physician will need to be notified for direction. Many regulatory bodies require detailed reconciliation of medications; if that is the case, the sleep program will need a plan to meet the specific accrediting body's regulatory statutes.

PATIENT ASSESSMENT

Physical assessment of the patient begins at the first encounter. One can readily assess affect, body habitus, and the patient's ability to communicate during the initial meeting. The technologist can then review the orders and conduct a short interview with the patient. The fact that the monitoring technologist has an extended period with the patient provides a perfect opportunity to have meaningful discussion and provide teachable moments. Practicing and learning **patient assessment** skills enables the technologist to gain improved knowledge of the individual patient. At a minimum, during the assessment, the technologist should take into account the patient's age, cultural issues, cognitive level, literacy, and current state of health, and should ascertain any concerns that the patient may want to discuss[6] (Table 9-1). The technologist should also perform a complete set of vital signs prior to testing (Table 9-2).

TABLE 9-1
Patient Assessment Options

Type of Assessment	When Assessment Should Occur
Vision	Assess on admission to the sleep center.
Hearing	
Mobility impairment	
Cognitive status	
Personal hygiene	
Cultural needs	
Facial symmetry	
Skin integrity	
Limb temperature	
Presence of edema	
Blood pressure	Assess on admission to the sleep bedroom.
Pulse	
Respiratory rate	
Temperature	
Neck size	
Weight	
Height	
BMI	
Readiness and willingness to accept treatment plan	Assess during pre-PAP training and education.

BMI, Body mass index; *PAP*, positive airway pressure.

TABLE 9-2
Normal Ranges for Adult Vital Signs

Adult Vital Signs	Normal Ranges
Blood pressure	90/60 mm Hg to 120/80 mm Hg
Respiratory rate	12-18 breaths per minute
Heart rate	60-100 beats per minute
Temperature	97.8° to 99.1° F
Pulse oximetry	95% to 100%

Data from Berry RB, Brooks R, Gamaldo CE, Harding SM, Marcus CL, Vaughn BV, Tangredi MM for the American Academy of Sleep Medicine: *The AASM manual for the scoring of sleep and associated events: rules, terminology and technical specifications, Version 2.0.* Darien, Ill, 2012, American Academy of Sleep Medicine.

One good way to conduct a patient assessment is to proceed by starting "head to toe." Although the technologist is not required to perform a comprehensive assessment, one can note the general physical condition of the patient. For instance, the technologist would note the orientation of the patient, general hygiene, and such things as hearing aids and dentures. Visual impairment should also be noted. In addition, observations should include assessment of respiratory status (respiratory rate, dyspnea, or wheezing), and skin should be assessed for color or overt skin problems such as psoriasis or acne.[12] Physical impairment should be documented. For example, what if, while shaking the patient's hand, the technologist notes tremors not mentioned in the available documents? Any new information relevant to testing that is gleaned by the technologist should be documented in the medical record.

TECHNICAL CONSIDERATIONS

This section describes the steps necessary to prepare the data acquisition system and the patient for the sleep recording. These steps and practices provide the basis for obtaining an optimal recording. The goal is to achieve an artifact-free, high-quality sleep recording. A proper diagnosis cannot be achieved without the efforts of the technologist to maintain an artifact-free recording. By understanding the importance of these preparations and the follow-through once conducting studies in the laboratory setting, the skills and prowess of a technologist will grow exponentially.

RECORDING MONTAGE

The **recording montage** is similar to a map. It is a map of the physiologic signals being collected via electrodes and sensors and the order in which they are being viewed. Recording montages may vary between sleep centers, but most include standard recording channels based on the American Academy of Sleep Medicine's (AASM) published guidelines.[13] Differences in recording montages are most often related to the study type (i.e., diagnostic or therapeutic). It is extremely important for the technologist to understand the importance of documenting any changes made to the recording montage not otherwise specified.

The recording montage is made up of individual channels that display the various signals. The electroencephalogram (EEG) output signal is determined from the electrode derivation.[14] The derivation shows from where the signals are being derived. In recording the sleep study, differential amplifiers are used. The amplifiers record from two different electrodes: inputs 1 and 2. For instance, a central EEG channel could be derived from electrodes placed at the anatomic locations C3 and M2. In this derivation, C3 and M2 represent input 1 and input 2, respectively. The display on the monitor is the amplified difference in electrical potential between the two sites. The AASM recommends three derivations for recording the EEG; these are F4-M1, C4-M1, and O2-M1.[13] These are called referential derivations because the active EEG electrode (e.g., C4) is referenced to an electrode overlying an area of little activity (e.g., M1), which optimizes the visualization of the desired wave form.

The varying data acquisition systems have proprietary software enabling the manipulation of the "map" depending on what and how the data are displayed; however, the basic principles are the same. In addition, depending on the type of diagnosis, alternative montages may be used to ascertain nocturnal epileptiform activity or unusual electromyogram (EMG) activity as might be found in rapid eye movement (REM) sleep behavior disorder.[15] It is important to review the orders to ensure that the correct type of recording is taking place to allow for an appropriate interpretation of the data leading to diagnosis.

EQUIPMENT CALIBRATIONS

Earlier chapters in this book describe the origins of bioelectric signals, electricity and electrodes, and the visual representation of the signals as they appear during a sleep study. This section discusses the importance of ensuring that the data collected are appropriate for the type of study being conducted.

Machine calibrations are the foundation that provides the knowledge of the veracity and validity of the data being collected. If the data acquisition system has inherent errors, the data that is collected will not be correct. These calibrations include assessment of the amplitude, decay, and morphology of each signal based on a known input voltage.[14]

The first step for calibration is to enter the same inputs (voltage and filter settings) to all of the channels; this is the all-channel calibration (Figure 9-1). The purpose of this step is to ensure that for the same input, the output signal amplitude, morphology, and decay time constant are the same on each channel, thereby confirming the integrity of the data acquisition system electronics. If the data acquisition system does not allow for an all-channel calibration, recording channels with like inputs (EEG, EMG, and respiratory variables) should be compared.

The next step to ascertain signal integrity is the montage calibration. As noted in this and previous chapters, the montage creates the map or graphical picture of the data on the screen. The varying physiologic signals are typically acquired using specific amplifier settings, which include high- and low-frequency filters, gain or sensitivity, and sampling rate. Each type of physiologic parameter is best viewed using prespecified settings. For instance, the EEG signals have a low-frequency filter setting of 0.3 Hz, and a high-frequency filter setting of 30-35 Hz.[16] The amplifier

settings for each physiologic parameter have nationally accepted recommendations published by the AASM[13] (Table 9-3).

Most data acquisition systems provide the ability to enter and store the montage and settings to be used for a specific study type. For instance, a CPAP titration study will require a different montage than a nocturnal seizure protocol. A particular montage can be reinstituted as needed without having to change individual settings. This option provides for ease of use and improves time management; nevertheless, the settings may have been altered by others. It is, thus, important for the recording technologist to reaffirm and assess the signals prior to each sleep study and ensure that the amplifier settings are appropriate for the type of study being undertaken. Physiologic calibrations are reviewed in another section.

The patient may require specialized equipment based on medical history or presentation. The technologist should note any equipment that might be needed such as a transcutaneous carbon dioxide monitoring system for a patient with chronic alveolar hypoventilation. A patient with a seizure history may need full EEG monitoring for the sleep study, requiring a different montage and more intensive electrode application. The sleep laboratory may have a protocol that requires enhanced video monitoring be performed for patients with a seizure history or sleep-related behavioral issues. The technologist must be prepared to adapt as needed to ensure that the patient receives the testing that provides the best opportunity to diagnose his or her sleep disorder.

ELECTRODE AND SENSOR APPLICATION

ELECTROENCEPHALOGRAM AND ELECTROOCULOGRAM ELECTRODE APPLICATION

The international **10-20 system** of electrode placement provides a standardized and consistent approach to collecting brain wave activity.[14] This task is important in that data can be compared to normative values in the literature. The head measurement is performed prior to electrode placement. Three primary measurements are taken: the head circumference, nasion to inion, and preauricular point to preauricular point. Electrode placements are then measured in 10% or 20% increments. In addition to the EEG, electrodes are placed to measure eye movements. These are placed 1 cm below the left outer canthus and 1 cm above the right outer canthus and are referenced to the M2 electrode.[13] The chin EMG can assist with determining REM sleep versus non–rapid eye movement (NREM) sleep, but should not be used to determine NREM sleep stages.

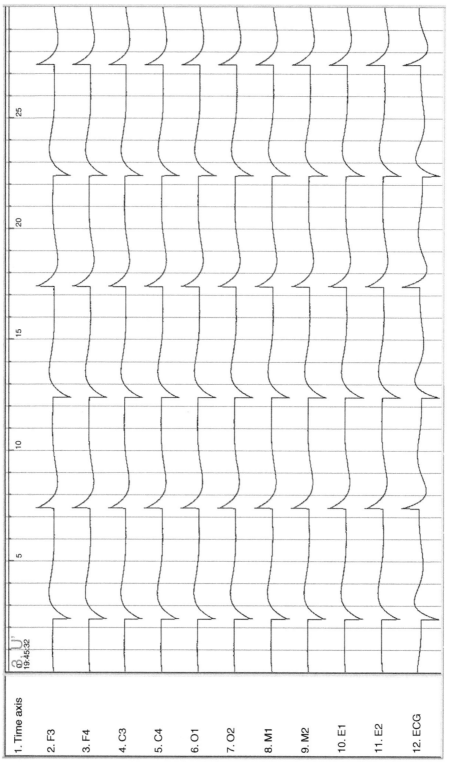

FIGURE 9-1 All-channel calibration.

TABLE 9-3
Recommended Amplifier Settings

Signal	Sampling Rates		LFF	HFF
	Desirable	Minimum		
EEG	500	200	0.3	35
EOG	500	200	0.3	35
EMG	500	200	10	100
ECG	500	200	0.3	70
Breathing Sensors	100	25	0.1	15
Oximetry	25	10	NA	NA
Snoring Sounds	500	200	10	100
Body Positions	1	1	NA	NA

ECG, Electrocardiogram; *EEG*, electroencephalogram; *EMG*, electromyogram; *EOG*, electrooculogram; *HFF*, high-frequency filter; *LFF*, low-frequency filter, *NA*, not applicable.
Data from Agency for Healthcare and Quality Research: Expanding patient centered care to empower patients and assist providers, 2012, retrieved April 23, 2012, from http://www.ahrq.gov/qual/ptcareria.htm.

ELECTROMYOGRAM AND NON-CEPHALIC SENSOR APPLICATION

The chin EMG recording can also be used to ascertain whether bruxism is present, and often snoring can be visualized. Placement of the chin EMG electrodes is as follows: one in the midline 1 cm above the inferior edge of the mandible, one placed 2 cm below the inferior edge of the mandible and 2 cm to the right of the midline, and a third similarly placed on the left side. In addition to the EEG, electrooculogram (EOG), chin EMG, and ground electrode placements, noncephalic sensors are used to collect other types of data. These include a modified lead II ECG, limb EMG, and measurements of respiratory activity.

The recommended placement for leg EMG electrodes is on the anterior tibialis muscle group, which runs along the outside of the tibia bone. Electrodes should be placed 2-3 cm apart. Data should be recorded from both legs. This signal is typically recorded in a bipolar manner.

RESPIRATORY MONITORING SENSORS

Recommended technology to measure respiratory status involves using thermal oral-nasal sensors for identification of apnea, a nasal pressure transducer to record hypopneas and RERAs, respiratory inductance plethysmography (RIP) for chest and abdominal effort, and pulse oximetry.[13] The pulse oximeter sensor is typically placed on the finger, with the diodes in direct opposition to each other. Other sites such as the

ear may be used. In infants, it is appropriate to place the sensor on the toe. The chosen sensor should be appropriate to the age of the patient. Nail polish or synthetic nails should be removed because these may hinder the ability of the oximeter to accurately sense and calculate the oxyhemoglobin saturation. A good rule is to read the manufacturer's specifications for the use of a pulse oximeter to better understand the principles of operation, sensitivity, and specificity.[16]

In other allied health fields, it has been documented that there is a dearth of understanding of pulse oximetry.[17] Because of its importance in providing a key diagnostic feature, it is vitally important for the sleep technologist to understand the use of oximetry and its associated limitations. The aggregate of these respiratory data provides for the visualization of waveforms and trending of oxygenation, which aid in the determination of respiratory status changes. Chapter 11 in this text discusses the cardiopulmonary anatomy and physiologic characteristics of the patient with possible sleep-disordered breathing.

Proper placement of respiratory monitoring equipment must be a priority, especially for patients receiving testing for sleep-related breathing disorders. The correct location and fit of the respiratory belts determine if the data is diagnostically viable. When calibrated correctly, RIP provides valuable information regarding flow volume loops and paradoxical breathing accuracy if the belts are applied to the proper location on the chest and abdomen, and maintained throughout the sleep study with integrity. Additionally, the proper placement of the thermal sensor and the pressure airflow transducer ensures that oral and nasal breathing are accurately recorded and maintained, allowing for respiratory event recognition.

SKIN PREPARATION

Electrode application technique is of the utmost importance. To ensure good signals, the skin should be adequately prepped. After carefully measuring the head using the 10-20 system, the skin is prepped at the site of electrode placement. The skin should first be cleaned with an alcohol wipe. Using a cotton-tipped swab, a slightly abrasive, gritty-type solution is used to lightly abrade the skin. The technologist must always be careful to maintain the integrity of the skin. This step ensures that recommended impedances of 5 kΩ are met at study commencement and maintained throughout the sleep study.[13]

Impedance is a measure of the resistance between an electrode and the skin that poses no appreciable risk to the patient. Many of the sleep data acquisition systems have built-in impedance measuring capabilities; however, if that is not the case, an impedance meter must be used to demonstrate that this criterion has been met.

ELECTRODE METAL RECORDING PROPERTIES

There are a variety of types of electrodes made from various metals including silver–silver chloride, gold, and tin.[18] In addition to the variety of electrodes, differing types of gels and pastes can be used that have differing conductive properties. Electrodes of the same type must be used within each recording derivation. When differing metals make contact, an electrical potential is generated. Using two dissimilar metals within a derivation results, at minimum, in artifact on the recording.

Numerous techniques are used to affix the electrodes to the head; these include the use of collodion, paste, and tape. Recently, collodion has been used less and a technique that uses a thick type of paste and gauze has replaced it. The electrodes are then affixed with the lead wires pointed toward the crown of the head. The facial electrodes can be attached in a similar fashion, using care not to get any paste or gel into the patient's eyes.

Good preparation technique is the surest route to a recording that is as artifact free as possible and provides for a robust sleep recording. The technologist will encounter numerous types of artifacts during the study. Such artifacts include sweat, muscle, respiratory, and ECG.[19] Chapter 10 in this text provides an in-depth review of artifact prevention, identification, and processes to minimize it.

RECORDING THE SLEEP STUDY

PREBEDTIME ACTIVITIES

Questionnaire

At some point prior to bedtime, the patient is asked to complete a prebedtime questionnaire. The purpose of the questionnaire is to help with the interpretation of data. The questionnaire provides an overview of the patient's day before the sleep study. Typically a presleep questionnaire has questions related to medications, caffeine use, and sleep information.[10] After completion of the application of electrodes and other sensors and the completion of questionnaires, the patient should finalize bedtime requirements.

Physiologic Calibrations

Physiologic calibrations are a tool for the technologist and physician to use to aid in the interpretation of the data collected over the course of the sleep study. This process provides for the examination of each parameter (i.e., EEG, EMG, and respiratory variables) in a controlled environment so that the technologist can determine whether the signal response is correct. This process also allows for a comparison between wake and sleep behavioral states. The primary purposes of this set of calibrations are to determine whether sensors are functioning properly and to provide baseline data specific to the particular patient. These commands should produce the expected response. The importance of this process cannot be overstated. For instance, without these comparative data, it may be impossible to differentiate between wake and N1, particularly in those patients who are low alpha producers.

Proper channel polarity must also be determined during physiologic calibrations. This is the opportunity for the technologist to verify EEG, EOG, and ECG polarity appropriateness. The channel input must be an indicator for polarity to properly record signals. A good example is the EOG channels. If the polarity is not correct, REMs will be in sync instead of as needed for recognition of REM sleep. Another example is the respiratory channels: These channels must have proper polarity determined during physiologic calibrations to determine in-phase versus out-of-phase (paradoxical) breathing.

The sequence of the maneuvers may be different from lab to lab, but should include the following: eyes open for 30 seconds, eyes closed for 30 seconds; movement of eyes to the left and right, and up and down; slowly blink the eyes five times; grit teeth or swallow; simulate a snore or hum; dorsiflex and plantarflex the great toe; and, normal breathing for at least three breaths followed by a 10-second breath hold. These maneuvers are done twice, once at the beginning of the recording and again at the end of the recording, to determine whether sensors are functioning properly and to establish baseline patient data.

Although physiologic similarities are present between patients, differences do exist. It is imperative to assess the physiologic signal of each individual channel and adjust the settings as appropriate to optimize signal display (Figure 9-2). Scoring procedures, a term used by the sleep field to describe tabulation and data review, can be used as a comparison during equivocal epochs of wake and the various sleep states.

At the completion of the physiologic calibrations, the patient is ready for "lights out." To understand what is outside of a normal parameter, the technologist must be well-versed in normal values for vital signs.[20] The implications for practice include the recognition of atypical heart rate and rhythm, respiratory patterns, and pulse oximetry values. For example, a baseline SpO_2 is 94% while awake. During sleep, as normal physiologic changes occur, there may be a significant change in baseline saturation. This may point to an underlying pulmonary disease.[21] Any parameter outside of the normal for the specific age ranges should be noted in the patient's medical record and technologist's documentation, even if further action is not immediately warranted.

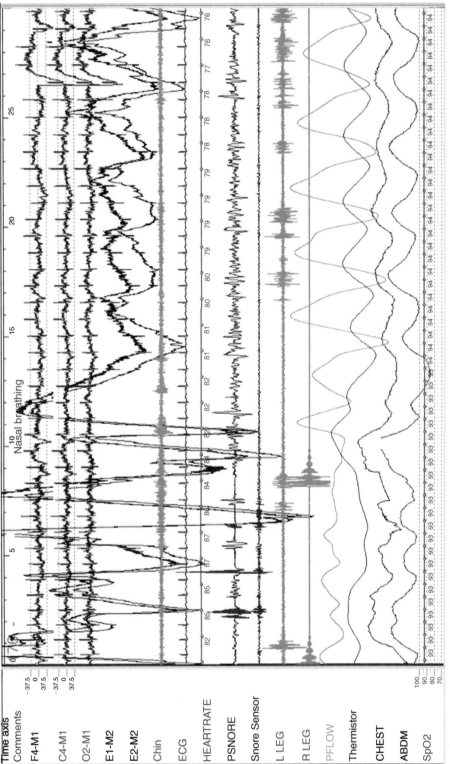

FIGURE 9-2 M2 electrode is unstable and must be securely attached prior to "lights out."

MONITORING AND DOCUMENTING

Once "lights out" has occurred, the patient tries to settle down and get to sleep. It is critical that the sleep study be performed as close as possible to the normal sleeping hours for that patient. Sleeping in a strange place with strange wires can be challenging, but trying to replicate the sleeping hours and the sleeping situation can be helpful. A comfortable bed and pillow should be available. Privacy is essential. Patients feel very vulnerable during a sleep study, and constant reassurance may be needed. The patient should be encouraged to relax and clear his or her mind.

The decision to have a sleep study may be a difficult one for the patient. It is also an expensive endeavor. The sleep technologist plays a vital role in the outcome of that decision and should not take the responsibilities lightly. Reassurance that the technologist will be readily available at all times can help the patient feel secure.

Audio and visual monitoring should be active from the moment the patient enters the sleep room to the moment they leave after completion. This is for the patient's safety as well as for the technologist's assistance. The technologist must correlate recorded physiologic data to the visual manifestation of the data. Obscuring body movements on the polysomnogram may be the patient experiencing a seizure. It could possibly be a confused geriatric patient attempting to get out of bed. Having visual and audio clues can help the technologist differentiate and respond when necessary.

The technologist must maintain constant vigilance throughout the sleep study. It only takes a few seconds for a cardiac dysrhythmia to occur and the technologist may only have a few minutes to respond appropriately to ensure best outcomes (refer to Figures 9-3 through 9-6).

QUALITY MONITORING

Failure to develop work habits that include a vigilant monitoring routine may prove a liability for the patient, the sleep program, and the sleep technologist. The technologist's primary duty is to maintain a study quality that will assist the physician with an accurate diagnosis. Failure of electrodes or sensors, failure to respond to artifacts in a timely manner, and failure to react to physiologic variances can affect the quality of the study and the resulting recording (refer to Figures 9-7 through 9-10).

RECORD-KEEPING

The technologist must keep an accurate record of everything that transpires during a sleep study. Normal and abnormal vital signs should be documented, body positions should be recorded through a position sensor device or by visual confirmation with documentation, and any variances from normal recording parameters must be noted (refer to Figures 9-11 through 9-13).

Modern computerized sleep acquisition systems time stamp changes to recording settings, and electronic documentation programs also record the exact time and date a comment was added. Gone are the days when a sleep technologist could wait until 5 a.m. to perform all of the documentation for the entire sleep study. This simply doesn't happen anymore, and if it does, the supervising personnel are quite aware of those performance issues. In addition, documentation is *not* just for that split-second of time. Any routine documentation such as "30-minute time checks," should clearly document exactly what has been happening for the previous 30 minutes. The monitoring technologist should also clearly document respiratory events; sleep disturbances; electrocardiogram (ECG) abnormalities, which are commonly referred to as dysrhythmias; body movements; therapeutic interventions; and any recording parameter changes in real time.

RESPONSE TO CLINICAL EVENTS

The patient may have physical needs that require the assistance of the sleep technologist during the study. Many patients need help using the restroom and certainly need help with the disconnection of equipment required to do so. The patient should be instructed to call or summon the technologist for any reason, and especially for getting out of the bed. With the acuity of sleep center patients higher than in the past, many patients have physical, emotional, and mental challenges that require significant time and effort by the technologist. If possible, having at least one additional staff member floating between patients can help the assigned technologist see to the patient with those significant needs.

The technologist must be prepared to respond to unexpected or life-threatening events. The technologist should be trained to recognize and respond to cardiac events such as ventricular fibrillation, epileptiform or seizure disorders manifested as abnormal EEG activity, parasomnia-related manifestations, and respiratory events (refer to Figures 9-14 through 9-16). The sleep program should have protocols to address each of these possibilities.

The technologist may also need to respond to fire; weather-related events; internal or external disasters; and violent behaviors by a patient, a visitor, or a co-worker. As many sleep technologists may be working alone, an emergency call button is a tremendous bonus, and security personnel making frequent rounds through the sleep center can also be a method to help the solo technologist. Regardless, there must be detailed protocols that identify what to do, whom to call, and how to ensure the patients' well being.

(Text continued on page 195)

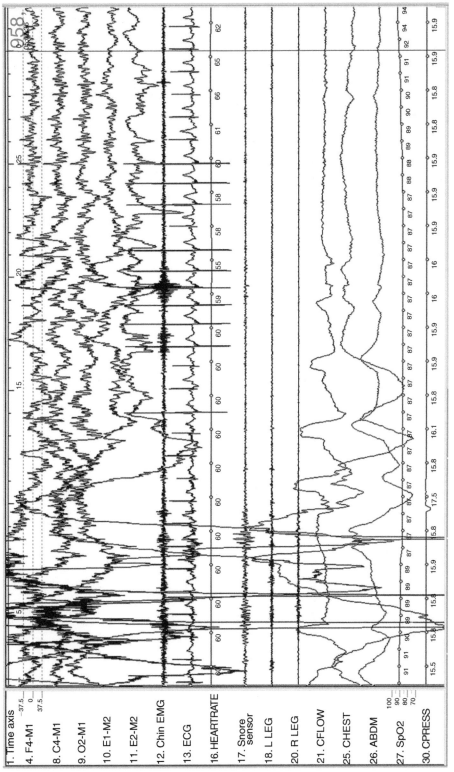

FIGURE 9-3 M2 is very unstable and should be investigated. The electrocardiogram shows a variance that could be artifactual in nature, but physiologic origin needs to be ruled out.

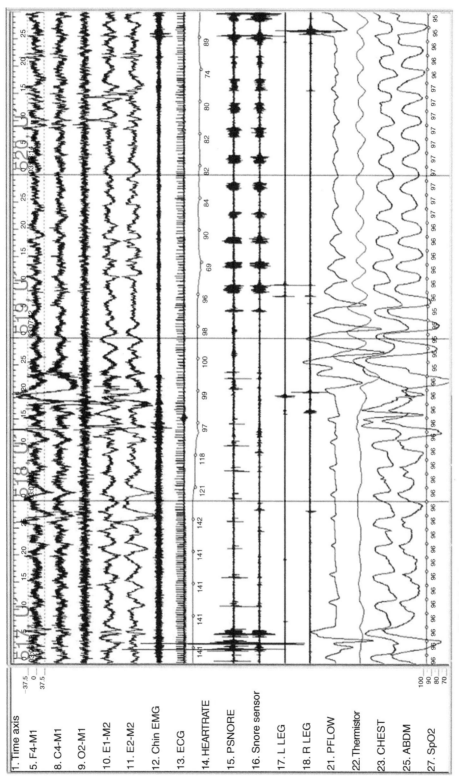

FIGURE 9-4 Heart rate variability is extreme. The technologist should investigate, document, and respond if indicated.

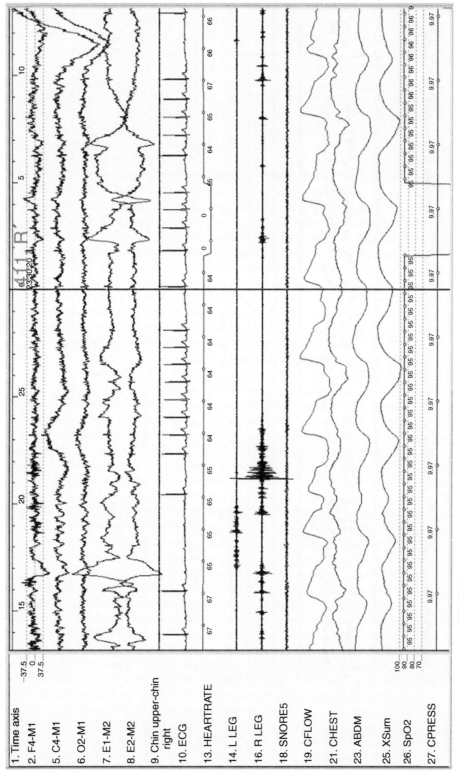

FIGURE 9-5 Electrocardiogram shows an atrioventricular block most consistent with a second-degree, type 2 block (normal atrial rhythm and normal ventricular rhythm except for nonconducted p waves). The technologist must recognize, document, and respond if indicated.

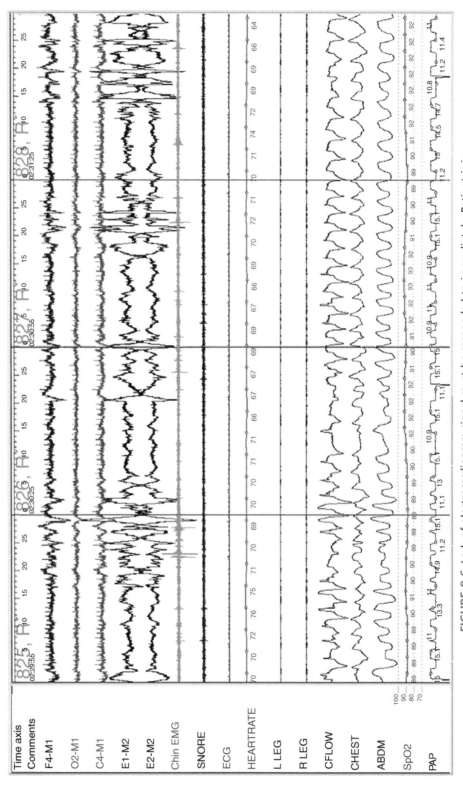

FIGURE 9-6 Lack of electrocardiogram signal must be responded to immediately. Patient is in rapid eye movement sleep and the decision must be made as to when is the appropriate time to correct artifactual reading.

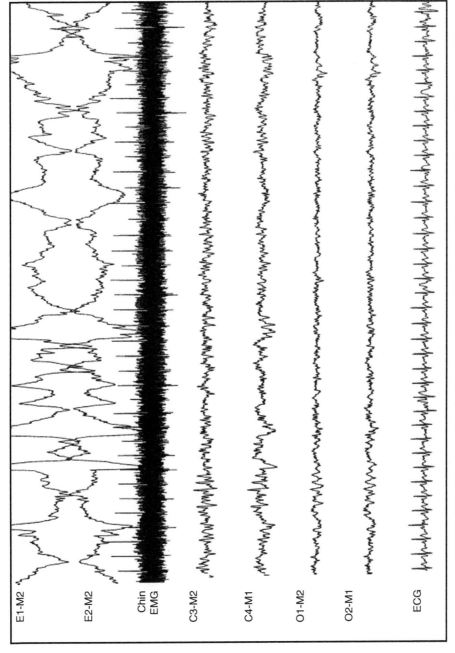

FIGURE 9-7 60-hertz artifact in chin electromyogram must be addressed as soon as rapid eye movement sleep period completes.

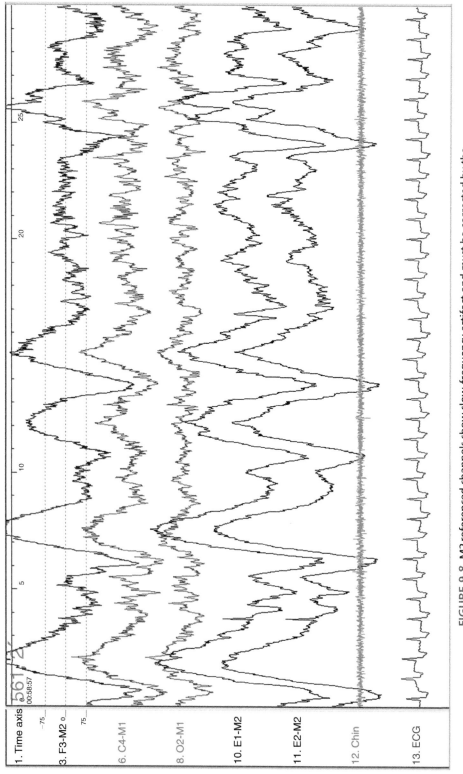

FIGURE 9-8 M2 referenced channels show slow-frequency artifact and must be corrected by the technologist.

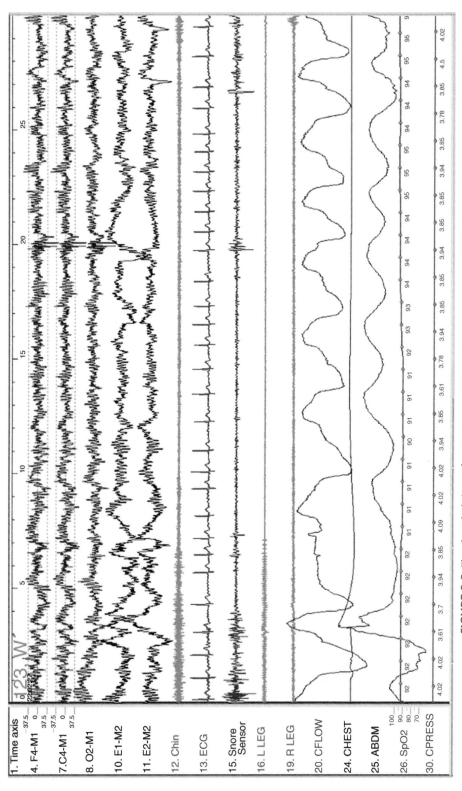

FIGURE 9-9 The chest belt is not functioning, making respiratory event type difficult to positively ascertain. This issue must be corrected. In addition, the technologist should be documenting dysrhythmia type and frequency.

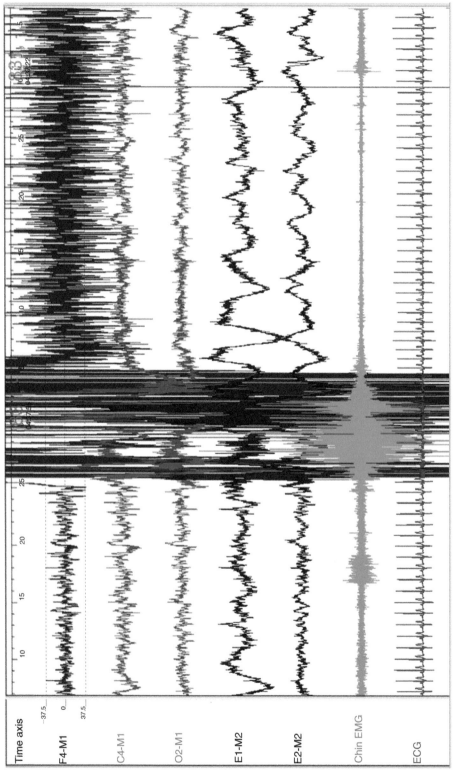

FIGURE 9-10 Disconnection of the F4 electrode following body movement and arousal. The technologist should make a decision to correct or re-reference based on patient's status.

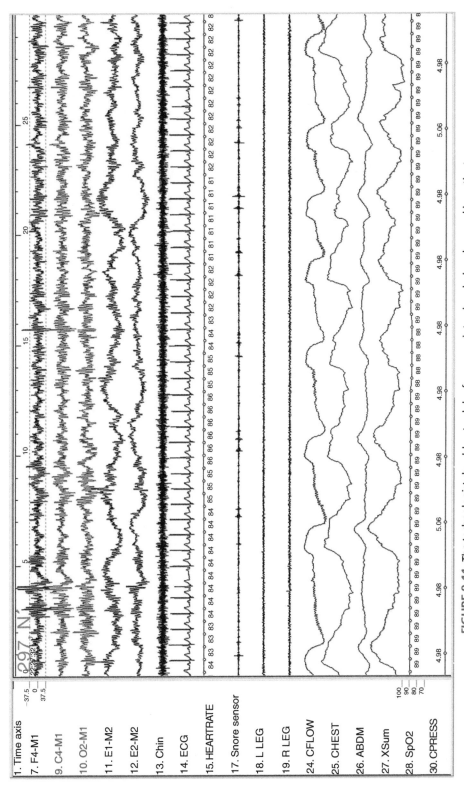

FIGURE 9-11 The technologist should note alpha frequency intrusion during sleep and investigate physiologic condition or medications that may be contributors.

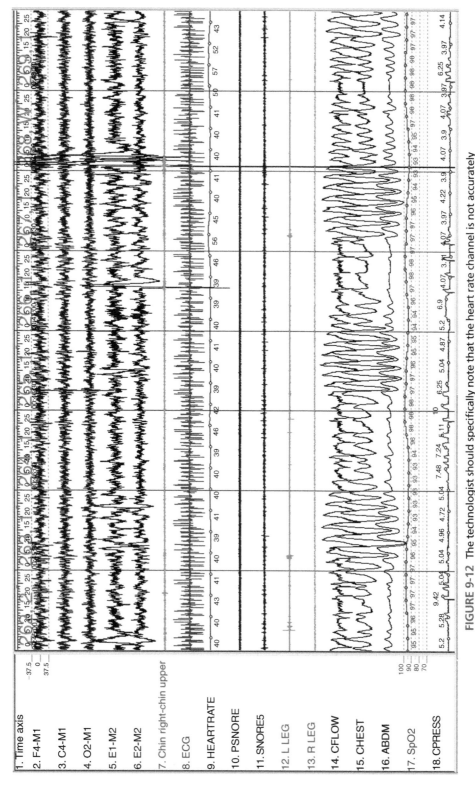

FIGURE 9-12 The technologist should specifically note that the heart rate channel is not accurately capturing the true heart rate because of atrial fibrillation or flutter noted on the electrocardiogram channel.

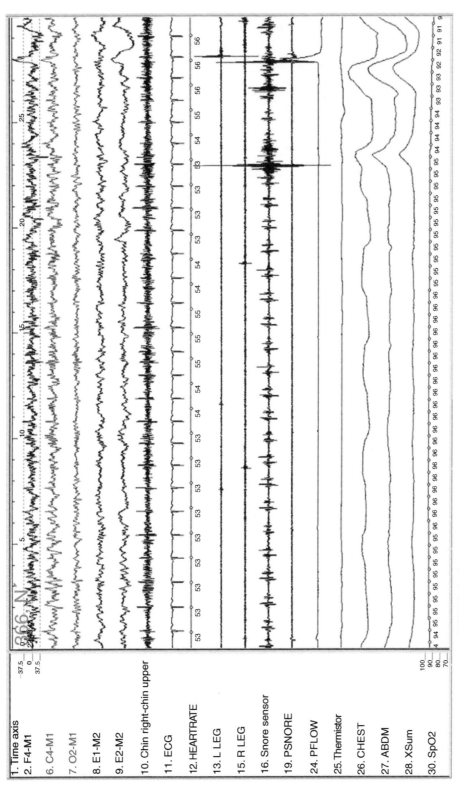

FIGURE 9-13 The technologist should note that the electrocardiogram signal is reversed and change the polarity on the recording channel. The technologist should also investigate the lack of signal on the pressure transduced flow (PFLOW) and the thermistor channels even when breathing resumes as evidenced by the effort channels.

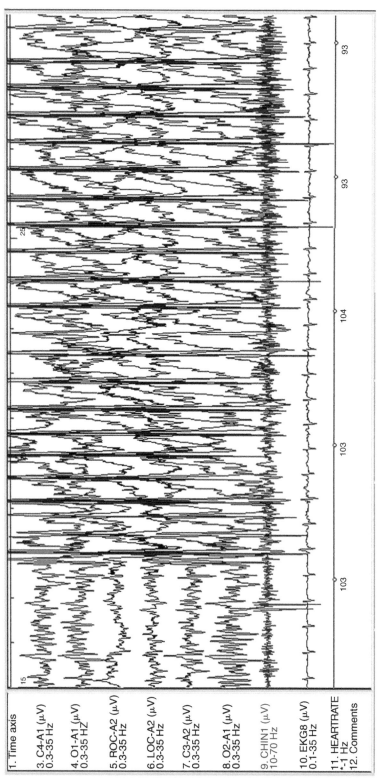

FIGURE 9-14 The technologist must evaluate and determine the distinction between epileptiform activity versus manifested seizure activity versus electrode artifact. The technologist must be able to differentiate and respond appropriately.

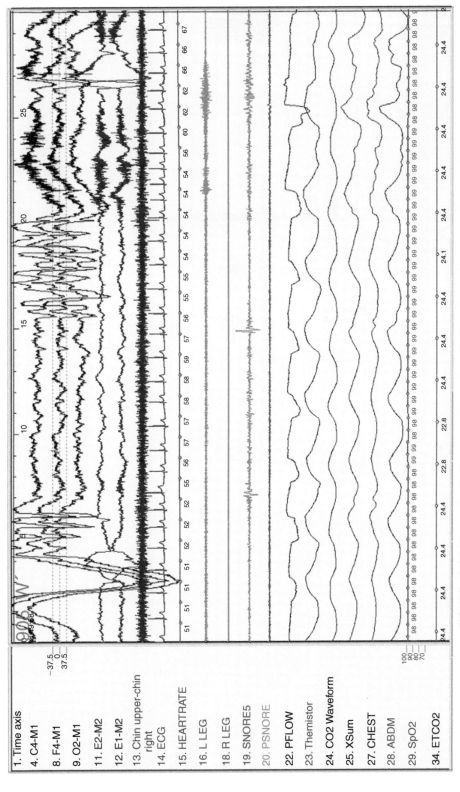

FIGURE 9-15 The technologist must determine if the observed abnormality on the electroencephalogram channels is physiologic or artifactual. This is an example of "head scratching," which emphasizes the need for correlation of audio and visual cues to physiologic recording.

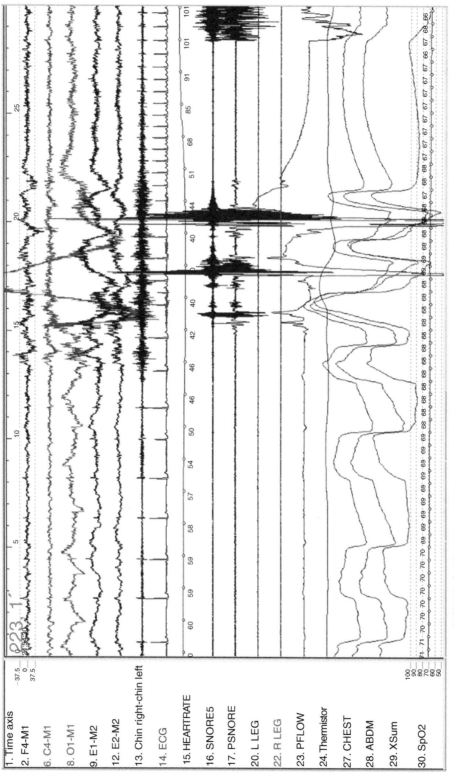

FIGURE 9-16 Patient demonstrating severe apnea with hypoxemia, bradycardia, and sleep fragmentation. This degree of severity warrants immediate positive airway pressure intervention.

CONCLUSION OF THE SLEEP STUDY

The completion of the sleep study depends on numerous factors. The patient may have identified a time for "wake up" if she needs to report to work or school or has family obligations. The technologist also needs to determine if the study requirements have been met. Has enough REM sleep been recorded? Did the patient agree to sleep supine for at least some portion of the sleep study? Was CPAP applied, and if so, has optimal PAP been achieved? Did the total sleep time replicate the patient's normal sleep time as closely as possible? Does the patient need to stay for a multiple sleep latency test (MSLT)? The technologist needs to weigh all relevant factors and information to make an informed decision regarding the time to end the sleep study.

POSTSTUDY ACTIVITIES

Physiologic Calibrations

Poststudy calibrations are very similar to prestudy calibrations. Once the patient is awakened and "lights on" is performed, the technologist should have the patient assume a supine position. Physiologic calibrations should be implemented exactly as performed prior to "lights out." A montage calibration should be performed to accurately record all amplifier settings as used at the end of the test. This may be followed by an all-channel calibration.

Electrode and Sensor Removal

The technologist has the responsibility to gently and completely remove all recording electrodes and sensors. This may be uncomfortable for a patient as the equipment has possibly been attached for longer than 8 hours and paste, gel, collodion, and tape can be a challenge to remove in a gentle manner. This may be especially true for pediatric and geriatric patients because their skin can be thin and sensitive. It may be necessary for the technologist to help the patient remove all excess paste and gel after electrodes and sensors have been removed to ensure no traces of testing remain. Most residues can be removed with a hot, soapy shower, and some vigorous shampooing of the hair and scalp.

Poststudy Patient Instructions

The patient and the family should be given verbal and written instructions regarding the next steps. If the patient was placed on CPAP during the test, it is possible that the physician will want the patient to begin therapy as soon as possible. If the practice of the sleep program is to start the patient on therapy right away, the patient should be informed of that possibility so

he or she understands that the criteria for PAP application have been met and the physician wants the patient to get started on therapy. The patient should be told that a durable medical equipment (DME) company or a home health care company will be in contact to set up a time to instruct the patient on the use of the PAP device in the home setting. The technologist has the responsibility to tell the patient to be sure to follow up with the physician to get complete sleep study results.

After answering all questions and ensuring that the patient has all personal belongings and understands exactly what to do next, the technologist can officially discharge the patient and provide assistance as the patient leaves. Discharge documentation should be completed, especially for pediatric patients, to ensure they are released to the care of a parent or guardian. It is likely that the parent or guardian has been present for the entire sleep test, but documentation is the best step for legal coverage of pediatrics.

The sleep program may also require that the technologist create a summary report of the sleep study. This document supplies information for the scoring technologist (if different than the monitoring technologist) and for the interpreting physician.

SCORING AND REPORT TABULATION

Scoring

The next step for the sleep study is scoring completion and report tabulation. **Scoring** is a term commonly used in the sleep medicine field to indicate an epoch-by-epoch examination and classification of the sleep data. Many sleep programs require technologists to score sleep studies while the data are being acquired. This helps improve the technologist's proficiency of sleep stage, respiratory event, body movement event, and ECG dysrhythmia recognition. A monitoring technologist will not have the necessary skills to effectively monitor and treat the patient during the sleep study if he or she is unable to recognize sleep stages and respiratory events. All technologists, whether their primary duty is scoring or monitoring, should participate in an interscorer reliability program. This helps maintain a level of competency necessary for the sleep program to confidently trust that scored data is diagnostically accurate.

Study Status Tracking

Some type of study tracking methodology should be used to monitor the status of a sleep study. The sleep program should be able to have a sleep study scored and ready for the physician's interpretation within 24 hours of completion of the study. A methodology to track unscored studies, scored studies, interpreted studies, and processed studies helps all members of the sleep program perform their duties in a timely manner. This also helps ensure that no patient "falls through the cracks." The status of each and every study should be apparent for any staff member who has a medical reason to be involved in that patient's care.

Data Tabulation and Report Elements

An important aspect of the scored data is the sleep study report. The report is only as accurate as the data generated by the software program and it is imperative that the scoring technologist manually review and edit each aspect of the report. The report will be used for interpretation purposes and *must* be accurate.

Data Tabulation

Components for the sleep architecture that need to be confirmed include "lights out" and "lights on" as those markers are used to determine total recording time (TRT); total sleep time (TST); sleep onset latency; sleep period; REM sleep onset latency; wake after sleep onset; each stage by total minutes and percentage of total sleep time to include stages N1, N2, N3, and R (REM); and percent **sleep efficiency.**[13] The sleep efficiency is a percentage of the amount of sleep accomplished during the allowable time allotment using the formula TST/TRT.

The sleep stage minutes and percentages may also be calculated for time spent in each body position. It is essential to accurately score and tabulate the arousals from sleep noted during the sleep test. This can give the interpreting practitioner insightful information regarding the disruption to the sleep architecture and correlation with event type. The AASM has published detailed sleep study scoring guidelines.[13]

Report components for respiratory event tabulation should minimally include an apnea and hypopnea index, which can easily be further subdivided into indices for each type of event; indices for each body position; and indices for NREM sleep, REM sleep, and wake. It may be important to calculate a respiratory disturbance index if the patient had numerous respiratory effort–related arousals because these events need to be captured on the report for diagnostic purposes but do not meet scoring requirements for an apnea or a hypopnea. TST is used to determine indices for events specific to sleep.

For respiratory event severity determination, it is important for the oxygen saturation recording to be accurate for the entire sleep test and for all artifactual data to be eliminated or accounted for in the scoring process; in addition, significant desaturations must be enumerated. Typically, the report should include total minutes of recording time with SpO_2 less than 90%

and then further accounted for with total minutes of recording time with SpO_2 of 88% or less.

Report Elements

Other significant factors that must be scored and tabulated include limb movements, body movements, epileptiform or seizure-related activity, parasomnia-related activity, and ECG abnormalities. Depending on the acquisition software capability, the techniques for reporting each of these may differ greatly. All limb movements that meet periodicity criteria should be counted and tabulated for reporting purposes. Any restless limb movement activity during wake episodes, especially when contributing to difficulty getting to sleep or staying asleep, must be accounted for in some manner, even if only by text documentation.

A patient being seen in a sleep center for abnormal activity during sleep such as sleep-walking, sleep-talking, sleep-eating, or violent behaviors should be closely monitored during the study with complete documentation. The documentation and correlation to video and audio recordings should be summarized and included in the interpretation for diagnostic purposes. ECG dysrhythmias must be noted, including bradycardic and tachycardic episodes, and abnormal ventricular or atrial rhythms. Dysrhythmias correlated to respiratory events or oxygen desaturations are particularly noteworthy.

Documenting Medication Use

The report should also include any information that would have a direct effect on the interpretive process. Patient medication dosage and frequency must be reported as accurately as possible. It should be emphasized to the patient by the ordering physician, prior to testing, which medications to continue and which medications to wean or discontinue for sleep testing to be diagnostically significant.

At the time of testing, medications must be documented and it should be specifically noted if the patient took medications the day of testing, immediately prior to "lights out," during the sleep test, or on awakening at the completion of the sleep test. Many medications affect sleep, breathing, cardiac function, and behaviors. Specifically for MSLT and maintenance of wakefulness testing, a urine drug screen may be indicated to assess for medications that contribute to difficulty getting to sleep or difficulty staying awake.

INTERPRETATION

The interpretive process should be timely and diagnostically significant. The interpreting practitioner should be a physician boarded or board eligible in his or her respective discipline's sleep medicine subspecialty. The sleep study data should be reviewed epoch by epoch for accuracy of scoring and completeness of summarization of events. This includes careful review of summarization data, especially if the data interfaces automatically with interpretation template macros, which many software programs now offer. The temptation to assume that the data are absolutely correct or the macro is uncorrupted can lead to erroneous data and a missed or inaccurate diagnosis.

A diagnosis and diagnostic code should be clearly outlined on the interpretation report using a crosswalk from the ICSD to the ICD. The interpretation should include all diagnostically significant data and all recommendations. The recommendations should outline treatment options, indicated behavioral modifications, medication deletions or additions, and potential consequences of failure to treat.

The interpretation should be timely, with many programs able to complete the entire process from sleep performance through interpretation in less than 24 hours. The sleep study should not be considered complete until this step is accomplished. This timeliness helps build rapport with referring practitioners and builds a level of confidence and satisfaction with the sleep program. Interpreting physicians must be held accountable for timeliness and many sleep programs have tied interpretive timeliness to financial incentives.

PATIENT FOLLOW-UP

The sleep program should have a method to not only track sleep study status but to also track the patient from initial referral to follow-up. With the recent trend toward EHR systems, many sleep programs have the electronic means to track referrals, scheduling attempts, testing procedures, scoring procedures, interpretation status, new orders for therapy or further testing, and follow-up recommendations, which may include a referral to another subspecialty such as cardiology or weight loss management. Most EHR systems have a billing component that can also track the status of insurance authorization, charge entry, and payments. The purpose of the EHR is to allow immediate access on a need-to-know basis for all members of the health care team who have a medically related need to view that data.

QUALITY MEASUREMENTS

INTERSCORER RELIABILITY

The sleep program should be evaluating and improving on quality measures. Nationally accredited sleep programs must use interscorer reliability as a measurement of scoring correlation between each technologist as one of their quality improvement markers. Performance improvement and quality assurance measurements should always include patient satisfaction. Using an independent, unbiased outside survey source can help distribute surveys, analyze data, compare with national averages for reporting purposes, and institute improvement initiatives.

THERAPY COMPLIANCE MONITORING

Therapy compliance monitoring is an important quality measurement for any sleep program. Tracking patients' **PAP therapy adherence** is now easy to manage with the aid of cloud-based technology. The PAP devices on the market track use, apnea and hypopnea indices, leak values, and pressure settings and needs. This tool helps the sleep program and dedicated clinical sleep educators work with patients to help them adjust to therapy and address any barriers to therapy in a timely manner. Patients often need mask adjustments or changes early in the therapy process, and often need additional instruction and education to continue therapy. The sleep physician assigned to the patient's care should be included in this responsibility to make changes to PAP settings by prescription and reinforce the need for therapy.

Many sleep programs have their own sleep-related DME to participate in the continuum of care for patients with sleep-disordered breathing, which is most likely a chronic condition with lifelong needs and support. Addressing the need for new PAP supplies, including masks, tubing, filters, and so on, is a part of this support. Even with proper maintenance, interface parts wear and can diminish effectiveness of therapy if replacements are not regularly available.

CHAPTER SUMMARY

- The technologist is responsible for review of the patient's history and indicated testing.
- Communicating with, and educating, the patient and the patient's family is a vital role for the technologist.
- Equipment preparation and calibration must be performed and verified prior to sleep testing.
- Patient preparation includes electrode and sensor application.
- The sleep study is composed of prestudy calibrations, the sleep study, and poststudy calibrations.
- The sleep study is a diagnostic and therapeutic tool, and the accuracy of the data is paramount.
- The patient needs instruction regarding next steps after completion of testing.
- The scoring and tabulation of the data is essential to provide an accurate diagnosis.
- The interpretation of the sleep study is performed by a physician; the sleep study must undergo a thorough review for accuracy of diagnosis.
- Quality measurements should include all activities related to patient care, including patient communication, sleep study accuracy, patient follow-up, therapy adherence, and continuation of care.

References

1. Grandi E: Personal communication, 2011.
2. Agency for Healthcare and Quality Research: *Expanding patient centered care to empower patients and assist providers* (website). www.ahrq.gov/qual/ptcareria.htm. Accessed April 23, 2012.
3. Behar-Horenstein LS, Guin P, Gamble K, et al: Improving patient care through patient-family education programs, *Hospital Topics* 83(1):21-27, 2005.
4. Institute of Medicine: *Crossing the quality chasm: a new health system for the 21st century*, Washington, DC, 2001, National Academies Press.
5. Keating SB: Components of the curriculum, In Keating SB, editor: *Curriculum development and evaluation in nursing*, ed 2 New York, 2011, Springer.
6. Paget L, Han P, Nedza S, et al: *Patient-clinician communication: basic principles and expectations*, Washington, DC, 2011, National Academies Press.
7. Beyea SC: Patient advocacy: nurses keeping patients safe, *Assoc Periop Reg Nurses J* 81(5):1046-1047, 2005.
8. Sorlie V, Torjuul K, Ross A, et al: Satisfied patients are also vulnerable patients: narratives from an acute care ward, *Iss Clin Nurs* doi 10.1111/j.1365-2702.2006.01352.x.
9. Irwin RS, Richardson ND: Patient-focused care: using the right tools, *Chest* 130;73S-82S, 2006.
10. Pressman M: *Primer of polysomnographic interpretation*, Boston, 2002, Butterworth-Heinemann.
11. De Ridder D, Geenen R, Kuiher R, van Middendorp H: Psychological adjustment to chronic disease, *Lancet* 372(9634):246-255, 2008.
12. Wolf L, Fiscella E, Cunningham H: 10-minute assessment for patient safety, *Nurse Educator* 33(6), 2008.
13. Berry RB, Brooks R, Gamaldo CE, et al., for the American Academy of Sleep Medicine: *The AASM manual for the scoring of sleep and associated events: rules, terminology and technical specifications, Version 2.0*, Darien, Ill, 2012, American Academy of Sleep Medicine.
14. Fisch BJ: *Fisch and Spehlmann's EEG primer, 3rd edition basic principles of digital and analog EEG*, Philadelphia, 2000, Elsevier.
15. Montplaiser J, Gagnon J, Fantini ML, et al: Polysomnographic diagnosis of idiopathic REM sleep behavior diagnosis, *Mov Dis* 2010, doi:10.1002/mds.23257.
16. Butkov N: Polysomnography recording systems in Butkov N, Lee-Chiong T, editors: *Fundamentals of sleep technology*, Philadelphia, 2007, Wolters Kluwer/Lippincott Williams and Wilkins.
17. Grap M: Pulse oximetry, *Crit Care Nurse* 22(3):69-74, 2002.
18. Tallgren P, Vanhatalo S, Kaila K, et al: Evaluation of commercially available electrodes and gels for recording slow EEG potentials, *Clin Neurophysiol*, 2005, doi:10.1016/j.clinph,2004.10.001.
19. Patil SP: Technical aspects of sleep testing, *ACCP Sleep Medicine Board Review*, ed 4, Northbrook, Ill., 2009.
20. Normal ranges for vital signs, *Medline Plus*, 2012, retrieved May 20, 2012, from http://www.nlm.nih.gov/medlineplus/ency/article/002341.htm.
21. Valdez-Lowe C, Ghareeb SA, Artiniean NT: Pulse oximetry in adults, *Am J Nurs* 109(6):52-59, 2008.

REVIEW QUESTIONS

1. Patient centeredness involves the concept of:
   a. Autonomy
   b. Behavioral theories
   c. Cultural competence
   d. Collaboration

2. According to the IOM, quality care includes the following:
   a. Safe, effective, patient-centered, timely, efficient, and equitable
   b. Direct, cost-effective, patient-centered, justifiable, evidence-based, and equitable
   c. Safe, patient-centered, cost-effective, evidence-based, timely, and physician-directed
   d. Medical home, efficient, safe, preventative care, highly trained care professionals, and timely

3. The international 10-20 system is used to:
   a. Calibrate the polysomnogram
   b. Measure the head for electrode placement
   c. Score sleep
   d. Classify sleep states

4. The technologist must review the order form to:
   a. Effectively conduct the study
   b. Engage in a discussion regarding the diagnosis
   c. Bill for the study
   d. Use the information for the final report

5. Which of the following is true regarding the use of medications during sleep testing?
   a. The patient does not need to bring their medications to the sleep lab
   b. The patient should self-administer all medications
   c. All medications should be stopped 3 days prior to sleep testing
   d. The sleep technologist should administer all medications

6. Communication is an important part of the role of the technologist and includes:
   a. Frequent telephone calls with the patient
   b. Engaging the family, if available
   c. Speaking another language
   d. Conducting reading assessments

7. The AASM recommends which of the following EEG locations for the recording of sleep?
   a. T3-C4
   b. O2-M1
   c. FZ-M2
   d. Fp1-M1

8. Optimum impedance for the electrodes is:
   a. 2 KΩ
   b. 20 KΩ
   c. 5 KΩ
   d. 10 KΩ

9. Using electrodes of dissimilar metals can cause:
   a. Electrocution of the patient
   b. Degradation of the signal
   c. A flat line
   d. Artifact

Chapter 10

Recognizing, Evaluating, and Minimizing Recording Artifacts

K. Wayne Peacock • Bonnie Robertson • Buddy Marshall

CHAPTER OUTLINE

LEARNING OBJECTIVES

After reading this chapter, you will be able to:
1. Identify physiologic signals related to specific recording channels.
2. Articulate the importance of impedance testing.
3. Define acceptable impedances for each recording site.
4. Assess an artifact source and appropriate technologist response.
5. Differentiate an electroencephalographic artifact.
6. Categorize an electromyographic artifact.
7. Assess a respiratory artifact.
8. Identify a beneficial artifact.
9. Identify and respond to unwanted artifacts.
10. Select appropriate electrodes to reference for artifact reduction.
11. Recommend interventions to eliminate or reduce various artifact types.
12. Differentiate beneficial versus unwanted artifacts.
13. Choose appropriate filters when assessing artifacts.

KEY TERMS

airflow signal artifacts	implanted electronic device	salt bridge
artifact isolation	line frequency artifact	short circuit
cardioballistic artifact	muscle artifact	signal processing
channel-blocking artifact	oximetry artifacts	slow-frequency artifacts
electrocardiographic (ECG) artifact	pulse artifact	sweat artifact
	respiratory artifact	system reference artifact
electrode popping artifact	respiratory effort sensor artifact	

According to *Webster's Medical Dictionary,* artifact is defined as "an electrocardiographic and electroencephalographic wave that arises from sources other than the heart or brain." This very basic definition is inadequate when dealing with a 6- to 10-hour polysomnogram (PSG) because artifact may arise from a variety of sources, both internal and external to the recording. Some artifacts, such as snoring and the muscle associated with bruxism, may be beneficial to the recording, but are still considered artifactual in origin. For the purpose of polysomnography, any data that appear on a channel in addition to, or in place of, the desired signal of interest, is considered artifact.

Early recognition and evaluation of various artifacts is an essential role of the sleep technologist, both during acquisition and review of data. Timely and accurate correction of the various types of unwanted signals leads to the acquisition of a high-quality and artifact-free recording. It is also important to determine when artifacts cannot be eliminated without jeopardizing signals of interest. Through careful assessment and analysis, one must either determine if ways to minimize the artifact exist, or document the justification for allowing it to remain part of the recording.

There are several ways to achieve a relatively artifact-free recording. This chapter addresses three basic processes to ensure that a quality recording is acquired: electrode and sensor application, signal processing, and artifact isolation.

An artifact-free recording begins with proper electrode preparation and placement techniques. The integrity of electrode and sensor application is the single largest determinant of the quality and accuracy of recorded data.[1] Ensuring electrodes and sensors are properly prepared and affixed to the patient helps reduce or even eliminate many of the artifact types discussed in this chapter.

The next step is to ensure accurate **signal processing** through the use of a quality acquisition system and optimal amplifier settings. In fact, identification of some artifacts depends entirely on a technologist's understanding of amplifier controls. The low-frequency filter (LFF) plays a large role in whether a particular artifact is seen on a channel type such as electroencephalography (EEG), electrooculography (EOG), breathing, and so on. Likewise, the LFF setting can affect the duration of a signal to make it appear more spikelike than its true morphology. This is why a popping electrode looks very different on an EEG channel as compared with an electromyography (EMG) channel. The gain and sensitivity setting can also have a profound effect on signal amplitude and can be the sole cause for amplifier blocking artifact.

Finally, vigilant maintenance of the recording integrity is essential. If adjustments are not made to amplifier settings, and artifacts corrected on an ongoing basis, data can become so confounded with problems that even the best, seasoned technologist may not be able to effectively sort out the issues.

These three processes may be performed independently or simultaneously, based on need and timing of artifact presentation. For the purposes of this chapter, artifact recognition is discussed in individual steps. Over time and with experience, the student-technologist will be able to call on these steps in various configurations and simultaneously, as needed.

The reader should realize that this chapter is not intended to be a comprehensive atlas of artifact identification and correction. That is beyond the scope of this publication. The intent of this chapter is to provide an overview of the most common artifact types and general recommendations for avoiding their occurrence, minimizing them when present, and offering acceptable options for maintaining the recording when unwanted data cannot be avoided. The reader is urged to review and analyze as many real-life and textbook examples of nonartifactual and artifactual recordings as are available. By applying the principles outlined in this chapter to other materials, these necessary skills will be further developed for application during patient testing.

ELECTRODE AND SENSOR APPLICATION

It is virtually impossible to discuss artifacts and recording quality without addressing electrode and sensor application; however, the following is not intended as comprehensive coverage of electrode site selection, preparation, and application.

Application of recording sensors and electrodes is the first step toward ensuring a quality recording with little or no unwanted artifact. The importance of this process cannot be overemphasized; without proper electrode and sensor application, it is not possible to produce a quality recording representative of physiologic data. The electrodes and sensors typically applied include EEG, EOG, electrocardiography (ECG), and EMG electrodes; respiratory inductance plethysmography bands; an airflow pressure sensor; a thermal airflow sensor; a snoring sensor; and an oximeter probe. A body position sensor is also used by many sleep-testing facilities, or the technologist may be responsible for documenting this parameter.

ELECTRODE APPLICATION METHODS

There are several methods used to attach cup electrodes to the scalp and skin; most commonly, collodion or paste is used. There are advantages and disadvantages to the use of each fixative.

Collodion

Although the collodion method offers the advantage of very stable electrode application with fewer recording artifacts, there are numerous disadvantages caused by the chemical properties of this substance. According to its material safety data sheet (MSDS), collodion is both highly flammable and an irritant.[2] At minimum, it is suggested that collodion be stored in a cool, dry area; however, many facilities require that it be stored in a vented, fireproof container, which may be required by local building code. Before planning construction of a new facility, requirements for storing collodion should be investigated.

Inhalation of this product may cause irritation to the upper respiratory tract and mucous membranes. The MSDS also recommends the use of personal protective equipment when using the chemical. Collodion should be applied in a well-ventilated area to reduce inhalation of fumes by both the patient and technologist. Local building code may require that the fumes that are generated during electrode application be expelled from the building and not be combined with the return air within the building's ventilation system. In this scenario, separate ductwork must be installed to divert the collodion fumes from the work area directly to outside air. This decreases the hazard of explosion and reduces the risk of irritation to the mucous membrane and respiratory system from exposure to concentrated fumes.

Conductive Paste

Applying electrodes with a conductive paste is considered advantageous by some testing facilities because it is a nontoxic substance that requires no special storage or air-handling procedures. Unfortunately, paste application does not provide the same electrode stability as adherence with collodion and it increases the likelihood for recording artifacts. To apply cup electrodes with a conductive paste such as Ten20, Elefix, or EC2, a small square of gauze or tape placed over the paste-filled electrode will hold it in place because of the adhesive qualities of paste. Applying electrodes around the face can be accomplished by using small squares of hypoallergenic tape with one end tabbed over for easy removal following testing. An alternate skin-friendly adhesive such as Cover-Roll stretch or Tegaderm may also be used.

ELECTRODE REMOVAL

Historically, at the conclusion of testing, acetone has been used to remove electrodes adhered to the skin with collodion. This process is still widely used, even though acetone is flammable and emits noxious fumes.[3] Like collodion, acetone should be stored in a cool, dry location and local code may require a vented, fireproof cabinet. The solvent should never be used near a source of ignition; care must be taken when working around the patient's eyes, nose, and mouth to avoid exposure of the mucous membranes.

Likewise, the technologist must be acutely aware of the patient being exposed to fumes, particularly when removing ECG, facial, and scalp electrodes. This is of particular concern for patients with a history of respiratory disease who may already be short of breath or may have hypersensitive airways. The proficient technologist will thoroughly communicate this issue with the patient and allow breaks between removing electrodes beneath or near the nose and mouth, as needed. Collodion remover is a more skin-friendly solvent that may be used in place of acetone for electrode removal.

Removal of paste requires no special chemicals, but it is difficult to eliminate all traces of the product following the overnight recording. This can be frustrating for both the technologist and the patient.

GLOVING

Regardless of the electrode application method employed, gloves should be used during all direct patient contact. For the protection of the patient, and the protection of the technologist from long-term exposure to chemicals and possibly blood resulting from skin abrasion, gloves must be worn throughout electrode-site preparation, electrode application, and electrode removal.

If latex gloves are routinely worn, nonlatex options should be made available when working with a patient who has a known latex sensitivity. Nonlatex gloves are fast becoming stock items in most facilities because of the increasing prevalence of latex sensitivities. Multiple layers of nonlatex gloves may need to be applied when working with collodion and acetone as these chemicals tend to break down the material of which they are constructed. Because the same gloves should never be worn between patients because of cross-contamination, it is a good practice to remove gloves any time the technologist leaves the patient's room or set-up area.

Reviewing the MSDS and local policy is always recommended when dealing with any chemical in the sleep testing facility. The MSDS for each chemical used within a given facility should be available for reference at all times in the event of an exposure, and for general reference.

ELECTRODE-SITE PREPARATION

The technologist should routinely assess the patient's skin before applying adhesives. Assessment should focus on sensitivity to adhesives and any skin condition that may be irritated by applying adhesives and tapes. If a patient is sensitive to the products being used, hypoallergenic tape and adhesive electrode options are available. The technologist should consult the policies of the facility to determine when the physician should be contacted in reference to skin sensitivities.

When applying electrodes and sensors, the skin must first be prepared using skin prep lotion or another abrasive material. These items must be used with care to avoid excessive skin abrasion. Some commercially available skin preps are gritty like sand, whereas others contain very small silicone beads.

With experience, the technologist can easily determine how much pressure should be used with a given product. Preparing the electrode site with a skin prep material helps remove oils, skin care products, and dead skin cells that can lead to high impedance values. Low electrical resistance between the electrode and skin results in optimal signal quality. The technologist should only apply skin prep material to the area intended for contact of the electrode to the skin, because skin is conductive. Preparing an area larger than the size of the electrode can lead to signal contamination and a **salt bridge** artifact. Salt bridging occurs when there is excessive conductive material and electrodes in close proximity to one another communicate.

ELECTRODE COMPOSITION

Well-constructed electrodes should be used and composed of a material that does not interact chemically with the electrolytes of the skin. Precious metal electrodes are highly reliable for recording the electrical biopotentials from which the EEG, EOG, EMG, and ECG channels of a PSG are derived. For this reason, it is generally acceptable to use electrodes composed of gold, silver, or silver–silver chloride.

Gold cup electrodes are actually gold-plated silver, which, when scratched or cracked, can become the origin of artifact regardless of patent electrode application.[4] This is true of electrodes made of any material and plated with another. For this reason, the technologist should inspect all recording electrodes and sensors before and after each use. Much artifact can be avoided by replacing worn and broken sensors as needed.

Electrodes composed of various materials are available today, either constructed of one solid material or plated with precious metal. Examples include gold-plated silver, bright silver, silver–silver chloride, and silver-plated tin. Acceptable recording electrodes couple the electrical potential changes at the recording site to the input of the recording device without significant distortion of the patient data.

It is important to note that mixing electrode materials within a derivation should be avoided, as it will result in distortion of the data being recorded. Because of inherent differences in the properties of metals used in electrode construction, a mixture of electrode types within a derivation will result in an electrical potential difference. As an example, mixing a gold-plated electrode and a silver–silver chloride electrode results in an electrical potential difference of 1.28 V.[4]

ELECTRODE IMPEDANCE

It is imperative that the sleep technologist check the electrode impedance value prior to, and often during, acquisition of the PSG if an impedance issue is suspect. Electrode impedance is measured after the electrode has been applied to evaluate contact between the electrode and the skin. For cephalic electrodes, impedance values should be between 1000 and 5000 Ω, and fairly equal.

When electrodes in a given derivation yield dissimilar impedance values, known as being imbalanced, the common-mode rejection feature of a differential amplifier becomes ineffective.[4] It is undesirable to have very low, or very high, impedance.

LOW IMPEDANCE VALUE

An electrode yielding very low impedance values may possibly be making contact with another electrode because of an excess of electrode gel, paste, or skin prep material. This could also be caused by sweat, or another liquid containing electrolyte, forming a conductive bridge between the electrodes. When electrodes have impedance values of less than 1 kΩ, they should be inspected as a potential cause for poor signal quality.

Any conductive material that communicates between two or more electrodes yields a falsely low impedance value. The electrode site may need to be cleaned or the electrodes may need to be reapplied to remedy the situation.

HIGH IMPEDANCE VALUE

When the impedance value is too high, additional conductive material may be needed between the electrode and skin, or elecrodes may need to be cleaned. In some instances, especially when high impedance values are intermittent or abrupt, electrodes must be replaced as the electrode may be making intermittent contact with the skin or the electrode wire may be fractured. This abrupt change in impedance results in electrode popping, which will be discussed later.

Very high or imbalanced electrode impedance values are undesirable because this makes the recording more susceptible to 60-Hz electrical interference or any other artifact introduced equally to both inputs within a recording derivation. As covered in a previous chapter, common mode rejection is only effective when electrode impedance values are fairly equal and relatively low.

Line noise, otherwise known as *60-Hz interference,* is usually minimized before the recorded signal reaches the amplifier output. When impedances are unequal or high, the electrical noise is not subtracted from the recorded signal and makes it to the recorder output as 60-Hz artifact, also known as line-frequency artifact. In countries outside of the United States, line frequency often runs at 50 Hz; therefore, 50-Hz artifact is recorded in those countries.

ELECTRODE IMPEDANCE SUMMARY

Balanced electrodes affected by line-frequency artifact should be inspected for compromised wiring and scratches to the surface coating of the electrode cup. Line-frequency artifact may also be the result of a loose connection anywhere in the patient circuit. Secure connections should be verified starting at the input board and ending at the amplifier or analog-to-digital converter. Derivations using electrodes with long wires and long interelectrode distances may be problematic by nature, as well. As noted previously, ensure low and equal impedances, patency of the electrodes and electrode wires, and secure connections throughout the patient circuit.

SIGNAL PROCESSING

The next step in ensuring a quality recording is proper processing of the input signals. To accomplish this, it is essential for the recording technologist to understand the basics of signal processing. This section covers key items that the technologist should become familiar with as a basic foundation for **artifact isolation**, and to ensure the recording of a high-quality, artifact-free PSG.

DIFFERENTIAL AMPLIFIER

The differential amplifier amplifies the difference between two input signals. Potentials shared between the two signals are minimized, leaving only the difference between them.[5] In other words, the output of a differential amplifier is the electrical difference between its two inputs. In many of today's PSG acquisition devices, the amplifier is housed in the head box (electrode board).

Common Mode Rejection Ratio (CMRR)

Common mode rejection ratio (CMRR) refers to the ability of an amplifier to reject in-phase potentials and amplify out-of-phase potentials. This is a defining feature of a differential amplifier. The CMRR is measured by connecting both channel inputs of the amplifier to the same signal source. Input 1 is the exploring electrode and input 2 is the reference electrode. For example, in the F3-M2 channel of the standard bipolar array, F3 is the exploring electrode and M2 is the reference electrode.

FILTERS

Filters allow manipulation of input signals to attenuate artifacts; however, they should be used only as a final option once all other measures have been exhausted.

The use of filters changes the appearance of both artifactual and physiologic data. In fact, with overuse of input filters, physiologic data can be made to appear nonphysiologic. Likewise, it is possible for artifact and nonphysiologic extraneous signals to be mistaken for physiologic data when filters are overused. In the latter case, these "clean" signals that may look ideal would be entirely meaningless.[5]

Low-Frequency Filter (LFF)

The LFF attenuates frequencies approaching, at, and below the assigned cut-off frequency. For example, if the LFF is set at 1 Hz, all activity approaching, at, or below 1 Hz is attenuated. A 1-Hz input signal is attenuated to exactly 80% of its original amplitude. A slightly faster input frequency is attenuated to greater than 80% and less than 100% of its original amplitude. An input signal with a frequency slower than 1 Hz will be attenuated to less than 80% of its original amplitude. The LFF setting changes the time it takes for the amplitude of an input signal to decay back to baseline. This setting can dramatically change the appearance of data, and is responsible for the difference between how **electrode popping artifact** looks on the EEG and

EOG channel as compared with the same artifact on an EMG channel.

High-Frequency Filter (HFF)

The high-frequency filter (HFF) attenuates frequencies approaching, at, or above the set cut-off frequency. For example, if the HFF is set to 35 Hz, frequencies approaching, reaching, and surpassing 35 Hz are attenuated. The effect of the HFF mirrors that of the LFF.[6]

50/60 Hz Filter

The 50/60 Hz filter is designed to minimize data associated with electrical current interference that has a frequency of 60 Hz in the United States. In many other countries, line current alternates at a frequency of 50 Hz. This filter is designed to "notch out" frequencies surrounding the frequency of line noise and is sometimes referred to as the *notch filter* or *line filter*.

ARTIFACT ISOLATION

Signal artifacts may result from various sources, several of which are covered in this chapter. The first, and possibly most important, step in the process of artifact correction is artifact isolation. Most artifacts can be distinguished from physiologic activity in that they differ radically from previously recorded data, and often seem to be superimposed on normal signals. Although this is often the case, it is not always the case, and some artifacts can actually resemble patient data.

The first step in artifact isolation is to determine if the issue is common in more than one channel. When artifact is suspected, look at the overall image and determine whether the activity in question is arising from a single derivation or multiple derivations using a common electrode. If the latter occurs, the common electrode is clearly problematic. In the event of the former, one of the two inputs is the issue. If one of the two inputs is used in another derivation for which the recording channel is unaffected, the other electrode is the cause.

Changing input derivations also assists in isolating the problematic electrode through the process of elimination. Once the affected input is isolated, the correction process begins by determining whether the source of artifact is mechanical or physiological.

In Figure 10-1, the primary artifact can be isolated by visually scanning the tracing and comparing each channel to identify the common denominator. It is evident that the first three channels are intact and appropriately acquiring data when compared with the exaggerated appearance of the fourth and fifth channels. On channels four and five the common denominator is input 2, the reference electrode

M2. Although the main issue is a popping M2 electrode on the EOG channels, note that there is also pervasive **ECG artifact** contaminating the three EEG channels.

If the impedance check on this electrode initially yielded acceptable results, the issue may be that the electrode has loosened and lost complete contact with the skin, or the electrode wire is fractured and intermittently losing contact. In this example, it is recommended for the technologist to first visually inspect the electrode and ensure it is making contact with the skin. If not, it may be possible to temporarily remedy the issue by adding tape or paste to the electrode application. If the impedance values are high, the technologist should first reapply conductive material. If neither of these actions correct the artifact, it may be necessary to replace the electrode.

A **short circuit** is an electrical circuit with lower resistance, or impedance, than intended. If a short circuit is suspected because of a fractured electrode wire, a continuity test may be performed using a multimeter (Ohmmeter) with the electrode disconnected from the patient and input board. If there is only intermittent or no signal continuity, the electrode is defective. Be aware that it is possible to have an intermittent short during data acquisition, and a continuous circuit while later testing the electrode. It is imperative that the electrode be disconnected from the patient during testing with a multimeter. Otherwise, polarization of the electrode from the direct current used by the meter can result in chemical burns to the patient's skin (refer to Figure 10-1).

LINE FREQUENCY ARTIFACT

Electrical current noise, or **line frequency artifact**, is a common artifact that originates from electrical wiring and equipment. In North America, electricity travels across the power lines and into homes and businesses alternating at 60 cycles per second. In many other countries, it alternates at a frequency of 50 Hz. This interference may be unavoidable if the current is inordinately strong. Sixty-hertz artifact is commonly seen in channels in which the electrode impedance is high or imbalanced, or the electrode is faulty. It is most readily present in bioelectric channels (EEG, ECG, EOG, EMG), but may also occur in transduced channels.[1] Typically, when 60 Hz artifact is present on channels recorded with a transducer, the device is either defective, or there is a break in the circuit or cable shielding.

This type of artifact may appear in only one channel or may be the same in all channels. When 50/60-Hz artifact is in all bioelectric channels, the most likely cause is a defective ground electrode that needs to be regelled, repositioned, or replaced, depending on the

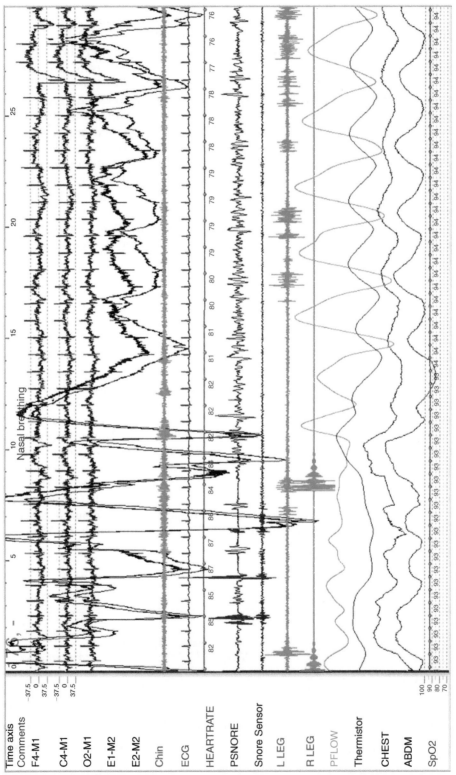

FIGURE 10-1 Artifact origin can often be traced to common signals in multiple affected channels.

issue. The artifact has a very uniform appearance. To identify accurately, the time base can be adjusted to a 1-second window and the peaks counted. This reveals a frequency of 60 cycles per second, with every other cycle having identical morphology and amplitude.

Another way to identify the artifact is to activate the 60-Hz filter. Following deactivation of this filter, the artifact will reappear. Application of the 50/60-Hz filter to recorded data should be the last alternative once all other options to correct the artifact have been exhausted without success because it attenuates data surrounding 60 Hz and may affect signals of interest. Most importantly, epileptiform spikes in the bandwidth affected by the filter are attenuated.

When electrical artifact is seen in one or more specific channels, one should check impedances of the affected electrodes to determine if there is a need to re-gel, reapply, or replace. If excessive artifact of this type is seen, the technologist should check all connections to ensure no input connections are loose, and inspect the lead wire for any cuts or breaks in the casing because these are conducive to excess electrical interference. When all bioelectric channels are affected by 60-Hz artifact, this is usually the result of a defective ground electrode, which may need to be regelled, reattached, or replaced.

If the electrode or electrodes in question yield acceptable impedance measures, this may indicate that the amplifiers are picking up ambient leakage current from nearby electrical sources. Typically, all channels are affected when this is the case. To reduce this problem, the technologist should assess electrical outlets in the area and ensure that no electrical cables are crossing or running parallel to the patient input cable. Excessive leakage current can contaminate the recording when an electrical plug is not properly seated in the outlet, or when the data acquisition system or one of its components is in close proximity to an electrical outlet. Electrical interference is also exacerbated by the use of long electrode wires. All measures should be exhausted to reduce the problem before applying the notch filter.

The American Academy of Sleep Medicine (AASM) recommends that the line filter not be used on an EMG channel because this may mask actual physiologic bursts of muscle activity recorded on these channels.[7] The notch filter significantly attenuates 60-Hz noise derived from electrical sources outside the body. This filter is designed specifically for this frequency, although it attenuates a range of frequencies around 60 Hz. When the filter is used, it will also attenuate, or reduce, any biopotentials in its range. This filter should, therefore, be used as a last resort after all other measures have been exhausted.

In Figure 10-2 high-amplitude, uniform, extraneous signals are recorded on the C4-A1 channel, among others. To confirm that the artifact is 60 Hz as suspected, the line filter is applied. Clearly, the signal is grossly attenuated by use of this notch filter. The same data displayed at a 1-second time base, and with the gain of channel C4-A1 reduced, is seen in Figure 10-3. Note that every other cycle is identical in frequency and morphology and 60 cycles exist on the 1-second example. This is the most effective test of whether high-frequency artifact is the result of line noise.

Not all fast artifacts are caused by 60-Hz line noise, but only 60-Hz data is effectively attenuated using a notch filter. The example in Figure 10-4 contains fast artifact for which a notch filter might work. When these data are viewed at a 1-second time base (Figure 10-5), the frequency and morphology can be easily determined. This example of high-frequency artifact is not the result of 60-Hz line noise. If a notch filter were applied, it would be ineffective.

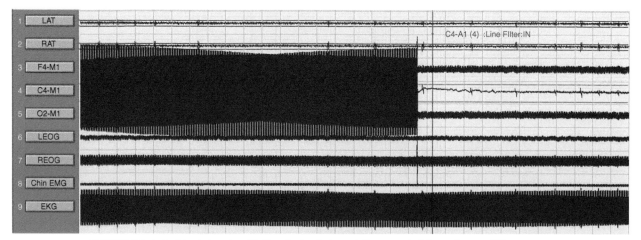

FIGURE 10-2 Ambient signals with the electrode board disconnected from the amplifier system.

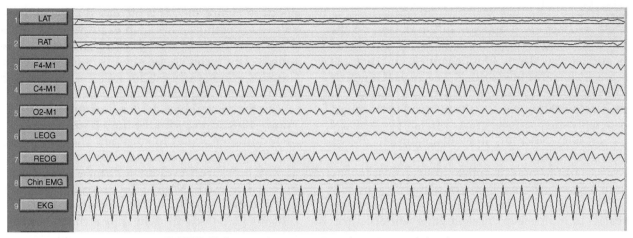

FIGURE 10-3 60-Hz line noise viewed at a 1-second time base.

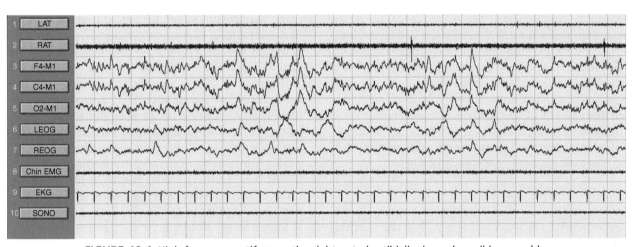

FIGURE 10-4 High-frequency artifact on the right anterior tibialis channel possibly caused by electrical noise.

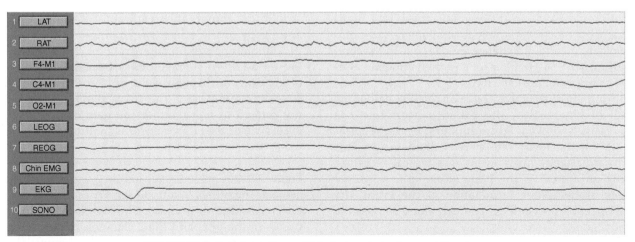

FIGURE 10-5 Data from Figure 10-4 displayed at a 1-second time base.

MUSCLE ARTIFACT

Muscle artifact often appears in the tracing on the EEG, EOG, and occasionally the ECG channels.[1] This artifact also affects EMG channels, but may not necessarily be unwanted artifact. The artifact is generated by localized muscle activity, which has a frequency of 20-200 Hz, close to the electrode placement. The activity may appear very similar to electrical noise artifact; however, it is distinguished by its irregular frequency and morphology.

Muscle artifact may disappear at sleep onset as the patient becomes more relaxed, because it is generally a sign of tension. At the beginning of the recording, especially prior to sleep onset, no intervention is necessary. If the artifact persists into sleep to a point that the EEG patterns are obscured and efforts to correct it fail, the technologist may have to rely on behavioral correlates to identify sleep.

Muscle Artifact Variants

Often, when muscle artifact persists, it is the result of pressure being exerted on the offending electrode. This typically happens when the side of the patient's head is against the pillow or mattress, putting pressure on either the reference or exploring electrode. When the source of the artifact is identifiable, then the derivation may be changed to a back-up configuration. When there is excessive muscle artifact, the recording may become completely obscured.

Respiratory Event

After termination of the respiratory event on the 30-second epoch, as seen in Figure 10-6, the scoring channels are obscured by high-frequency muscle artifact. Lower amplitude artifact, embedded on wanted physiologic signals, persists throughout the example. Note the random nature of muscle artifact in contrast to the rhythmic frequency and consistent amplitude of 60-Hz artifact seen in Figure 10-2. It is sometimes difficult to differentiate these two high-frequency artifacts, especially for the novice technologist. When uncertain, a change in time base to 1 second or turning the 60-Hz filter on and then off again confirms or negates the suspicion.

During the obstructive apnea on the first half of the epoch in Figure 10-6, the patient's heart rate has progressively slowed. At termination of the respiratory event, the heart rate speeds dramatically. This bradycardia-tachycardia event is a typical response during an apnea, as the body attempts to conserve oxygen stores. After termination of the event, the heart speeds up to deliver as much blood as possible to reoxygenate tissue cells.

Leg Cramps

Note the long bursts of muscle activity on the left anterior tibialis (*L LEG*) EMG channel of the 120-second epoch in Figure 10-7. This increased activity is the result of leg cramps. This is an example of physiologic EMG activity for which no corrective action is warranted. The technologist should note the time and duration of muscle bursts for later review by the physician and scoring technologist.

Another example of leg cramps is seen in Figure 10-8. Along with the limb EMG activity, there are additional issues to consider. The airflow signal (CFLOW) was recorded directly from the positive airway pressure (PAP) device while 8 cm H_2O was being delivered. Notice the unusual, multiphase morphology of the CFLOW signal, indicating significant variations in delivered airflow. Because of rainout in the breathing circuit, condensation accumulated in the tubing through which air was "bubbling" with each breath. This can be disruptive to the patient's sleep, particularly if the water travels far enough to reach the nasal or oral interface. In the same way PAP is measured by the amount of water it can displace, the valve created by the column of water in the circuit causes fluctuations in the pressure being delivered to the patient.

There are many benefits to the use of heated humidification along with PAP. The general rule of thumb is to increase the temperature setting as high as possible without significant rainout in the tubing. Once rainout is observed, reduce the heater to the next lower setting. When condensation accumulates in the tubing, as in this example, the technologist must drain it to ensure the patient is not awakened by a nose full of water.

Abdominal Effort

The abdominal effort channel presents another consideration. The series of epochs was sleep-stage scored as N1 sleep, so breathing should be stable. A vigilant technologist will adjust the gain or sensitivity on the abdominal effort channel to obtain consistent amplitude among the respiratory parameters. The amplitude of the other two channels is appropriate: prominent enough for interpretation without intruding on adjacent signals. Likely because of the noise of air flowing through water in the PAP circuit, the baseline amplitude of the snore signal is elevated. If not related to noise, either the gain or sensitivity is excessive, or the snore sensor is malfunctioning.

Bruxism

Figure 10-9 represents yet another variant of muscle artifact. The bursts of muscle activity on this 30-second epoch are due to bruxism. The simultaneous muscle bursts in the EEG and EOG channels are an example of when artifacts can be potentially beneficial. Although the bursts are pronounced on the chin EMG channel in this example, if they were less dramatic, the artifact might support event identification and scoring.

(Text continued on page 215)

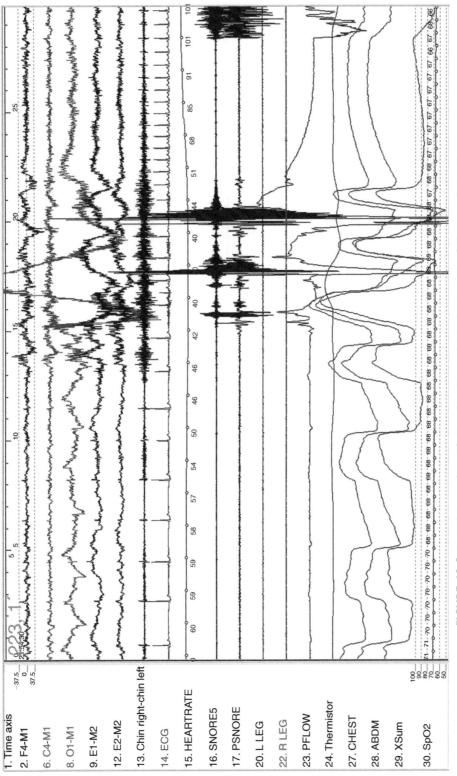

FIGURE 10-6 Excessive muscle artifact and oxyhemoglobin desaturation follow an obstructive apnea and electroencephalogram arousal.

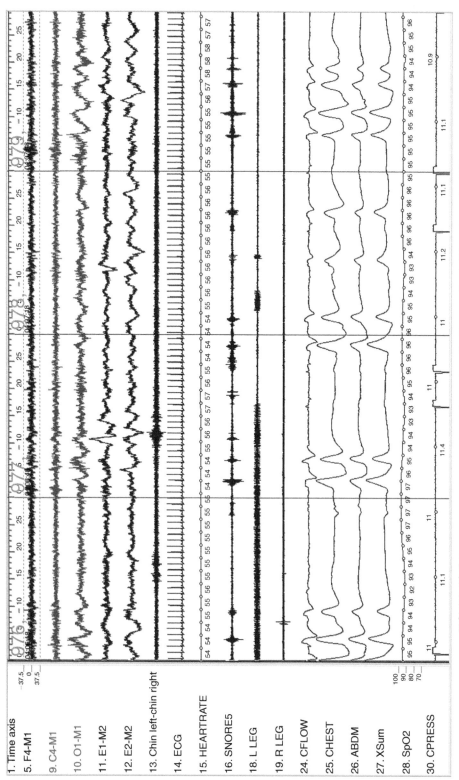

FIGURE 10-7 Leg cramp seen as prolonged muscle activation on the left-leg channel of this 120-second epoch.

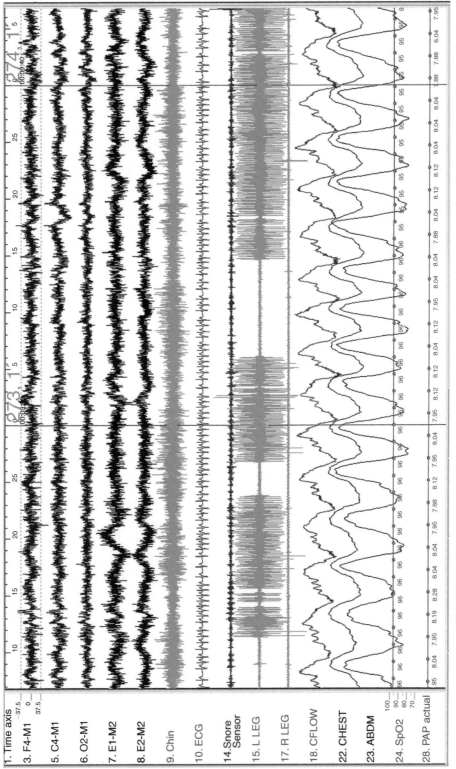

FIGURE 10-8 The patient is having leg cramps, and there is an unusual airflow signal on the 60-second epoch.

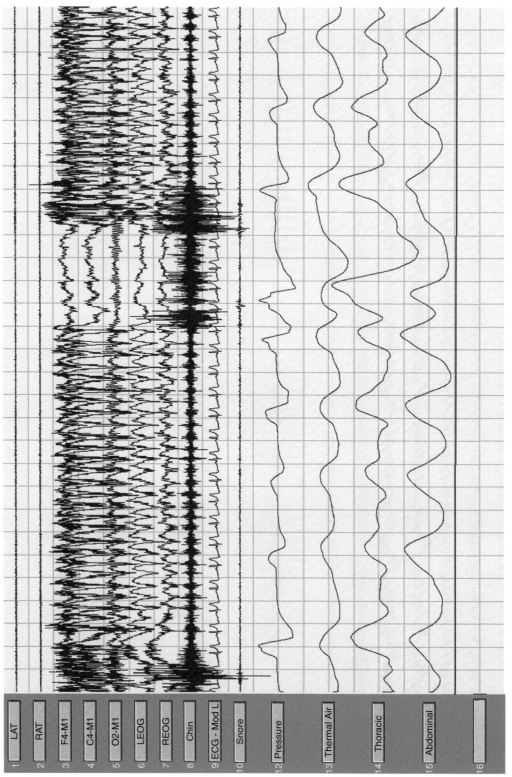

FIGURE 10-9 The bursts of electromyographic activity on the 30-second epoch represent bruxism.

EEG Arousal

In Figure 10-10, an EEG arousal begins at approximately second 7 of the 30-second epoch. Arousal scoring rules require an abrupt shift in EEG frequency lasting at least 3 seconds. The high-frequency activity superimposed on all EEG channels during and following the arousal is muscle artifact. When data are obscured by artifact for greater than 15 seconds, a major body movement is scored rather than an arousal.

If any alpha is present on the major body movement epoch, it is assigned a score of stage wake. If there is no alpha on the epoch, the previous epoch is considered. If it was staged as wake, the current epoch is assigned a stage of wake. If neither of these conditions are met, the epoch is assigned the stage of the epoch that follows.

Note that the EOG channels do not contain high-frequency muscle artifact, although the signals on these channels do appear erratic. This is an example of overuse of the HFF, likely at a setting of 15 Hz. Excessive filtering produces a "clean," artifact-free recording, but the data obtained are often meaningless.

Body Rocking

Another form of muscle artifact, body rocking, is more specifically a type of rhythmic movement disorder. In Figure 10-11, the rocking motion obscures the EEG and EOG channels of the 30-second epoch and is also responsible for distortion of the snore and respiratory channels, and increased activity of the limb EMG.

ELECTROCARDIOGRAPHIC ARTIFACT

ECG artifact is common and can be seen in all other channels recording biopotentials (EEG, EOG, and EMG). Strong ECG voltages may be detected from almost any location on the body.[1] Its amplitude may be increased because of impedance imbalance between the exploring (input 1) and reference (input 2) electrodes. This should always be considered because reapplying conductive material to the electrode with the higher impedance value may reduce the imbalance.

In some cases, particularly with patients who are obese, some amount of ECG artifact will be present in spite of low and balanced impedances. The reason for this is that adipose tissue is a much better conductor of electrical activity than muscle. To reduce the probability of ECG artifact contaminating the recording, care should be taken to avoid placing reference electrodes M1 and M2 on soft, fatty tissue. Mastoid electrodes should be placed on top of the bony protrusion, as far away from soft, fatty tissue as possible. Even then, ECG artifact may be unavoidable. In practice, when this placement is routinely used, less ECG artifact is recorded.

If ECG artifact remains, the technologist may link or "double reference" the two reference electrodes. This can be accomplished either with jumpers or by using a derivation that allows the M1 to be linked electronically with M2 (M1 + M2). This method, called "double referencing" and "linking the mastoids," was accomplished via the electrode selector panel on traditional analog systems. Although an acceptable means of minimizing ECG artifact, it should only be used after attempting to prevent and minimize the artifact through proper electrode placement and low, balanced impedance measures. When the mastoids are linked, signals of common phase and voltage are minimized or eliminated from the recording channel; thus, data are distorted. Many of today's digital recording systems have provisions allowing double referencing, which may be as simple as the click of a mouse.

ECG Artifact Variants

To determine whether artifact suspected to be the result of the electrical activity from the heart is ECG artifact, place a straight edge perpendicular to the bottom of the screen aligned with the spikelike R waves on the ECG channel.

In Figure 10-12, for example, when this is done, it is evident that the spikes embedded on the top channels of the epoch are aligned with those of the ECG. Because the left and right anterior tibialis electrodes are linked to record movements from both legs on one channel of this recording, the interelectrode distance is excessively long. A long interelectrode distance invariably results in recording excessive ECG artifact. The other four channel derivations use either M1 or M2 as the reference electrode. The mastoid electrodes, particularly when placed over tissue surrounding the mastoid process, are notorious for introducing ECG artifact into the recording channel. Also note the consistent amplitude and frequency of the chin EMG recording. This occurs because 60-Hz artifact is embedded over the actual chin EMG recording. Occasionally, higher amplitude EMG spikes appear from behind the solid block of line-noise artifact, but the EMG data is obscured by the artifact most of the time. Muscle activity is never this consistent in amplitude and frequency.

SLOW-FREQUENCY ARTIFACTS

Slow-frequency artifacts seen in the EEG or EOG channels are usually the result of either perspiration or body movements associated with breathing. They are not present on EMG or ECG channels because of the standard LFF setting used. These artifacts are often very high amplitude, may be 1-2 Hz or slower in frequency and, to the inexperienced technologist, may have the appearance on the EEG of stage N3 sleep.

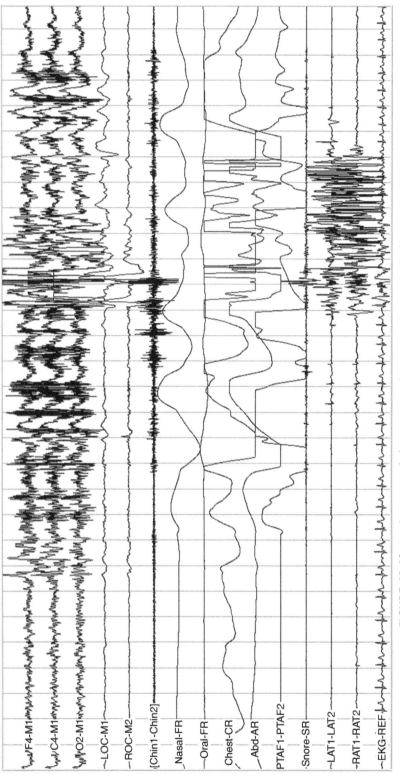

FIGURE 10-10 An electroencephalogram arousal progresses to a major body movement event.

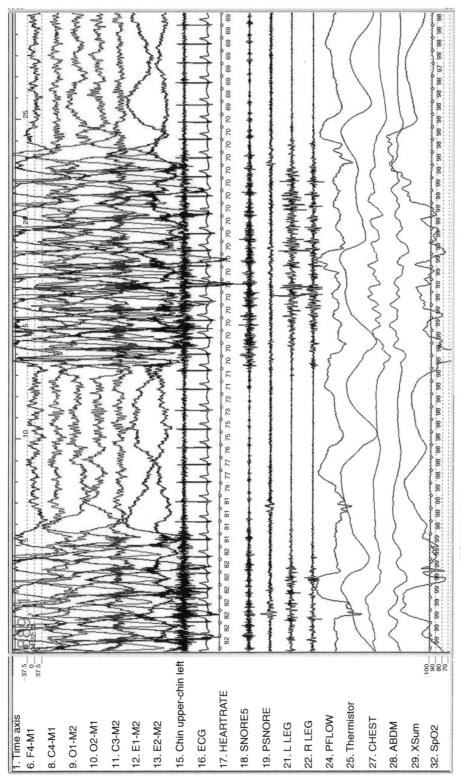

FIGURE 10-11 Body rocking, a type of rhythmic movement artifact.

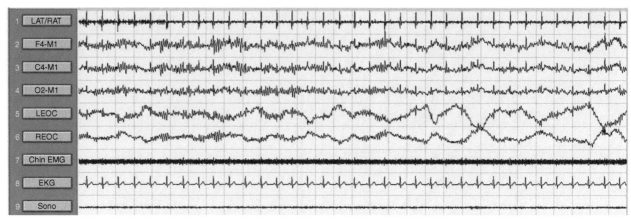

FIGURE 10-12 Electrocardiogram artifact in the top six channels of this 30-second tracing

Sweat Artifact

It is very important for a technologist to distinguish **sweat artifact** and other slow-frequency artifacts from normal physiologic EEG. Perspiration can loosen electrodes and dilute the conductive media (gel or paste) between the electrode and the skin. Loosening of the electrodes can result in artifact as the electrodes move on the skin. In addition, the dilution of conductive media by sweat can result in chemical instability of the electrode-skin interface.

When sweat artifact occurs (see Figure 10-18), electrodes may need to be reaffixed or regelled, and the patient's skin must be cooled. This can be accomplished by removing bed covers or reducing the temperature in the room. Keep in mind that cooling the skin may take several minutes. Because of the severe nature of sweat artifact, it is a good practice to maintain a relatively cool testing environment.

Respiratory Artifact

Respiratory artifact is also a slow-frequency artifact, typically recorded from electrodes around the scalp and face; it is distinguishable by its synchronous occurrence with the patient's breathing rate and rhythm. Respiratory artifact may be the result of the bed moving along with patient breathing, an unstable input board moving in synch with breathing, or electrode wires next to the patient moving with each breath. Often, a patient is lying on the affected electrode, which is moving up and down on the pillow along with breathing. The underlying cause may also be attributed to, or exacerbated by, chemical and/or mechanical instability of the electrode.

In some cases, especially when caused by movement of electrode or sensor wires, respiratory artifact may resolve with patient repositioning. Repositioning of one or more of these items or fixing the problematic electrode should resolve the issue. If the artifact persists, the technologist may choose to reference the electrodes to the opposite side of the head away from the side resting on the pillow.

Replacing electrodes may also be effective in eliminating this artifact if mechanical instability exists. Sometimes respiratory and sweat artifact cannot be differentiated. In fact, the two often coexist and the distinction between them is only helpful for identification and correction of the cause of the artifact.

Typically, slow-wave artifact is a combination of both respiratory-generated movement and sweat-related loosening of electrodes. The input board and extra lengths of electrode wiring should always be placed on a stable surface and the testing room kept cool to minimize the problem of slow-wave artifact. Slow-frequency artifact related to respiratory movement appears on the last half of the 60-second epoch, as seen in Figure 10-13. Each wave of the wandering baseline on the O2-M1 channel appears to line up with breathing. During the first 30 seconds of the recording, prominent ECG artifact is present in all EEG and EOG recordings. After termination of the respiratory event, muscle artifact obscures the EEG and EOG data, with the exception of the O1-M2 channel on which the prominent slow-wave artifact exists. This is suspect that the offending electrode became loosened, suggesting that the problem is, in fact, both respiratory and sweat-related in origin.

Slow-frequency artifact apparently caused by respiratory movement is seen in all three EEG channels in Figure 10-14. Because it affects the EEG channels and not the EOG channels, the artifact must arise from an electrode common to all EEG channels. When assessed against the breathing channels, it is clear that there is a 1:1 relationship between the artifact waves and breath cycles. For this reason, the slow-wave artifact is subclassified as respiratory artifact. Because the EOG derivations use M2 as a reference and the EEG channels use M1, the artifact clearly arises from M1. Respiratory artifact may be the result of the M1 electrode wire swaying back and forth in synch with breathing.

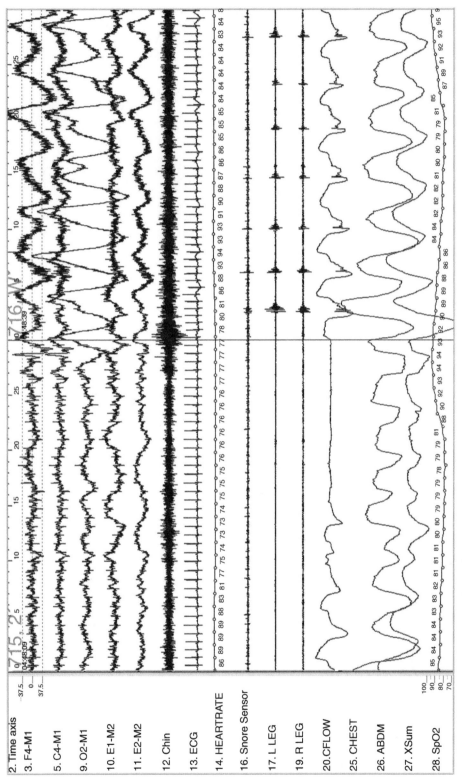

FIGURE 10-13 Slow-wave artifact related to respiratory movement appears after termination of the obstructive apnea on this 60-second epoch.

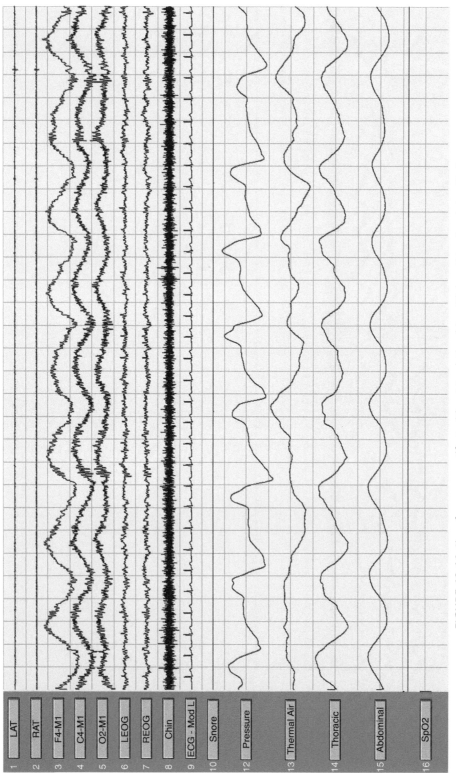

FIGURE 10-14 Slow-frequency artifact with a 1:1 relationship with breathing is subclassified as respiratory artifact.

Pulse Artifact

Pulse artifact is another type of slow-frequency artifact that may be recorded in one or more EEG or EOG channels. This phenomenon occurs when an electrode is placed over a pulsating blood vessel. As with ECG artifact, the rhythmic activity will line up with the R wave of the QRS, but it produces a sinusoidal slow wave rather than a spike. The existence of pulse artifact is confirmed by matching the R wave of the ECG with the slow wave on the EEG (Figure 10-15). If possible, a back-up derivation can be used in place of the affected signal until the opportunity arises to fix the issue. The problematic electrode must be relocated as soon as practical to remedy the issue of pulse artifact. The technologist should note that the electrode was repositioned and whether the opposite correlate was adjusted for symmetrical effect.

Following AASM guidelines, only one hemisphere of the EEG is needed, so the technologist may choose to hide this channel if the artifact is too severe and obscures the underlying EEG activity while displaying the back-up configuration. In the event that only three channels are displayed, the technologist may select the opposing derivation.

Cardioballistic Artifact

Cardioballistic artifact is also a slow-wave artifact generated by cardiogenic oscillations, resulting in movement from intrathoracic pressure changes caused by the contraction and relaxation of the heart within the thorax. It is also referred to as *ballistocardiographic artifact* (refer to Figure 10-16). This is not an electrical artifact, but it will line up with the QRS waveform on the ECG channel similarly to pulse artifact. This type of artifact is typically recorded on pressure and respiratory effort channels during a sleep-disordered breathing event of central origin. It is most often seen during prolonged central apneas and can be misinterpreted as

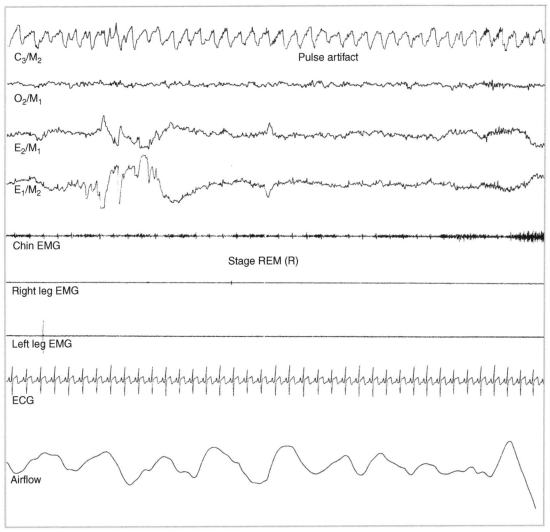

FIGURE 10-15 The slow-frequency artifact on the top electroencephalogram channel aligned with the electrocardiogram QRS is pulse artifact. *From Butkov N:* Atlas of clinical polysomnography, *ed 2, Medford, Ore, 2010, Synapse Media. Reprinted with permission.*

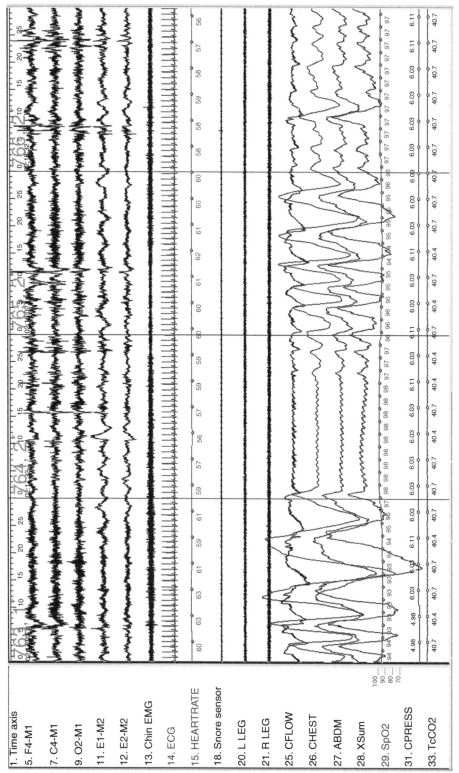

FIGURE 10-16 Cardioballistic artifact on the respiratory channels of this 120-second epoch.

rapid breathing effort. The technologist should recognize this artifact as normal and document its presence. There is no need to attempt to eliminate it.

An example of cardioballistic artifact during a PAP-induced central event can be seen in Figure 10-17. The artifact on the thoracic channel is present throughout this central apnea during REM sleep, and is even embedded on the channel during the hypopnea that precedes the apnea. PAP was being titrated for obstructive apnea. When a pressure of 11 cm H_2O was reached, PAP-induced central apneas and hypopneas emerged. The pressure was reduced to 10 cm H_2O and the central events dissipated.

Channel-Blocking Artifact

Slow-frequency baseline sway artifacts often affect EEG, ECG, and EOG channels when recording a diaphoretic patient. This artifact is differentiated from respiratory artifact by comparing the artifact with breathing signals and noting the misalignment. It is often difficult to determine whether the issue is respiratory or sweat-related in nature, however, and it is sometimes the result of both.

Sweat artifact results when electrodes are physically loosened from the skin because of sweat combining with the fixative material. A salt bridge may also occur when sweat, or any other conductive material, communicates between two electrodes. If a patient is severely diaphoretic, electrodes may become completely dislodged and cause electrode popping that is severe enough to cause amplifier-blocking artifact.

Amplifier blocking, also known as **channel-blocking artifact,** occurs when the amplitude of the recorded signal is higher than can be recorded within the physical limitations of the channel. When this happens, signals intrude on adjacent channels and distort the data, or are clipped because of the recorded voltage potential exceeding the range of the channel's display capability. This is most often the result of a faulty lead wire, popping electrode, or an excessive gain or sensitivity setting.

Depending on the software and available settings, channel-blocking artifact may appear with the positive and negative extremes of the signal being "chopped off," causing a flat appearance, or the signal may intrude on adjacent channels. When caused by profuse sweating, the technologist should attempt to cool the patient and reaffix electrodes. When this does not resolve the issue and no back-up options exist, the affected electrode or electrodes must be replaced to maintain the integrity of the recording. Good documentation to support actions is always necessary to properly communicate with the scoring technologist and interpreting practitioner.

As an absolute last resort, the LFF may be adjusted to 1 Hz on an EEG channel affected by sweat artifact, keeping in mind that this will attenuate delta frequencies and may cause misinterpretation of sleep staging data.[1] Many physicians and laboratory managers require that the recording technologist never raise the LFF setting to 1 Hz on EEG channels, as this can be done in a digital world after the fact and without compromising the raw data. This change should only be used as a temporary measure when it is counterproductive to awaken the patient. The problem should be resolved and the filter reset at the first patient awakening.

The channel-blocking artifact on the respiratory signals of Figure 10-18 is due to a signal with excessive amplitude, but that is otherwise intact. To correct this, the technologist only needs to reduce the amplifier gain or sensitivity setting. Respiratory variables should be adjusted during stable breathing throughout the recording to ensure that each variable has adequate amplitude for interpretation, but does not block or intrude on other channels.

The channel-blocking artifact seen in Figure 10-19 can be traced to the C4 electrode because other channels sharing the M1 reference are unaffected. A back-up central derivation may be employed temporarily, but the C4 electrode must be repaired or replaced as soon as practical to ensure a back-up option remains available throughout testing. Figure 10-20 provides an example of channel-blocking artifact for which the signals do not appear "blocked" or "clipped." This is due to a software selection available on many PSG platforms. Whether the clipping feature is selected is simply a facility or personal preference. Because the F4-M1 channel is obscured by artifact, the problem must be corrected.

Of interest, the patient from Figure 10-20 has phrenic nerve dysfunction, which is responsible for the odd breathing pattern. A technologist unaware of this patient's medical history would most assuredly believe the respiratory signals were artifactual. The medical record, or other test-related information that is available to the technologist, should always be reviewed prior to patient arrival in preparation for testing.

ELECTRODE POPPING ARTIFACT

Electrode popping artifact is the result of an abrupt shift in electrode impedance. This may be due to mechanical instability of the electrode, an intermittent short in the electrode wire, or an intermittently disconnected circuit. Depending on the cause, reaffixing the electrode, securing the circuit connection, or replacing the electrode entirely may be warranted to repair the issue.

When a popping electrode generates extremely high amplitude, the signal meets the physical upper and lower limitations of the recording channel. This is known as *channel-blocking* or *signal-blocking artifact*. In the days of paper and ink writer units, this was referred to as *pen-blocking artifact*. Any high-amplitude signal can cause it and, depending on the digital acquisition system and its settings, the signal will either "block" or intrude on adjacent channels, as seen in Figure 10-21.

(Text continued on page 229)

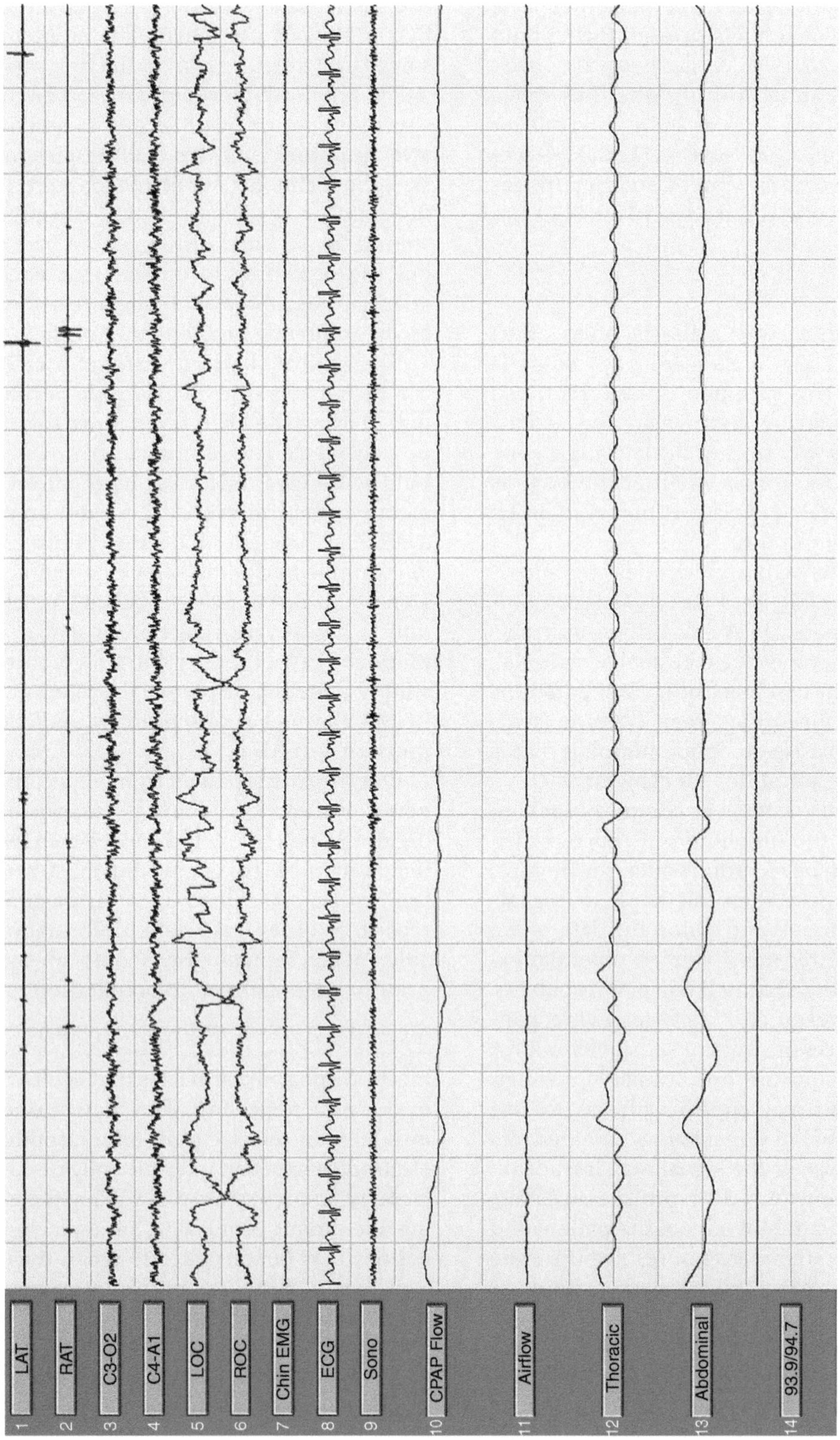
1 LAT
2 RAT
3 C3-O2
4 C4-A1
5 LOC
6 ROC
7 Chin EMG
8 ECG
9 Sono
10 CPAP Flow
11 Airflow
12 Thoracic
13 Abdominal
14 93.9/94.7

FIGURE 10-17 Another example of cardioballistic artifact on the thoracic channel throughout this central apnea during rapid eye movement sleep.

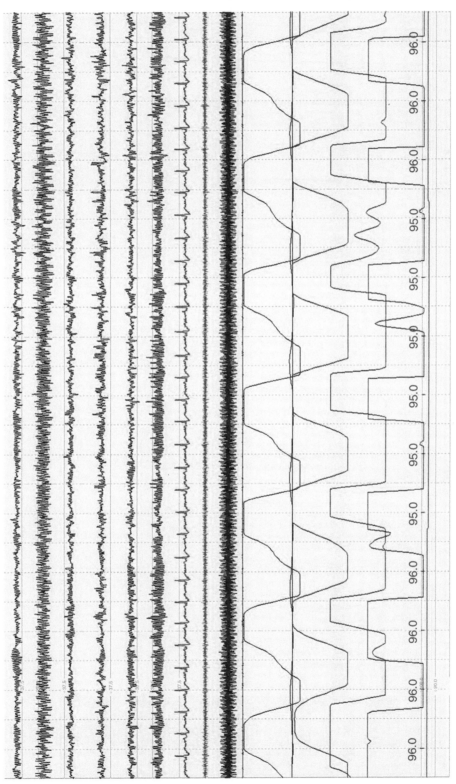

FIGURE 10-18 Prior to physiologic calibrations, this record is rich with artifacts, including channel blocking on the respiratory channels.

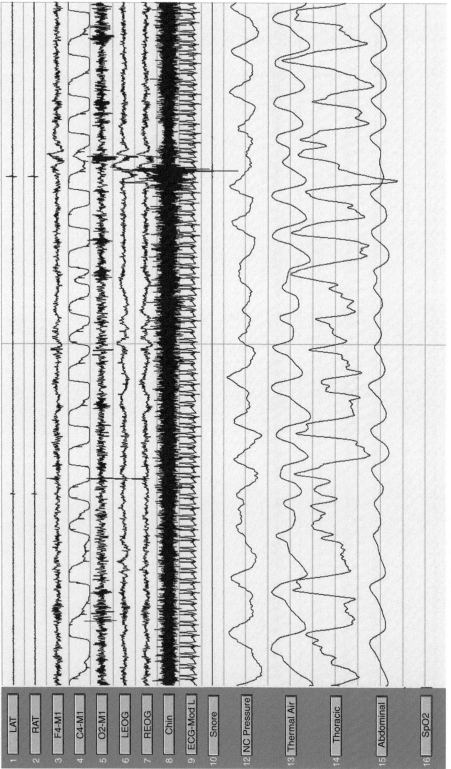

FIGURE 10-19 Channel-blocking artifact on the central electroencephalogram channel.

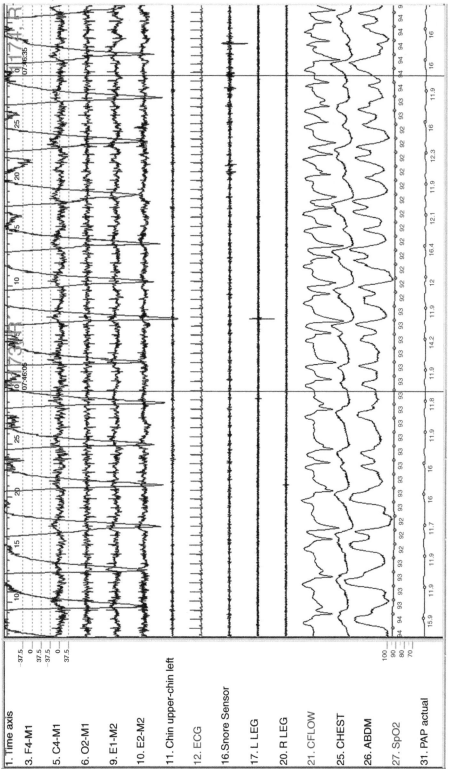

FIGURE 10-20 Slow-frequency artifact results in a signal intruding on other channels.

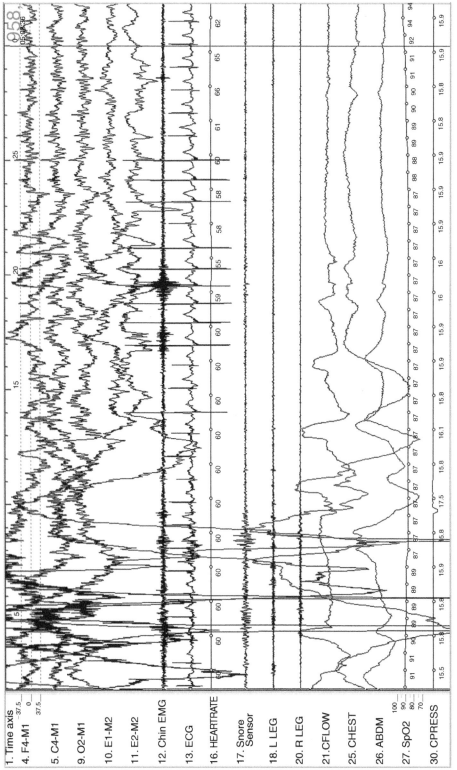

FIGURE 10-21 An extreme example of electrode popping on this 30-second epoch.

Differences in the morphology of electrode popping may be noted when recorded on various channel types. This is the result of the LFF setting, which alters the duration of the artifact. The decay time constant determines how quickly or slowly a signal decays. A longer time constant means a slower return to baseline, whereas a shorter time constant means a faster decay. A lower LFF setting in hertz results in a longer decay time constant in seconds; a higher LFF results in a slower time constant.

An extreme example of electrode "popping" can be seen in the EOG channels using the M2 reference on the 30-second epoch illustrated in Figure 10-21. By the process of elimination, it is evident that the faulty electrode is M2. Because this montage contains a back-up occipital EEG channel, it may be acceptable to turn this redundant channel

off until an opportunity arises to fix the offending electrode.

Electrode popping artifact on the right anterior tibialis channel can be seen on this 30-second epoch in Figure 10-22. With the relatively high LFF setting of 10 Hz, the decay time constant is short. This explains the speed with which the artifact returns to baseline.

Consider Figure 10-23 in which the popping artifact on an EEG channel is wider. This is the result of an LFF setting of 0.3 Hz and the relatively slow decay time constant that results. This example of electrode popping is on the F3-M2 channel. Clearly the F3 electrode is problematic because other channels with derivations using M2 remain unaffected. Either a back-up frontal derivation must be used, or the F3 electrode must be reattached or replaced. If F4 is used

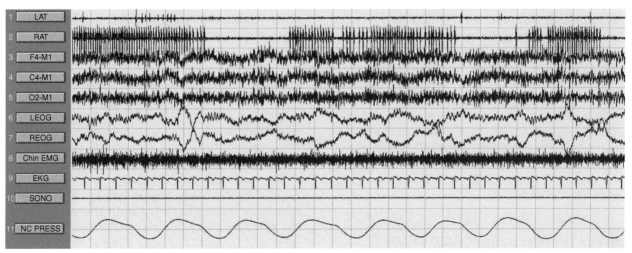

FIGURE 10-22 Electrode popping artifact with a fast return to baseline on this 30-second epoch.

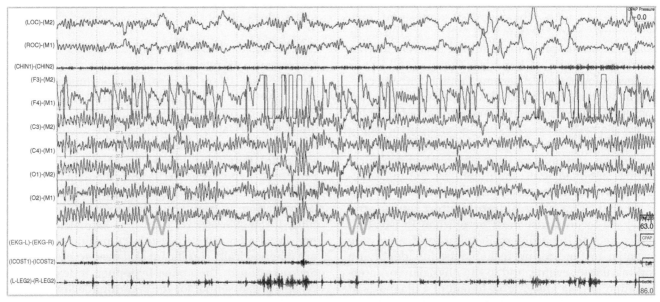

FIGURE 10-23 Electrode popping artifact with a relatively slow return to baseline on this 30-second epoch.

as a back-up, the issue with F3 must be resolved at the first practical opportunity to in order maintain a back-up option throughout recording.

AIRFLOW SIGNAL ARTIFACTS

Airflow signal artifact may occur when the signal from a thermistor or themocouple degrades because of patient movement, the sensor being dislodged from the direct path of airflow, oral breathing, or when the sensor comes in contact with the skin. Anything that reduces the relative change in temperature between inspired and exhaled air at the thermal sensor degrades the quality of its signal.

The degraded signal seen in Figure 10-24 is potentially the result of a mechanical issue, or the need to adjust amplifier gain or sensitivity. The technologist noted that the thermal sensor was displaced and the patient's skin was touched prior to fixing the issue on subsequent epochs. In this example, adjusting the signal amplitude would have only increased the size of the artifactual signal. Amplifier controls are only beneficial when the underlying signals are intact.

A nasal pressure transducer signal may be lost or diminished because of patient movement, cannula displacement, or the cannula becoming completely or partially occluded with moisture or organic material. When these signals are lost or distorted, the technologist must make every effort to correct the malfunction, as they are imperative for respiratory event scoring and subsequent patient qualification for the treatment of sleep-disordered breathing

RESPIRATORY EFFORT SENSOR ARTIFACT

Artifact on the thoracic and abdominal effort channels may be due to one or more issues. The sensor may be faulty, but more often this is the result of the band being displaced, over-tightened, or under-tightened. As with other signals, connections may become unplugged or damaged. When an external or in-line power supply is required, the problem may be the result of depleted batteries. These are all issues the technologist should become familiar with. As consistent with all other technical aspects of polysomnography, the technologist's most valuable tool is his or her knowledge of the type of equipment being used, how it operates, and how it interfaces with the acquisition system. The user's manual or technical manual supplied with equipment by the manufacturer is a great place to find this information.

When dealing with **respiratory effort sensor artifacts**, the technologist must be efficient in isolating and correcting the problem. Respiratory channels are essential to the scoring technologist for identifying and tabulating events, and to the physician for interpretation of data and establishment of a diagnosis of sleep-disordered breathing. A high-quality study has minimal loss of respiratory channel, among other data. The most important variables in troubleshooting loss of these data are technologist vigilance and knowledge of the equipment. The technologist should always be aware whether the sensors have separate battery packs, additional adaptors, filters, or even a separate or specialized amplifier. Proper knowledge of the equipment allows the technologist to quickly and accurately assess artifact and develop a plan of action for correction.

Figure 10-25 illustrates contamination of the abdominal effort channel by high-frequency artifact. The normal adult breathing rate is typically reported as 12-20 breaths per minute. Here, the rate is approximately 16 breaths per minute. On this 30-second epoch, the high-frequency artifact is well above the expected frequency range for normal adult breathing of 0.2-0.33 Hz. The artifact is possibly the result of a malfunctioning sensor, but is much more likely caused by an over-tightened or under-tightened respiratory belt, or a belt that has slipped out of place. Note, however, that the respiratory signals are in phase with one another and they have fairly consistent amplitude, which is high enough for clear assessment of the data. Although impractical to always maintain consistent amplitude and phase during patient movement and periods of transition, a vigilant technologist closely monitors these parameters and makes changes for consistency during periods of stable breathing.

The artifact on the chest effort channel in Figure 10-26 likely represents a malfunctioning sensor or intermittent break in the sensor cable. If the problem persists, the device should be removed from service until it can be further assessed for adequate function. Also, consider the amplitude of the snore sensor recording. The gain or sensitivity should be adjusted to reduce the amplitude so the signal does not obscure other recording channels.

OXIMETRY ARTIFACTS

Oximetry artifacts must be quickly identified and corrected to ensure all respiratory events are scored and quantified according to standards. In fact, faulty oximetry recordings may significantly alter sleep study interpretation.[8] According to the recommended rules of *The AASM Manual for the Scoring of Sleep and Associated Events* for scoring adult sleep-disordered breathing, hypopneas can be scored only if there is an associated EEG arousal or a $\geq$ 3% oxyhemoglobin desaturation as compared with the pre-event baseline.[7] If the oximeter is faulty, or if oximetric data are missing, it may not be possible to include events that are diagnostically significant and need to be validated for inclusion in the apnea-hypopnea index. For this reason, it is essential for the recording technologist to quickly correct any malfunctions or excessive artifacts on the oximetry channel.

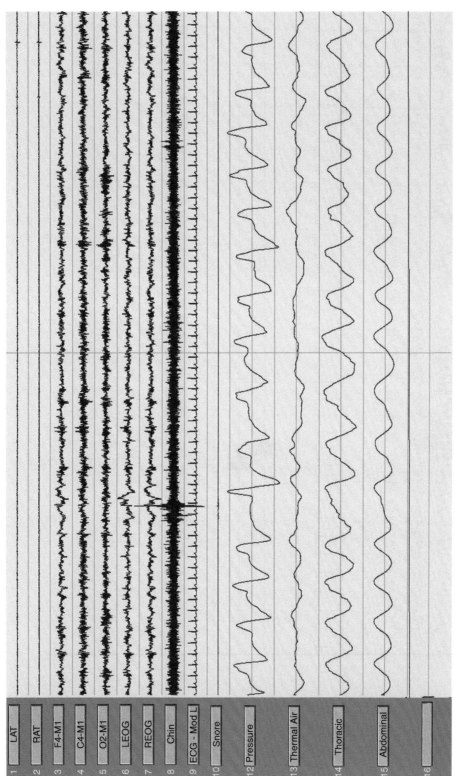

FIGURE 10-24 An example of a degraded thermistor signal on a 60-second epoch.

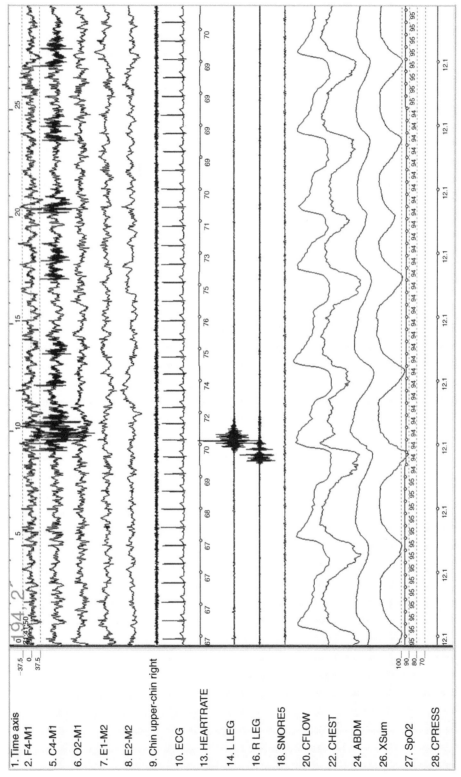

FIGURE 10-25 Abdominal effort channel artifact on the 30-second epoch.

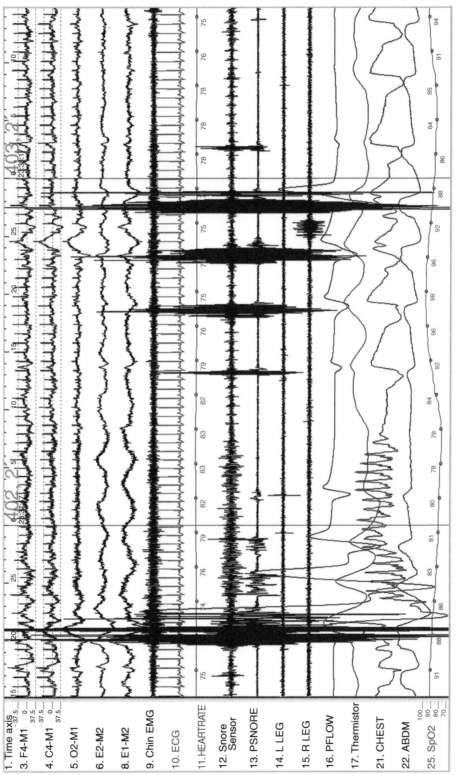

FIGURE 10-26 Artifact on the chest effort channel following an EEG arousal on this 60-second epoch.

Inaccurate data may be collected from the oximeter if the probe is not attached properly, or has become dislodged from either the equipment or the patient. Poor perfusion, severe hypoxemia, nail polish or nail coverings, and movement may also lead to the acquisition of artifactual data on the recording. Because the heart rate channel, when recorded, is derived from the oximeter, these data will be simultaneously lost, or erroneously recorded, along with faulty oxyhemoglobin saturation values.

The oxyhemoglobin saturation and heart rate data are abruptly lost for almost 5 seconds on the 30-second example in Figure 10-27. A complete loss of signal is most likely the result of a loose sensor or oximeter input cable; poor connection between the oximeter and acquisition system; or patient movement. Because other parameters are unaffected on this epoch, patient movement is unlikely. With the loss of data being only temporary, no corrective action is necessary, as long as the issue does not return. The technologist should, however, document that he or she recognized the issue, and describe any occurrence that might explain the signal loss.

SYSTEM REFERENCE ARTIFACT

Currently, most digital acquisition systems used in polysomnography and electroencephalography are referential recorders. A referential recorder stores the data of every electrode plugged into the electrode board as the exploring electrode of a derivation with a common reference electrode routed to each input 2. The common reference electrode is applied to a site such as Cz or Fz, considered electrically neutral because it is midline and toward the top of the head. When a back-up option exists, the two system reference electrodes are typically placed at Cz and Fz, as well.

The referential recorder allows recording of an almost unlimited number of channels, but, more importantly, for polysomnography it makes it possible to manipulate derivations and montages after the fact. Because each electrode is recorded in its own derivation linked to a common, or system, reference, any two stored derivations can be selected to display a channel in real time, or after the fact, because the common reference electrode will be subtracted out of the data.

In practical terms, consider that the recording technologist maintains the AASM-recommended channels throughout the night. During physician review the following day, it is noted that the M1 electrode became dislodged in room 1, resulting in a 20-minute loss of all EEG channel data while the technologist was assisting the patient in room 2. Data from all electrodes was being acquired, even data not being displayed during recording, so the physician selects C3-ref for input 1 and M2-ref for input 2 of a channel derivation. With (C3-ref) – (M2-ref), the reference electrode data cancel out, and, therefore, a derivation of C3-M2 remains to be displayed as the central EEG. The same is done for other EEG derivations.

For clinical EEG, derivation and montage options are endless. A traditional bipolar recorder provided quality data, but was limited to the number of physical channels it possessed. These recorders are sometimes referred to as *what you see is what you get (WYSIWYG) technology.* Whatever was recorded was permanent. There was no way to go back and retrieve lost data, correct technologist errors, or apply a filter or sensitivity change.

Referential recorders are not without limitations and still require that a technologist make ongoing adjustments to yield a quality recording. Because they are not very good at recording certain types of data, most systems still have bipolar channels dedicated for sensor input. Referential channels are reserved for recording data obtained from electrodes. For this reason, bioelectric data are typically obtained using a recorder's referential capability. Because the entire system relies on one or two reference electrodes, patency is critical. If the system reference electrode becomes dislodged or is contaminated by significant artifact, all bioelectric channels will be affected by **system reference artifact.** The example in Figure 10-28 shows signal distortion in all bioelectric channels caused by a faulty system electrode connection. When system referencing is used, the system reference electrode requires special attention because all bioelectric inputs are routed through this single electrode.

VARIOUS OTHER ARTIFACTS

Even the most proficient technologist will be faced with artifact identification, troubleshooting, and minimization on occasion during PSG acquisition. The following examples contain various artifact types that do not necessarily fit neatly into the previously described categories.

An abrupt shift or flattening of all traces is usually indicative of a disconnected amplifier system or electrode board. When this happens the technologist simply needs to inspect all connections to ensure they are secure. The high-amplitude and erratic artifact on the first two-thirds of the 60-second example (Figure 10-29) represents a disconnected electrode board. The last third represents the connection being reestablished and the signals returning to baseline.

Some digital acquisition systems can produce surprising patterns when no input board is attached. One amplifier currently on the market displays data in all channels that looks very much like human EEG when the head box is disconnected. Some recorders also display high-amplitude, erratic signals when the amplifier system or electrode board is disconnected, whereas others display only minimal ambient noise (Figure 10-30). It cannot be overemphasized: Know one's equipment.

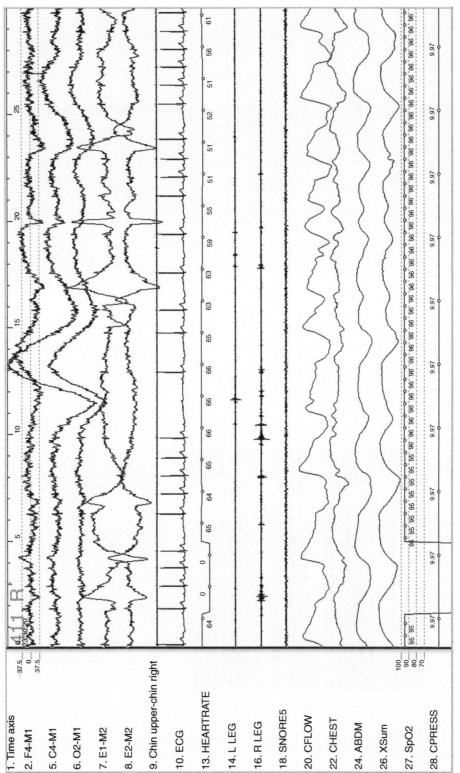

FIGURE 10-27 Complete loss of oximetry data.

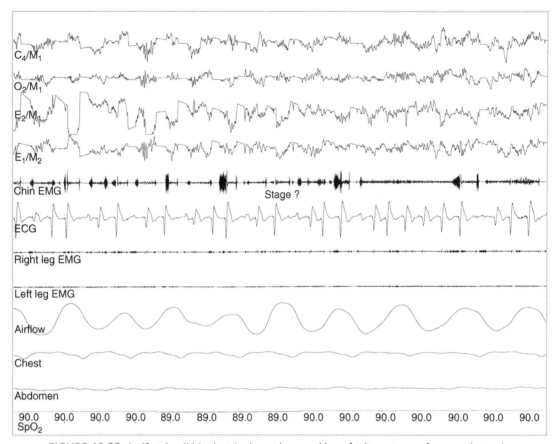

FIGURE 10-28 Artifact in all bioelectric channels caused by a faulty system reference electrode. *From Butkov N: Atlas of clinical polysomnography, ed 2, Medford, Ore, 2010, Synapse Media. Reprinted with permission.*

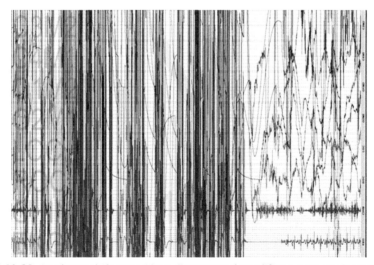

FIGURE 10-29 An abrupt shift caused by a disconnected amplifier system or electrode board.

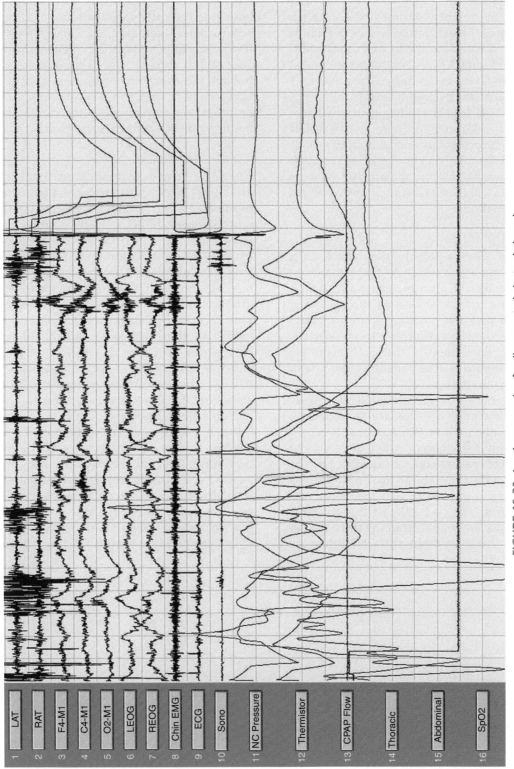

FIGURE 10-30 Another example of a disconnected electrode board.

IMPLANTED ELECTRICAL DEVICES

Patients may arrive for an overnight PSG with an **implanted electronic device**. Occasionally patients may have cranial implants and stimulators. These may cause electrical interference at times when electric charges are being delivered. Some devices constantly discharge electrical signals and may obscure the PSG completely. It is important to recognize this and document on the sleep study as discharges are witnessed. If a device that continuously emits electrical energy cannot be turned off for the study, much of what is recorded for later interpretation may be completely inaccurate. The interpreting physician may rely solely on accurate and thorough technologist observation and documentation of behavioral correlates of sleep and wake. The EEG, and other data, may be rendered useless in this situation.

Cardiac Pacemakers

In an ideal world, when a patient arrives for testing, the technologist will already know if that patient has a cardiac pacemaker. Unfortunately, such details sometimes do not get passed on to the recording technologist who may not have access to the entire medical record. When the recording technologist is unsure based on assessment of the ECG recording, the technologist should ask the patient whether he or she has a cardiac pacemaker.

The following examples are intended to provide only the basic information necessary to identify a cardiac rhythm with characteristic "pacer spikes."

Figure 10-31 is a histogram of data from a patient with an implanted pacemaker responsible for the consistent heart rate throughout the duration of a 6- to 7-hour sleep study. Note that the heart rate rarely waivers from the set rate of the patient's pacemaker. In fact, the only deviations from the set rate likely represent movement artifact. During the first portion of the recording, the patient experiences frequent oxyhemoglobin desaturation events, consistent with sleep-disordered breathing. Later, PAP is applied. During episodes of sleep-disordered breathing, especially obstructive sleep apnea, the heart rate typically varies wildly.

A cardiac pacemaker is a small, battery-operated device typically implanted in the chest just below the right or left clavicle. An electrode wire is threaded through the subclavian vein, vena cava, and into the right atrium or ventricle.[9] Various configurations exist for providing a stimulus to the cardiac muscle, depending on the needs of the patient.

Atrial Pacemaker

When the heart's anatomical pacemaker, the sino-atrial (SA) node, fails to consistently generate an impulse, and the circuitry to carry the signal throughout the heart is intact, only an atrial pacemaker may be needed. The electrode for an atrial pacemaker rests in the right atrium and stimulates the atrium similar to how the SA node normally performs. The impulse travels throughout the heart to generate atrial contraction followed by ventricular contraction. Figure 10-32 represents atrial pacing of the cardiac rhythm. Keep in mind that the traditional ECG paper speed is 25 mm/second as compared with the PSG speed of 10 mm/second. This means that the time base of the example ECG tracings is spread out 2.5 times as compared with how the data look on a sleep study recording.

When a pacemaker "fires" to generate the cardiac stimulus, a high-amplitude spike will be seen prior to the P wave, the QRS complex, or both, depending on whether the atria, ventricles, or both the atria and ventricles are being paced. In this example, only the atria are being paced, as evident by the large spike prior to each P wave. The pacemaker-generated impulse is responsible for the spike, which causes atrial

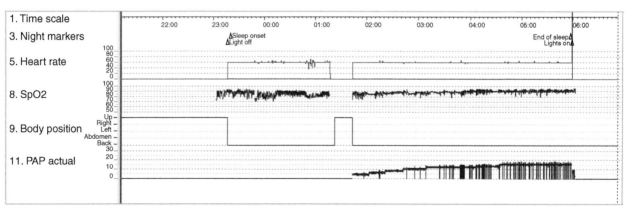

FIGURE 10-31 Histogram of data from a patient with an implanted pacemaker.

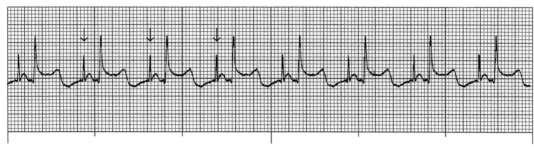

FIGURE 10-32 Atrial pacing. *From Aehlert B: ECGs made easy, ed 4, St Louis, 2011, Mosby JEMS-Elsevier.*

contraction as denoted by the P wave. The signal travels through the heart, causing ventricular contraction, represented by the QRS complex.

Ventricular Pacemaker

Sometimes the path between the atria and ventricles becomes blocked and impulses cannot travel from the atria to the ventricles, or the atrial signal is ineffective for some other reason. In the event the atria are functioning properly, the physician may only place a ventricular pacer that will fire after each P wave. A ventricular pacer might also be placed and set to fire at a specified frequency in absence of supraventricular stimulation when the atrial signal is unreliable. Figure 10-33 is the ECG rhythm one would expect during ventricular pacing. In this example, a P wave is not evident, and the atria may contribute little, if any, to the work being done by the heart. The patient has a ventricular pacemaker, as can be seen by the "pacer spike" prior to each QRS complex. When conduction spontaneously arises from within the ventricle, or is generated by an electronic pacemaker stimulating the ventricle, the QRS complex will be abnormally wide.

Atrioventricular (AV) Sequential Pacemaker

When the patient's heart requires stimulation of both the atria and the ventricles, an atrioventricular (AV) sequential pacemaker is placed. The AV sequential

pacer has an electrode that resides in the atrium and one that rests in the ventricle. Since the signal does not travel normally between the atria and ventricles of the patient's heart, a ventricular impulse is generated by the pacemaker following each atrial impulse (Figure 10-34). An AV sequential pacemaker generates a spike prior to both the P wave and the QRS complex.[9] Because the ventricles are being paced, and the origin of the stimulus is within the ventricle, the QRS complex is abnormally wide.

When a bipolar pacemaker electrode is in use, it can be difficult to see pacer spikes. The patient should be routinely asked whether she or he has an indwelling electronic pacemaker during the evaluation prior to testing or by the technologist on the evening of testing. With the various configurations of pacemakers available, this means that depending on the type of pacemaker, a spike may be seen only before each P wave, only before the QRS complex, or before both the P wave and QRS complex.

Fixed-Rate and Demand Pacemakers

Fixed-rate pacemakers generate an impulse at a specified rate and do not wait to sense if the heart spontaneously generates its own rhythm. Demand pacemakers sense whether the heart is generating an impulse and only fire when the rate drops below programmed settings.[9] For some individuals, therefore, every cardiac impulse is paced, whereas for others a pacer spike is observed only periodically.

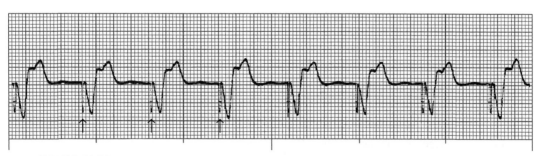

FIGURE 10-33 Ventricular pacing. *From Aehlert B: ECGs made easy, ed 4, St Louis, 2011, Mosby JEMS-Elsevier.*

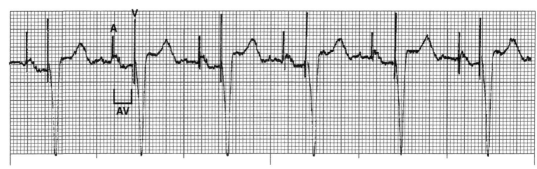

FIGURE 10-34 Atrioventricular sequential pacing. *From Aehlert B:* ECGs made easy, *ed 4, St Louis, 2011, Mosby JEMS-Elsevier.*

ARTIFACT RESPONSE

Recognizing artifacts and responding to them are only the first steps toward developing strategies to ensure that the overnight technologist acquires an optimal recording. The technologist must also determine when it is essential to disrupt the patient's sleep to correct artifacts and when it is prudent to wait until the next arousal or awakening to resolve an issue. Some things to consider are sleep stage, how long the patient has been asleep, the initial sleep latency, total sleep time, time remaining, and whether back-up electrodes are available. Although this may sound simple to the inexperienced technologist, all of these actions, along with the patient's medical and sleep history, must be considered when making these value judgments.

If a patient has been referred for evaluation of sleep terrors and has only just entered stage N3 sleep, it may be beneficial to let the patient sleep and attempt to temporarily correct an artifact, either by using back-up electrodes or filters, until the patient returns to a lighter stage of sleep and the underlying issue can be resolved.

As another example, it is potentially detrimental to the study to awaken a patient who has been asleep for 30 minutes following a 4-hour sleep latency in order to repair a faulty C4 electrode. The thoughtful technologist will re-reference to C3-M2 and repair the faulty electrode at the first patient awakening.

The possible scenarios for making these judgment calls are numerous; however, each is based on common sense and knowledge of the patient history, physician orders, equipment, and recording protocols. Regardless of the patient scenario, if both the primary and back-up derivations are contaminated with artifact, the technologist must repair the issue. Any time the patient is awake, the technologist is expected to correct the source of artifact. When the patient enters sleep, there should always be patent primary and back-up derivation options.

For the experienced technologist, each step of artifact isolation is assessed almost simultaneously, but for the novice technologist it is suggested that each question be pondered individually, in a linear path (see Figure 10-35). An example might be, "Is the artifact generated by the patient, or does it exist in the environment?" For each answer that is "no," the technologist moves to the next question until the artifact has been isolated. Often the isolation process suggests the required corrective action. Keep in mind that every cable, sensor, and interface in the patient-testing circuit is a potential route for introduction of artifact, loss of signal, or the actual source of artifact contamination.

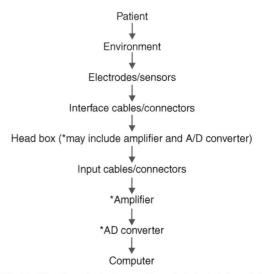

FIGURE 10-35 When isolating artifact, it is helpful to follow a linear pathway, beginning at the patient. This patient pathway model approach helps determine what the artifact is, where it originates, and why it is present.

CHAPTER SUMMARY

- Artifact can arise from the patient's body, the recording equipment, or an external source.
- Recognition of expected physiologic data is essential to the recognition of unwanted signals.
- Artifacts are typically unwanted signals, but at times can be beneficial to the recording technologist, scoring technologist, or the individual interpreting the sleep study.
- Knowledge, training, and skills developed through practice are necessary to differentiate normal versus unwanted signals and beneficial, but unexpected, data.
- The quality, quantity, and significance of recorded data all assist in the determination of whether data is artifact.
- Unwanted artifacts must be categorically identified and assessed to determine if correction is warranted.
- Artifact correction requires mastery of physiologic data collection, and detailed knowledge of the equipment interface and limitations and capabilities of amplifier controls.
- There is no valid excuse for allowing artifact to persist at lights out or any time the patient is awake.
- The failure to correct unwanted artifact can lead to misinterpretation of patient data.
- Misinterpretation of data may result in misdiagnosis of the patient, failure to qualify the patient for treatment, or inappropriate therapeutic intervention.

References

1. Butkov N: *Atlas of clinical polysomnography*, vols 1 & 2, ed 2, Medford, Ore, 2010, Synapse Media.
2. Material Safety Data Sheet, Collodion.
3. Material Safety Data Sheet, Acetone, Rev 2, 1997.
4. Tyner FS, Knott JR, Mayer WB: *Fundamentals of EEG technology: basic concepts and methods*, vol1, ed 1, Philadelphia, 1983, Lippincott, Williams & Wilkins.
5. Geyer JD, Carney PR, Payne TA: *Atlas of polysomnography*, ed 2, Philadelphia, 2010, Lippincott, Williams & Wilkins.
6. Fisch BJ: *Fisch and Spehlmann's EEG primer: principles of digital and analog EEG*, ed 3, Amsterdam, 1999, Elsevier.
7. Berry RB, Brooks R, Gamaldo CE, et al., for the American Academy of Sleep Medicine: *The AASM manual for the scoring of sleep and associated events: rules, terminology and technical specifications*, ed 2, Westchester, Ill, 2012, American Academy of Sleep Medicine.
8. Davila DG, Richards KC, Marshall BL, et al: Oximeter's acquisition parameter influences the profile of respiratory disturbances, *Sleep* 1;26(1):91-95, 2003.
9. Aehlert B: *ECGs made easy*, ed 4, St Louis, 2011, Mosby JEMS-Elsevier.

REVIEW QUESTIONS

1. Just following lights out, the technologist notes artifact apparently caused by increased muscle activity in the channels using the F4-M1, C4-M1, and O2-M1 derivations. The patient is lying on the left side and appears to remain awake. Which of the following is the *best* corrective action to *first* attempt?
   a. Move the patient to the right side.
   b. Allow the patient time to relax.
   c. Re-reference all named channels to M2.
   d. Replace the affected electrode or electrodes.

2. During the recording, the technologist determines that both the F3 and F4 electrodes are popping to the point that the frontal EEG channel is obscured. The technologist should *first* take which of the following measures?
   a. Record an additional central derivation.
   b. Reapply both frontal electrodes.
   c. Allow time for the patient to relax.
   d. Decrease the HFF setting to 15 Hz.

3. Using good site preparation and electrode application techniques along with high-quality amplifiers and electrodes, ensuring appropriate impedances, and avoiding placement of electrodes over soft, fatty tissue reduces the likelihood of which of the following artifacts?
   a. Cardioballistic
   b. Muscle tension
   c. Pulse-generated
   d. Electrocardiographic

4. The patient turns to the left side 2 hours after lights out, after which the technologist notes artifact caused by increased muscle activity in the F4-M1, C4-M1, and O2-M1 channels. The patient appears to remain asleep following the movement. Which of the following is the *best* corrective action to *first* attempt?
   a. Move the patient to the right side.
   b. Allow the patient time to relax.
   c. Re-reference all named channels to M2.
   d. Replace the affected electrode or electrodes.

5. When ECG artifact is present in all derivations sharing a mastoid reference (M1 or M2), what is the *best* corrective or preventative action to first attempt?
   a. Reposition or replace the mastoid reference electrode.
   b. Use a combined M1 and M2 reference (linked mastoids).
   c. Decrease the HFF setting on affected channels.
   d. Reposition or replace the system reference electrode.

6. ECG artifact in the EEG channels is best confirmed by comparing which of the following?
   a. Alignment of the QRS complex to the artifact
   b. Patient's pulse rate to that recorded on the EEG
   c. Abnormalities on the ECG recording with the artifact
   d. Affected EEG channel or channels with an unaffected channel

7. If 60-Hz artifact is in multiple channels recording bioelectric potentials, but does not affect channels derived from transducers, which cause is *least likely*?
   a. High impedance on the system ground
   b. Excessively high leakage current
   c. A poorly applied or defective ground
   d. High mastoid reference impedance

8. Which of the following is most often caused by poor electrode contact or a broken electrode wire?
   a. Respiratory artifact
   b. Cardioballistic artifact
   c. Pulse artifact
   d. Popping artifact

9. If 60-Hz artifact is isolated to one channel, which cause is *most likely*?
   a. Excessively high leakage current
   b. High or imbalanced impedances
   c. A poorly applied or defective ground
   d. An input cable parallel to power cords

10. After the patient returns from a restroom break, the technologist determines that the resumed recording contains no physiologic data. Which of the following is *most likely* disconnected?
    a. Both mastoid inputs
    b. Exploring electrode or electrodes
    c. The patient input cable
    d. The patient ground

Chapter 11

The Cardiopulmonary System: Essentials for the Polysomnographic Technologist

Carolyn Campo

OUTLINE

LEARNING OBJECTIVES

After reading this chapter, you will be able to:
1. Identify the physical components of the respiratory system.
2. Describe the physical components of the cardiovascular system.
3. Explain ventilation and diffusion.
4. Explain perfusion and gas exchange.
5. Describe lung volume measurements in detail.
6. Apply arterial blood gas values to sleep states.
7. Monitor an electrocardiogram and identify dysrhythmias.
8. Correlate response to dysrhythmia type.

KEY TERMS

antegrade

arteries

atria

carbon dioxide transport

central chemoreceptors

depolarization

diaphragm

diffusion

dysrhythmia

exhalation

expiratory reserve volume (ERV)

functional residual capacity (FRC)

hypercapnic

hypoxemic

inhalation

internal respiration

inspiratory capacity (IC)

inspiratory reserve volume (IRV)

modified lead II derivation

nasopharynx

oropharynx

oxygen transport

peripheral chemoreceptors

residual volume (RV)

retrograde

thorax

tidal volume (V_T)

total lung capacity (TLC)

veins

ventricles

vital capacity (VC)

ANATOMY AND PHYSIOLOGY OF THE RESPIRATORY SYSTEM

THE THORAX

The **thorax** is the region of the chest formed by the sternum, the thoracic vertebrae, and the ribs. The thoracic cavity contains the heart, the greater and lesser blood vessels, lungs, trachea, esophagus, thymus gland, lymphatic structures, and many nerves[1]. These structures are protected by the thoracic cage. The thoracic cage is composed of the sternum, ribs, intercostal muscles, and thoracic vertebrae.

Thoracic Cage

There are twelve vertebrae attached to twelve ribs. The top seven ribs are attached to the sternum via cartilage. The lower five are not attached to the sternum and are sometimes referred to as "floating" ribs. The ribs connect anteriorly to the sternum, which is composed of the upper portion called the *manubrium*; the central portion called the *body*, and the lower portion, a small fingerlike protrusion known as the *xiphoid process* (Figure 11-1).

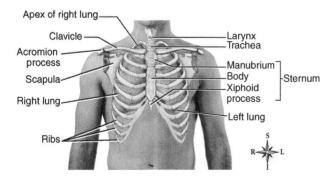

FIGURE 11-1 Bony structures of the chest. These structures form a protective and expandable cage around the lungs and the heart. *From Patton KT, Thibodeau GA:* Anatomy & Physiology, *ed 8, St. Louis, 2013, Mosby.*

Lungs

The lungs perform external respiration and, in the adult, provide more than 70 square meters of epithelial tissue surface area necessary for gas exchange. The right lung is composed of three lobes: the upper, middle, and lower. The left lung has only two lobes: the upper and lower. The lungs lie somewhat free in the thoracic cavity and are functionally very elastic, or dynamic.[2]

For ventilation to occur, the airway into the body must be open, or patent. The airway is broken into two basic areas: the extrathoracic or upper airway and intrathoracic or lower airways. When the airway drawing is inverted, it takes on the appearance of a leafless tree. This is why it is sometimes referred to as the *bronchial tree* or *tracheobronchial tree* (Figure 11-2).

Air moves into and out of the lung via the upper airway through the nose and **nasopharynx** and the mouth and **oropharynx**. The nasopharynx is the uppermost area of the back of the throat (pharynx) beginning with the superior level of the soft palate extending into the posterior portion of the nasal cavity. The oropharynx is the oral portion of the pharynx, which is the back of the throat from the soft palate down to the upper edge of the epiglottis.

On inspiration, air moves down through the space between the vocal cords, known as the glottis, and into the trachea, where it enters the intrathoracic or lower airway region. The large trachea bifurcates, or splits, into two bronchi, the left mainstem and the right mainstem. Each mainstem bronchus further divides into lobar bronchi and then into segmental bronchi.

The airways continue to divide, eventually becoming bronchioles which lack cartilage and have a diameter measuring less than one millimeter. Bronchioles terminate into small clusters of air sacs called *alveoli* (alveolus, singular). The sacs are encased in microscopic blood vessels known as *capillaries*. The alveolar sacs and abutting capillaries are where gas transfer to the body occurs. It is

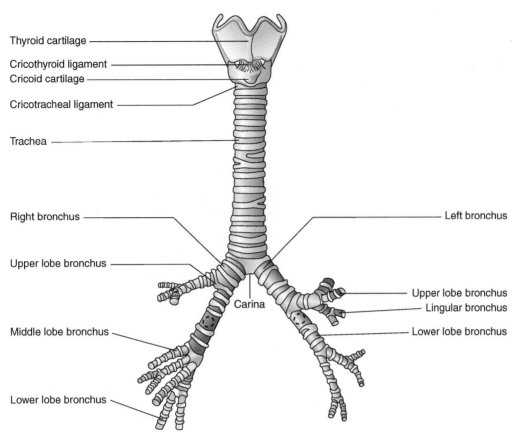

Thyroid cartilage

Cricothyroid ligament

Cricoid cartilage

Cricotracheal ligament

Trachea

Right bronchus

Upper lobe bronchus

Carina

Middle lobe bronchus

Lower lobe bronchus

Left bronchus

Upper lobe bronchus

Lingular bronchus

Lower lobe bronchus

FIGURE 11-2 Major airways of the tracheobronchial tree. *From Hicks GH:* Cardiopulmonary anatomy and physiology, *Philadelphia, 2000, Saunders.*

estimated that approximately 300,000,000 of these units are present in a normal adult human lung. This is where oxygen (O_2) and carbon dioxide (CO_2) are exchanged in a process known as **diffusion**. This process is further discussed later in this chapter.

Each lung is encased by a double-layered serous membrane, called the *pleura* (Figure 11-3). The visceral pleura are attached to the surface of the lung. The parietal pleura line the wall of the thorax and the slim space between the visceral and parietal pleurae is the *pleural cavity* or *pleural space*. It contains a small amount of serous fluid that is produced by the pleura to reduce friction as the two layers slide against each other during breathing.[3]

THE MUSCLES OF VENTILATION

Mechanical movement of air into and out of the lung is an active-passive muscular event. The **diaphragm** is located below the lungs and is the primary muscle of ventilation. **Inhalation** is an active muscular event, with the diaphragmatic muscle contracting downward, thus pulling the lung tissue or *parenchyma* with it. This downward movement physically increases the size of the lungs by stretching them into a larger space in the thorax. Contraction of the

muscle fibers causes the segments of the diaphragm to be pulled down and the lower ribs to move up and outward, thereby increasing the volume of the thoracic cavity. When the lungs physically become larger during inspiration, the pressure inside the thorax becomes relatively negative as compared to the ambient pressure exerted upon the outside of the body. Because nature abhors a vacuum, air from the outside atmosphere is now "sucked" into the body. Ambient air contains 21% oxygen necessary to maintain human life.

Exhalation occurs when the diaphragm relaxes from the contracted state, and the lungs recoil back to their resting state and push the gases out into the atmosphere. Exhalation is generally a passive muscular event. Figure 11-4 shows that the shape of the relaxed diaphragm in the exhalation phase is domed. During contraction or the inspiratory phase, it is flattened.

The diaphragm is the primary muscle of ventilation, but certainly not the only one. Accessory muscles (Figures 11-5 through 11-7) are recruited when the body needs additional ventilation for gas exchange over baseline respiration.[1] Such recruitment might occur during exercise or when an individual's physical condition is rapidly deteriorating during an asthma attack.

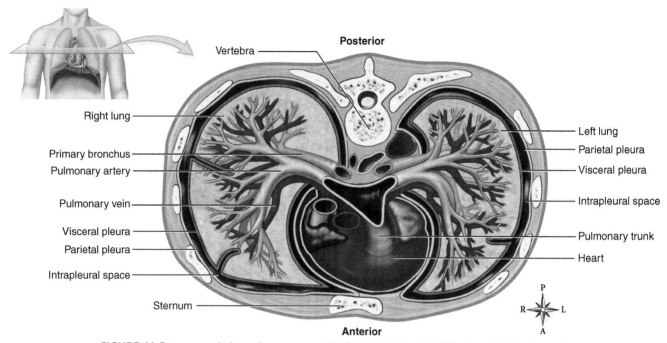

FIGURE 11-3 Lungs and pleura (transverse section.) *From Patton KT, Thibodeau GA:* Anatomy & Physiology, *ed 8, St. Louis, 2013, Mosby.*

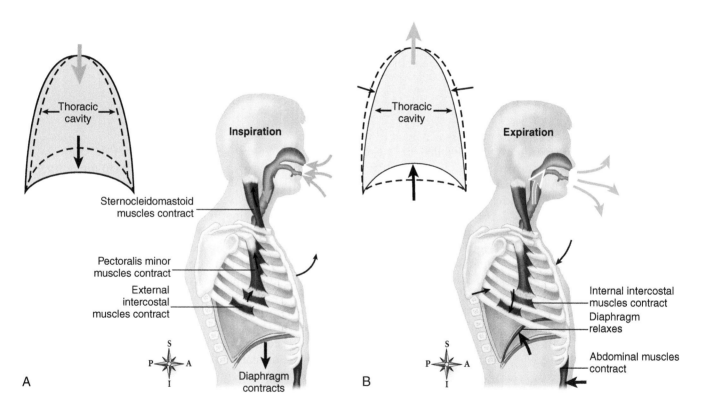

FIGURE 11-4 Inspiration and expiration. **A,** Mechanism of inspiration. Note the role of the diaphragm and the chest-elevating muscles (pectoralis minor and external intercostals) in increasing thoracic volume, which decreases pressure in the lungs and thus draws air inward. **B,** Mechanism of expiration. Note that relaxation of the diaphragm plus contraction of chest-depressing muscles (internal intercostals) reduces thoracic volume, which increases pressure in the lungs and thus pushes air outward. *From Patton KT, et al:* Essentials of anatomy and physiology, *St Louis, 2012, Mosby-Elsevier.*

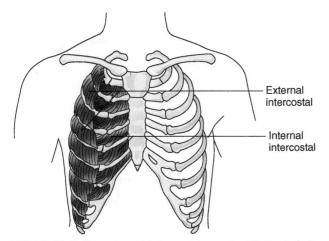

FIGURE 11-5 The external intercostal muscles lift the inferior ribs and enlarge the thoracic cavity. The internal intercostal muscles compress the thoracic cavity by pulling together the ribs. *From Hicks GH:* Cardiopulmonary anatomy and physiology, *Philadelphia, 2000, Saunders.*

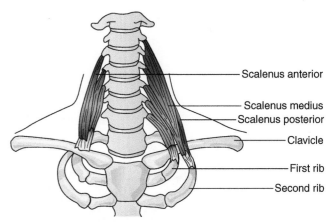

FIGURE 11-6 The scalene muscles originate from the lower cervical vertebrae and lift the clavicle and first two ribs. *From Hicks GH:* Cardiopulmonary anatomy and physiology, *Philadelphia, 2000, Saunders.*

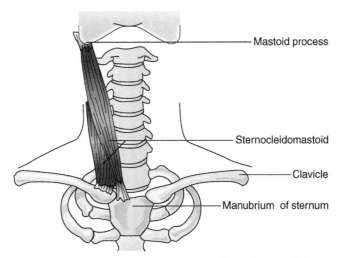

FIGURE 11-7 The sternocleidomastoid muscles originate from the manubrium and clavicle and insert on the mastoid process of the temporal bone. They lift the upper thorax when the trapezius stabilizes the head. *From Hicks GH:* Cardiopulmonary anatomy and physiology, *Philadelphia, 2000, WB Saunders.*

ANATOMY AND PHYSIOLOGY OF THE CARDIOVASCULAR SYSTEM

HEART

The adult heart is approximately the size of an individual's closed fist and sits in the thorax on the left side of the chest in front of the lungs. The heart is a mechanical pump with four chambers designed for specific functions. The four chambers are known as the *right atrium, right ventricle, left atrium,* and *left ventricle.* The **atria** are the smaller, less muscular upper chambers of the heart and the two **ventricles** are the larger, more muscular lower chambers of the heart. The muscular wall of the left ventricle is approximately twice as thick as the right ventricle because it needs to generate enough force to push blood through the entire body, whereas the right ventricle needs to generate only enough force to push blood about 6 inches through the lungs.

The heart has four valves. The *tricuspid valve* sits between the right atrium and right ventricle. The *pulmonary valve* is located between the right ventricle and the pulmonary artery. The *bicuspid* or *mitral valve* is between the left atrium and the left ventricle, and the *aortic valve* is between the left ventricle and the aorta.[1,3] The valves are in these locations to assist the forward movement of blood and to prevent blood from flowing backward during the contraction phase of the heartbeat (Figure 11-8).

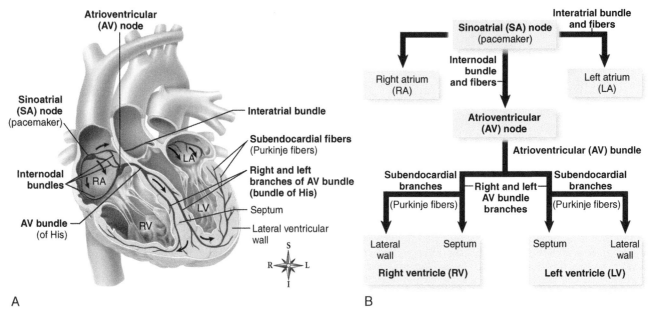

A   B

FIGURE 11-8 Conduction system of the heart. Specialized cardiac muscle cells (*boldface type*) in the wall of the heart rapidly initiate or conduct an electrical impulse throughout the myocardium. Both the sketch of the conduction system (*A*) and the flowchart (*B*) show the origin and path of conduction. The signal is initiated by the sinoatrial node (pacemaker) and spreads directly to the rest of the right atrial myocardium. From there, it travels to the left atrial myocardium by way of a bundle of interatrial conducting fibers, and then to the atrioventricular (AV) node by way of three internodal bundles. The AV node then initiates a signal that is conducted through the ventricular myocardium by way of the AV bundle (of His) and subendocardial branches (Purkinje fibers). *From Patton KT, et al: Essentials of anatomy and physiology, St Louis, 2012, Mosby-Elsevier.*

OXYGENATION OF THE BLOOD

In the arterial system, red blood cells (RBCs) carry oxygen throughout the body via hemoglobin (Hb). The oxygen is used by muscles and organs to sustain life. The venous system carries the deoxygenated blood back to the right side of the heart. The right ventricle then pumps blood into the pulmonary artery to both lungs, terminating in the pulmonary capillaries. The pulmonary capillaries are spread across the surface of the alveoli where the blood can pick up oxygen diffusing through the alveolar-capillary membranes. The freshly oxygenated blood is then returned to the left side of the heart to be pumped throughout the body for use by muscles and organs in the body.

Vessels carrying deoxygenated blood to the heart are called **veins**. Vessels carrying oxygenated blood away from the heart are called **arteries**. The pulmonary artery is the only artery carrying deoxygenated blood. The pulmonary artery supplies blood to the lungs to be reoxygenated. The pulmonary veins are the only veins carrying oxygenated blood. The pulmonary veins move the freshly oxygenated blood from the lungs to the left side of the heart to be pumped throughout the body.[1] Except as noted above arteries always carry pressurized blood away from the heart, whereas veins carry blood under less pressure toward the heart.

VENTILATION AND DIFFUSION

Respiration also occurs at the cellular level and is sometimes referred to as **internal respiration**. The body needs oxygen to convert sugars into energy for the cell to function. The result of this cellular metabolism produces carbon dioxide, a highly acidic waste product. The cardiopulmonary system transports the oxygen to the cells but, just as importantly, it transports this waste product, carbon dioxide, back to the lungs and kidneys to be processed out of the body. The backbone of this transport is the RBCs and plasma in the blood.

Oxygen is inspired from the atmosphere, diffused across the alveolar-capillary bed into the bloodstream, and delivered to the cells. Carbon dioxide is transported at the cellular level and returns to the alveolar-capillary bed where it off-loads and is exhaled. Gas diffusion takes place when an area of high concentration is exposed to an area of low concentration. In the alveoli, the blood is rich in oxygen and low in carbon dioxide. The oxygen moves from the alveoli into the deoxygenated blood and the carbon dioxide moves from the blood into the alveoli where carbon dioxide levels are lower (Figure 11-9).[2,5]

OXYGEN TRANSPORT

RBCs are responsible for **oxygen transport** in the blood. This occurs when oxygen attaches to the Hb

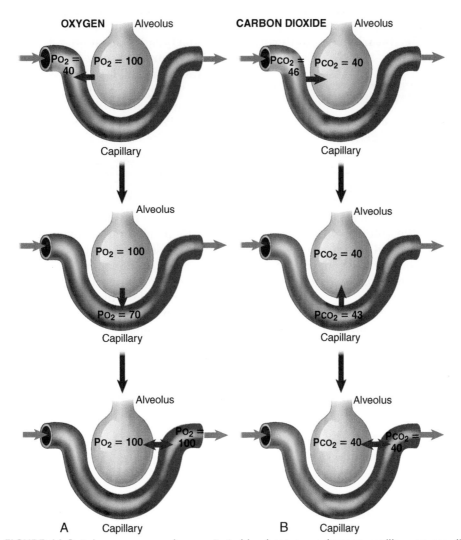

FIGURE 11-9 Pulmonary gas exchange. **A,** As blood enters a pulmonary capillary, oxygen diffuses down its pressure gradient (into the blood). Oxygen continues diffusing into the blood until equilibration has occurred (or until the blood leaves the capillary). **B,** As blood enters a pulmonary capillary, carbon dioxide diffuses down its pressure gradient (out of the blood). As with oxygen, carbon dioxide continues diffusing as long as there is a pressure gradient. PO_2 and PCO_2 remain relatively constant in a continually ventilated alveolus. *From Patton KT, et al: Essentials of anatomy and physiology, St Louis, 2012, Mosby-Elsevier.*

molecule via diffusion across the alveolar-capillary membrane in the lungs. A normal RBC has four Hb binding sites. Each Hb binding site can carry one molecule of oxygen. If each RBC is fully saturated with four molecules of oxygen, it is said to be 100% saturated. Normal oxygen saturation is between 95% to 100%. Measurement of oxygen saturation is essential in monitoring respiratory status. Blood oxygen levels are measured by sampling arterial blood and testing the amount of oxygen being carried by the plasma. Oxygen saturation can also be estimated by pulse oximetry.

The percentage saturation of Hb with oxygen is affected by (1) the amount of oxygen being delivered to the blood, (2) the acid-base balance (pH) of the blood, (3) the temperature of the blood, (4) the amount of Hb in the blood, and (5) the amount of oxygen required by the tissues.

CARBON DIOXIDE TRANSPORT

Carbon dioxide transport is the process of transporting carbon dioxide dissolved in blood plasma, RBC, or plasma protein in order to be released by the lungs. Approximately 5% of the produced carbon dioxide that is transported is dissolved in the blood plasma to be released at the lungs. Carbon dioxide is also transported bound to the RBC Hb or to a plasma protein in the blood. This method accounts for approximately 25% of carbon dioxide transport. The remaining approximately 70% is transported through the bicarbonate buffering system.[5]

LUNG VOLUMES AND CAPACITIES

Lung volumes and capacities are measured in liters. Two or more volumes added together are expressed as a *capacity* (Figure 11-10). A fundamental understanding of the volumes and capacities of the lungs is necessary for the technologist to fully appreciate how and why the application of positive airway pressure (PAP) as a therapeutic intervention is performed.

- **Tidal volume (V_T)** is the volume of gas inspired and expired with each normal breath.
- **Inspiratory reserve volume (IRV)** is the maximum volume that can be inspired *above* the tidal volume or normal breath.
- **Expiratory reserve volume (ERV)** is the maximum volume that can be expired after a tidal breath exhalation.
- **Residual volume (RV)** is the volume that remains in the lungs after a maximal expiration. This is the volume of air that holds the lungs open and that can never be exhaled.
- **Inspiratory capacity (IC)** = V_T + IRV
- **Vital capacity (VC)** = V_T + IRV + ERV

- **Functional residual capacity (FRC)** is the amount of gas remaining in the lungs following a normal tidal breath exhalation = ERV + RV
- **Total lung capacity (TLC)** = IRV + V_T + ERV + RV (the sum of all four lung volumes)

Technologists applying PAP are fundamentally changing the patient's FRC. This concept is important during PAP titration and is discussed later in this chapter in relation to the drive to breathe.

ARTERIAL BLOOD GAS INTERPRETATION AND MANIPULATION

Arterial blood gas (ABG) measurement is the gold standard for monitoring adequacy of ventilation and gas exchange. A deeper look at ABGs reveals that the acid-base balance in the human body has significant influence on the regulation of breathing, as well as implications for treatment of sleep-disordered breathing

As mentioned earlier, the body continually monitors all chemical systems to maintain homeostasis. Human beings function in a rather narrow range of pH. For cells to properly metabolize nutrients and perform their specific functions, the concentration of free hydrogen ions must be prevented from accumulating in the organism because this will result in an acidic environment. When carbon dioxide is exposed to water, it rapidly reacts to form carbonic acid (H_2CO_3),

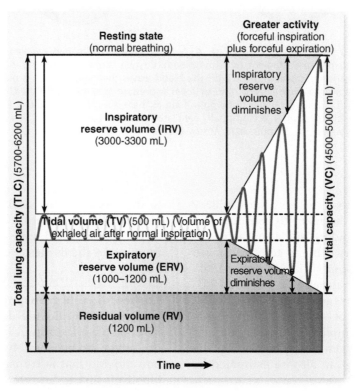

FIGURE 11-10 Pulmonary ventilation volumes and capacities. A spirogram. *From Patton KT, et al:* Essentials of anatomy and physiology, *St Louis, 2012, Mosby-Elsevier.*

TABLE 11-1

Arterial Blood Gas Values

pH	The acidity or alkalinity of the blood	Normal value = 7.35 − 7.45
$PaCO_2$	The partial pressure of dissolved CO_2 in the blood	Normal value = 35 − 45 mm Hg
PaO_2	The partial pressure of dissolved O_2 in the blood	Normal value = 80 − 100 mm Hg
HCO_3	Plasma bicarbonate calculated from pH and PCO_2	Normal value = 22 − 26 mmol/L
BE	Base excess (deficit) buffer produced by body	Normal value = +3 to −3

BE, Base excess; *CO₂,* carbon dioxide; *HCO₃,* hydrogen and bicarbonate ion; *O₂,* oxygen; *PaCO₂,* partial pressure of carbon dioxide; *PaO₂,* partial pressure of oxygen; *PCO₂,* partial pressure of carbon dioxide; *pH,* acid-base balance.

which further dissociates into hydrogen and bicarbonate ions (HCO_3^-), thus rendering the environment more acidic. One can summarize this process by understanding that the more carbon dioxide that is in the body (lungs), the more acidic the blood.[2,5]

For the sleep technologist, the normal values listed in Table 11-1 are a starting point. Note that the convention for reporting ABGs delivers the values in the following order: pH, partial pressure of carbon dioxide ($PaCO_2$), partial pressure of oxygen (PaO_2), HCO_3^-, base excess, and arterial oxygen saturation (SaO_2).

To interpret ABG data, the technologist should go through each of the five parameters and determine if the value is normal or abnormal. If everything falls into the range of normal, the ABG is said to be "normal."

- A **pH less than** 7.35 is acidotic and a **pH greater than** 7.45 is alkalotic.
- A **$PaCO_2$ greater than** 45 is acidotic and a **$PaCO_2$ less than** 35 is alkalotic.
- A **HCO_3^- less than** 22 is acidotic and a **HCO_3^- greater than** 26 is alkalotic.

Compare the pH with the $PaCO_2$ and the HCO_3^-. If both the pH and $PaCO_2$ are the same, for instance both are acidic, this results in respiratory acidosis. If the pH and the HCO_3^- are the same, the problem originates from a metabolic source such as kidney failure or diabetic acidosis.

To determine if this is an acute problem or a chronic problem, look at whether the pH falls in the normal range (7.35 to 7.45). If all other measures are outside normal but the pH is in the normal range, this is called a compensated or chronic acid-base balance (example shown in Table 11-2). If the pH is outside of the normal range, it is acute or uncompensated.

REGULATION OF BREATHING

The new technologist should expand his or her knowledge of the autonomic nervous system (ANS). The function of the ANS is fundamental to the neural control of ventilation and oxygenation. The ANS regulates the respiratory function via two primary components: the **central chemoreceptors** and **peripheral chemoreceptors**. Microscopic stretch receptors attached to the lung parenchyma also play a small role in providing biofeedback to the brain regarding the size and depth of each breath.[1] See Box 11-1 for key points of breathing regulation.

CENTRAL CHEMORECEPTORS

A region in the midbrain houses the respiratory center (Figure 11-11). This area of the brain is thought to contain at least three sites sensitive to carbon dioxide in the cerebral spinal fluid (CSF).[6] Central chemoreceptors in the medulla, and perhaps other areas of the brain, detect the levels of carbon dioxide in the blood, as the CSF that protects the brain and spine takes on the pH of the blood in the body. Increased carbon dioxide in the CSF results in an increase in the concentration of hydrogen ions. The increased hydrogen ions cause a decrease in CSF and blood pH. The decreased pH of the blood is a direct result of the raised carbon dioxide concentration.

In response to a decrease in pH (acidosis) of the CSF, the central chemoreceptors stimulate the inspiratory center, which in turn sends signals to the respiratory muscles. Thus, the normal neurochemical control of the ventilatory cycle is that of arterial

TABLE 11-2

Normal Ranges Compared with Values from a Patient with COPD

	pH	$PaCO_2$	PaO_2	SaO_2	HCO_3^-
Normal	7.35-7.45	35-45	80-100	94%-99%	22-26
COPD example	7.42	66	60	86%	38

COPD, Chronic obstructive pulmonary disease; *HCO₃,* hydrogen and bicarbonate ion; *PaCO₂,* partial pressure of carbon dioxide; *PaO₂,* partial pressure of oxygen; *pH,* acid-base balance; *SaO₂,* oxygen saturation level.

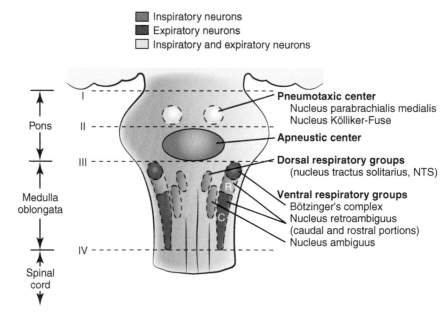

Inspiratory neurons
Expiratory neurons
Inspiratory and expiratory neurons

Pons

Medulla
oblongata

Spinal
cord

I
II
III
IV

Pneumotaxic center
Nucleus parabrachialis medialis
Nucleus Kölliker-Fuse

Apneustic center

Dorsal respiratory groups
(nucleus tractus solitarius, NTS)

Ventral respiratory groups
Bötzinger's complex
Nucleus retroambiguus
(caudal and rostral portions)
Nucleus ambiguus

FIGURE 11-11 Dorsal view of the brainstem. Phase I to IV refer to transections at different levels. *From Beachey W: Respiratory Care Anatomy and Physiology, ed 3, St. Louis, 2013, Elsevier.*

$PaCO_2$ and its effect on CSF pH.[6] The normal response to an increase in $PaCO_2$ is first an increase in tidal volume depth and then an increase in respiratory rate. This will likely trigger another signal to the brain that increases the heart rate (cardiac output) to move more blood and off-load more carbon dioxide.

PERIPHERAL CHEMORECEPTORS

Other chemoreceptors are located on the aortic arch and at the bifurcation of the internal and external carotid arteries. These are the peripheral chemoreceptors, also known as *aortic* or *carotid bodies*. They are extremely sensitive to decreases in the blood oxygen level. When the amount of oxygen traveling by these tissues decreases, the respiratory center is stimulated, resulting in inspiration (Figure 11-12).

MICROSCOPIC STRETCH RECEPTORS

During inspiration, the lungs become distended, activating the *stretch receptors*. Muscle spindles are located on the muscle fibers and are stretch sensing (Figure 11-13). As the degree of stretch increases, these receptors fire more frequently. The impulses that they send to the brainstem inhibit the medullary cells, decreasing the inspiratory stimulus.

Breathing during wakefulness is controlled by several factors, including voluntary and behavioral elements, chemical factors (e.g., low oxygen levels or high carbon dioxide levels) and mechanical signals from the lung and chest wall (stretch receptors).

BOX 11-1
Key Points of Breathing Regulation

- Increases in carbon dioxide stimulate the central chemoreceptors in the midbrain, which in turn stimulates breathing.
- Decreases in oxygen stimulate the peripheral chemoreceptors, which stimulates breathing.
- Stretch receptors fire impulses to the brainstem as the stretch increases, which inhibit the inspiratory stimulus.

CHANGES DURING SLEEP

During sleep, there is a loss of voluntary control and a decrease in the usual ventilatory response to both low oxygen and high carbon dioxide levels. Both **hypoxemic** (low oxygen) and **hypercapnic** (high carbon dioxide) responses are most depressed during rapid eye movement (REM) sleep. Many respiratory problems during sleep are related to an abnormal control of ventilation.

Much is known about the control of breathing during wakefulness, but less is known about how breathing is controlled in the healthy sleeping person or in patients with a sleep disorder. Breathing during sleep depends entirely on the autonomic respiratory control system. In normal persons, during both REM and non-REM (NREM) sleep, clear alterations are noted in tidal volume, alveolar ventilation, blood gas values, and respiratory rate and rhythm.

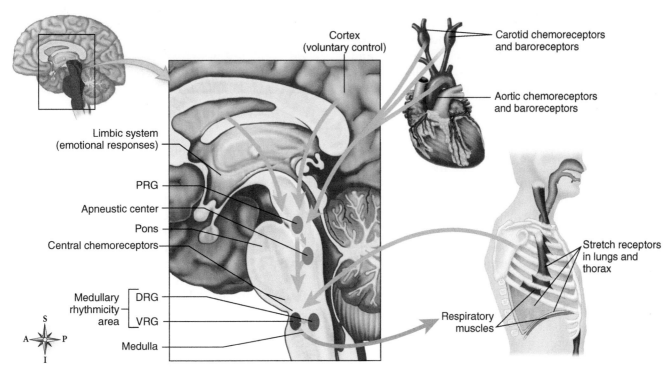

FIGURE 11-12 Regulation of breathing. The dorsal respiratory group (DRG) and ventral respiratory group (VRG) of the medulla represent the medullary rhythmicity area. The pontine respiratory group (PRG, or pneumotaxic center) and apneustic center of the pons influence the basic respiratory rhythm by means of neural input to the medullary rhythmicity area. The brainstem also receives input from other parts of the body; information from chemoreceptors, baroreceptors, and stretch receptors can alter the basic breathing pattern, as can emotional (limbic) and sensory input. Despite these subconscious reflexes, the cerebral cortex can override the "automatic" control of breathing to some extent to do such activities as sing or blow up a balloon. Green arrows show flow of information to the respiratory control centers. The purple arrow shows flow of information from the control centers to the respiratory muscles that drive breathing. *From Patton KT, Thibodeau GA:* Anatomy & Physiology, *ed 8, St. Louis, 2013, Mosby.*

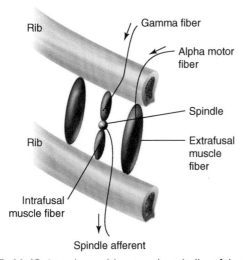

FIGURE 11-13 Stretch sensitive muscle spindle of intercostal muscle fibers. Spindle afferent fibers synapse with alpha motor fibers in the spinal chord, creating a single synapse reflex arc. *Modified from Berne RM, Levy MN:* Physiology, *ed 3, St. Louis, 1993, Mosby.*

CHANGES IN TIDAL VOLUME AND ALVEOLAR VENTILATION

During NREM sleep, breathing is very regular in both frequency and amplitude, although minute ventilation falls by 0.4 to 1.5 liters per minute secondary to a reduction in tidal volume, frequency, or both, as compared with wake values. In fact, breathing apparently declines progressively between wakefulness, stage N1 sleep, stage N2 sleep, and stage N3 sleep.[7] REM sleep is marked by irregular breathing, consisting of sudden changes in both frequency and amplitude, which is occasionally interrupted by central apneas.[7] As compared with NREM sleep, there is a similar reduction in minute ventilation, particularly during phasic REM sleep. The following factors may be responsible for "hypoventilation" during sleep:

1. Absence of tonic influence on the brain (wakefulness stimulus)
2. Reduced chemosensitivity (reduced sensitivity to hypoxemia and hypercapnia)
3. Increased upper airway resistance caused by reduced activity of pharyngeal dilator muscles during sleep
4. Decreases in oxygen consumption and decreases in carbon dioxide production

CHANGES IN BLOOD GAS VALUES

As a result of the fall of alveolar ventilation during sleep, the $PaCO_2$ rises by 3 to 7 mm Hg and PaO_2 decreases by 3.5 to 9.4 mm Hg. Significantly, SaO_2, the calculated oxygen saturation reported by ABG, decreases by less than 2%.[7]

CHANGES IN HEART RATE AND RHYTHM

In NREM sleep the respiratory rate primarily decreases. There is also waxing and waning of the tidal volume at sleep onset. During the deepening stages of NREM sleep, breathing becomes more stable and rhythmic. The decrease in minute ventilation is most likely linked to active sleep mechanisms rather than a decrease in metabolic rate. In REM sleep breathing becomes irregular, especially during phasic REM. Although it has been determined that the chemical control system during REM sleep is not abolished, it has been suggested that the irregular breathing pattern is produced by activation of the behavioral respiratory control system of REM sleep processes.[7]

Decreased ventilatory response to hypoxemia and hypercapnia, as well as inspiratory resistance during sleep, results in REM-related hypoxemia in patients with chronic obstructive pulmonary disease (COPD), chest wall disease, and neuromuscular abnormalities affecting the respiratory muscles. The hypoxemia is actually secondary to hypercapnia, which goes largely unnoticed during testing because most laboratories do not continuously monitor carbon dioxide. This dynamic may also contribute to the development of the sleep apnea-hypopnea syndrome.

VISUAL ASSESSMENT OF CARDIOPULMONARY STATUS

RESPIRATORY STATUS

The normal resting respiratory rate in an adult varies according to the institution or physician who describes it, but is often quoted as 12-20 breaths per minute.[4] The consensus of the normal adult heart rate seems to remain between 60 and 100 beats per minute (bpm), although the normal range is considered 40 to 90 bpm during sleep.[8] Most pulmonologists consider an oxyhemoglobin saturation obtained by ABGs or pulse oximetry of 90% or more adequate for adult patients.

The inspiratory (I) to expiratory (E) time, or I:E ratio, of a normal tidal breath is often expressed as 1:2 or 1:3. At rest, this means that for every 1 second spent inhaling, 2 to 3 seconds are spent exhaling. The time between breaths is expressed as total cycle time (TCT). For example, using easy math, if the adult is breathing 10 breaths per minute, on average, the TCT is 6 seconds long. If this is a normal healthy adult with a 1:2 I:E ratio, 2 seconds are spent inhaling and 4 seconds are spent exhaling.

BODY HABITUS

Another aspect of assessment that should be taken into consideration is a patient's body habitus (Figure 11-14). *Body habitus* means "physique" or "build." An adult can

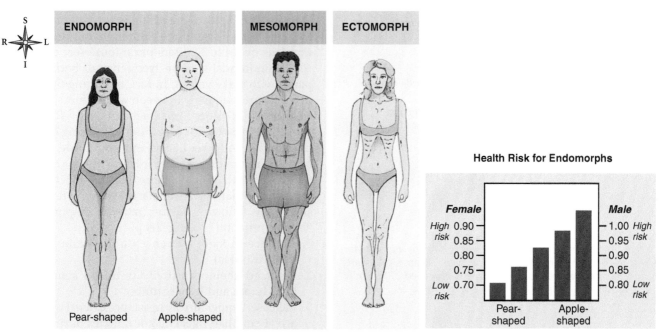

FIGURE 11-14 Body habitus. *From Patton KT, et al:* Essentials of anatomy and physiology, *St Louis, 2012, Mosby-Elsevier.*

be considered overweight (endomorphic), normal weight (mesomorphic), or underweight (ectomorphic). Excess body weight can affect the normal breathing patterns of an individual. Perhaps as importantly, the shape of the thorax can lend clues to physiologic conditions associated with a given disease process.

For example, if a patient presents to the sleep center with a large, barrel-shaped chest, one may consult the medical history or inquire from the patient about a diagnosis of COPD because the barrel chest can be the result of long-standing air trapping in the small airways. With small-airways trapping, these patients tend to have a short amount of time for inhalation and spend a longer amount of time exhaling. This is because obstructive respiratory disease makes it difficult to exhale; patients have difficulty getting air out of the lungs.[4]

A patient may present with the physical appearance of a "hunchback." This presentation should trigger a conversation or review of medical records to determine if he or she has a diagnosis of kyphoscoliosis or another condition of spinal curvature. Kyphoscoliosis is the classic restrictive lung syndrome, although many others exist. Restrictive lung disorders impede the lungs, making the patient unable to inhale to the capacities of someone without lung disease. The inhalation phase of breaths is longer for these patients and exhalation is much faster; they have difficulty getting air into the lungs.[4]

SKIN TONE

The skilled assessor must be aware of skin color. Color, or the lack of color, may direct the practitioner to the correct pathway for identification of issues. First, look at the sclera (whites) of the eyes. If they are yellow tinged, be sure to note this finding because this could indicate a possible liver problem.[9] For lighter-skinned individuals, observe the skin tone to assess whether the skin is pink or if it has a bluish discoloration, known as *cyanosis.* When assessing a patient with dark skin pigmentation, observe that normal brown skin appears to be yellow-brown, and black skin appears to be ashen-gray.[9] Cyanosis is often an indication of tissue hypoxia.

Assessment for cyanosis should include inspection of the oral mucosa, lips, nail beds, gums, palpebral conjunctivae, base of the tongue, and palms. It is possible for cyanosis to result from vasoconstriction caused by exposure to the cold, although it could lend credence to an acute or chronic respiratory disorder, such as COPD or heart disease.[9] Cyanosis typically occurs at or below an oxyhemoglobin saturation of approximately 60%. Given the opportunity, check for capillary refill in the patient's finger by squeezing the finger and then releasing to allow for "pinking up." Good capillary refill is a reflection of the patient's healthy cardiovascular system.

MONITORING THE ELECTROCARDIOGRAM

MODIFIED LEAD II DERIVATION

Cardiac monitoring during sleep testing should be performed using the **Modified Lead II derivation.** This is a method of recording ECG using the right upper chest region and the left lower thorax region for electrode placement.[8] Placement of the leads is the first step; proper placement yields the most useful tracings. The leads are polarized and if not placed properly will invert the tracing. For a three-electrode configuration, the mnemonic of "white to the right, smoke over fire" will assist memory. The white lead is most often placed just below the right clavicle or "collarbone." The black lead or "smoke" is placed on the left just below the clavicle, and the red lead or "fire" is placed on the left ribs on the midaxillary line approximately 6 inches below the armpit.

Many acquisitions systems require placement of only two chest electrodes: the right subclavicular placement and the left mid axillary electrode at the level of the lower ribs (Figure 11-15). For a system with inputs designated as negative (−) and positive (+) for electrocardiogram (ECG) electrode lead connection in the electrode board, the right subclavicular electrode is usually connected to the negative input and the left midaxillary electrode lead is connected to the positive input. At the beginning of the recording, an upright P wave should be confirmed. If inverted, reverse the ECG inputs.

THE ELECTRICAL PATHWAY

The heart functions automatically because it is composed of specially designed muscle cells that are fired rhythmically more than 2.5 billion times in a 70-year lifetime. These muscle cells are triggered via electrical

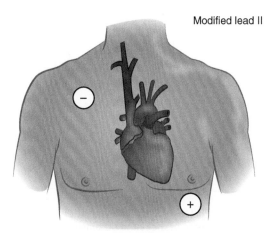

Modified lead II

FIGURE 11-15 Modified lead II electrode placement.

nerve impulses that follow specially designed pathways to meet up with other groups of special cells.

Depolarization is the fundamental electrical event of the heart. The cardiac contractions are regulated primarily by fluctuations of electrolytes moving into and out of the cells. The primary ions are potassium, sodium, and calcium. These molecules are electrically charged particles that create a difference or slope of change between the electrical charge inside and outside of each cell. The outside of the cardiac cell is more positively charged than the inside in its resting state (Figure 11-16).

To stimulate a contraction, the sodium potassium pump allows more sodium and potassium to enter the cell, causing a change in electrical balance between the inside and the outside of the cell. This process is called depolarization and is considered the beginning of a cardiac muscle contraction. When the contraction is complete, repolarization occurs when the "pump" expels sodium and potassium back out of the cell to return to the resting state.

The sinoatrial (SA) node is considered the pacemaker of the heart as the electrical impulses in a normal heartbeat all originate from this location high in the right atrium. The node has an inherent rate of between 60-100 bpm.[10] This rate varies from person to person and can be affected by ANS activation. This means that if a person becomes anxious (perhaps as a result of being startled or scared) and epinephrine, also known as adrenaline, is present, the rate will be higher. Conversely, vagal stimulation results in a lower rate.

The electrical heartbeat begins in the atria in the SA node and the "wave" of electrical charge flows across Bachmann bundle to the left atrium and through the intranodal pathways to the atrioventricular (AV) node. This part of the process results in the P wave of the complex.[1] The electrical charge collects and briefly "rests" in the AV node area. It is important to note that the AV node has an inherent rate of approximately 40-60 bpm. If there is a failure of the SA to conduct, the fail-safe "back-up rate" of the AV node is in place to protect the organism.[10]

The electrical impulse then proceeds from the AV node downward through the bundle of His and eventually bifurcates into the left and right bundle branches. The charge continues down these pathways until they are discharged at the end of the Purkinje fibers. These charges enervate the cardiac muscle in the ventricles, causing them to contract. Notable is that the ventricular tissue also has an inherent rate, which is between 20 and 40 bpm.[10] This, alone, is not sufficient to sustain long-term life in the organism. The ventricular contraction squeezes blood to the lungs and the body tissues via the great vessels and is represented on the ECG tracing as the QRS complex.

THE PQRST COMPLEX

The P wave (Figure 11-17) denotes depolarization, and contraction, of the atria, and typically originates from the SA node.

The QRS complex represents depolarization, which in a healthy heart stimulates contraction of the ventricles. The third wave on the ECG is the T wave, which represents *ventricular repolarization* and relaxation. *Atrial repolarization* cannot be seen because it occurs at the same time the ventricles are depolarizing and is "hidden" within the QRS complex.

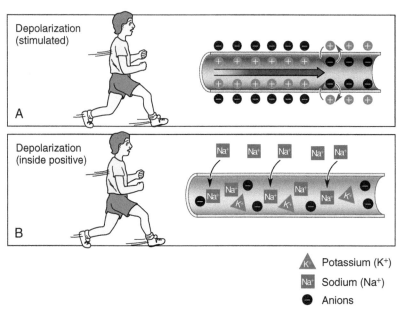

FIGURE 11-16 Depolarization is the movement of ions across a cell membrane causing the inside of the cell to become more positive. *From Aehlert B: ECGs Made Easy, ed 4, St. Louis, 2011, Mosby-Jems.*

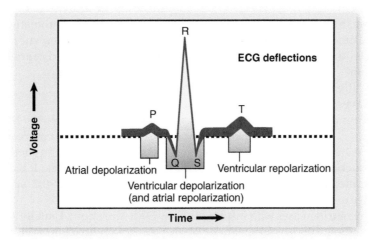

FIGURE 11-17 Electrocardiogram (ECG). Idealized ECG deflections represent depolarization and repolarization of cardiac muscle tissue. *From Patton KT, et al:* Essentials of anatomy and physiology, *St Louis, 2012, Mosby-Elsevier.*

DYSRHYTHMIA INTERPRETATION

THE TECHNOLOGIST'S GUIDE TO DYSRHYTHMIAS

Different types of heart disease or other illness can disrupt the normal contraction-relaxation cycle of the heart. Dysrhythmias cause the heart to beat less effectively and can reduce blood flow to vital organs, which can cause fainting, chest pain, or even sudden death. Dysrhythmias can be broken down into five sections: (1) sinus mechanisms, (2) atrial rhythms, (3) junctional rhythms, (4) ventricular rhythms, and (5) AV conduction delays. Even when the cardiac rhythm appears normal, it is prudent to contact the attending physician if at any time the patient becomes symptomatic (e.g., the patient exhibits confusion, dizziness, lethargy, or syncope).

Evaluating ECG rhythms requires much practice. Using a step-wise methodology is the key to proper interpretation *after* assessing that the tracing is valid. Proper electrode placement is imperative. This technique can guide detection of abnormal heart rhythms known as **dysrhythmias**.

Adhere to the following steps to assess and evaluate the rhythm, including steps for physician notification and follow-up:

1. What is the rate?
2. Is the rhythm regular?
3. What are the atria doing?
4. What are the ventricles doing?
5. What is the relationship between atria and ventricles?

Additional material summarizing technologist response is located in a later chapter.

SINUS MECHANISMS

Normal Sinus Rhythm

- Rate: 60-100 bpm
- Rhythm: P-P interval regular; R-R interval regular
- P waves: Upright in modified lead II; one precedes each QRS complex; P waves look alike
- PR interval: 0.12-0.2 seconds and constant from beat to beat (refer to Figure 11-18)
- QRS duration: Usually 0.1 seconds or less, unless an intraventricular conduction delay exists
- Conduction: A QRS complex follows each P wave

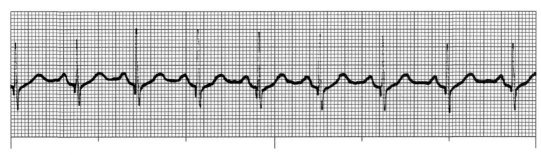

FIGURE 11-18 Normal sinus rhythm. *From Aehlert B:* ECGs made easy, *ed 4, St Louis, 2011, Mosby, Inc., an imprint of Elsevier, Inc.*

Sinus Arrhythmia

- Rate: Usually 60-100 bpm, but variable
- Rhythm: Irregular; phasic with breathing; heart rate increases gradually during inspiration and decreases with exhalation
- P waves: Upright in modified lead II; one precedes each QRS complex; P waves look alike
- PR interval: 0.12-0.2 seconds and constant from beat to beat
- QRS duration: Usually 0.1 seconds or less, unless an intraventricular conduction delay exists
- Conduction: A QRS complex follows each P wave

The sinus arrhythmia (Figure 11-19) is initiated at the SA node as a normal beat. The rate increases with inspiration and decreases with expiration. This is a normal finding in children and young adults, and is typically benign.

Sinus Bradycardia

- Rate: Less than 60 bpm
- Rhythm: P-P interval regular; R-R interval regular
- P waves: Upright in modified lead II; one precedes each QRS complex; P waves look alike
- PR interval: 0.12-0.2 seconds and constant from beat to beat
- QRS duration: Usually 0.1 seconds or less, unless an intraventricular conduction delay exists
- Conduction: A QRS complex follows each P wave

Sinus bradycardia (Figure 11-20) is common in athletes and is usually observed but not treated. For physically fit individuals, this should be documented at the beginning of the study to ensure it is not later misinterpreted. Some subjects have a normal resting heart rate that would represent an emergent event for the average patient.

Sinus Tachycardia

- Rate: Greater than 100 bpm
- Rhythm: P-P interval regular; R-R interval regular
- P waves: Upright in modified lead II; one precedes each QRS complex; P waves look alike
- PR interval: 0.12-0.2 seconds and constant from beat to beat
- QRS duration: Usually 0.1 seconds or less, unless an intraventricular conduction delay exists
- Conduction: A QRS complex follows each P wave

Sinus tachycardia (Figure 11-21) is a normal response to exercise and other stressors. It may accompany hypoxia, infection, fever, a heart condition, caffeine ingestion, nicotine use, or decongestant administration. It is important to treat the cause of the tachycardia. Sinus tachycardia may cause inefficient blood circulation, inducing palpitations or dizziness.

If the patient is cyanotic, or has labored breathing or chest pain, the technologist should contact the physician immediately or activate the emergency services per protocol; however, sinus tachycardia during a sleep study is usually benign and only warrants that the technologist documents its occurrence and continues monitoring.

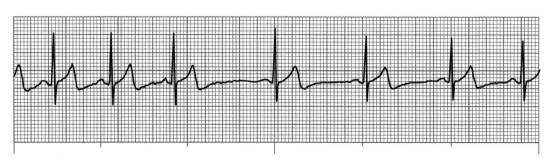

FIGURE 11-19 Sinus arrhythmia. *From Aehlert B:* ECGs made easy, *ed 4, St Louis, 2011, Mosby, Inc., an imprint of Elsevier, Inc.*

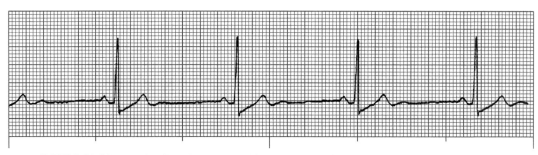

FIGURE 11-20 Sinus bradycardia. *From Aehlert B:* ECGs made easy, *ed 4, St Louis, 2011, Mosby, Inc., an imprint of Elsevier, Inc.*

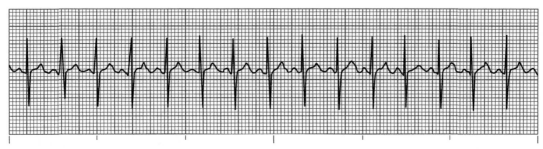

FIGURE 11-21 Sinus tachycardia. *From Aehlert B: ECGs made easy, ed 4, St Louis, 2011, Mosby, Inc., an imprint of Elsevier, Inc.*

Sinoatrial Block (Sinoatrial Pause)

- Rate: Usually normal but varies because of the pause
- Rhythm: Irregular because of the pauses caused by the SA block; the pause is the same as, or an exact multiple of, the distance between two other P-P intervals
- P waves: Upright in modified lead II and look alike; when present, one precedes each QRS
- PR interval: 0.12-0.2 seconds and constant from beat to beat
- QRS duration: Usually 0.1 seconds or less, unless an intraventricular conduction delay exists
- Conduction: A QRS complex follows each P wave that is present

When SA block occurs (Figure 11-22), exactly one PQRST will be missing, or an exact multiple of this distance. The technologist should contact the physician in the event of an SA block and document its identification on the recording.

Sinus Arrest

- Rate: Usually normal, but varies because of the pause
- Rhythm: Regular except for the event; pause is of undetermined length and not a multiple of other P-P intervals
- P waves: Upright in modified lead II when present; one precedes each QRS
- PR interval: When present 0.12-0.2 seconds
- QRS duration: Usually 0.1 seconds or less, unless abnormally conducted
- Conduction: A QRS complex follows each P wave that is present

Sinus arrest is differentiated from SA block because it is not the exact distance of other P-P intervals (Figure 11-23). More than one PQRST is missing and the absence of activity is not a multiple of other P-P intervals.

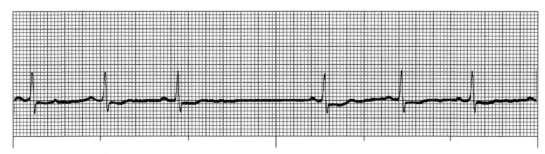

FIGURE 11-22 Sinus rhythm at a rate of 36 to 71 beats/min with an episode of sinoatrial block. *From Aehlert B: ECGs made easy, ed 4, St Louis, 2011, Mosby, Inc., an imprint of Elsevier, Inc.*

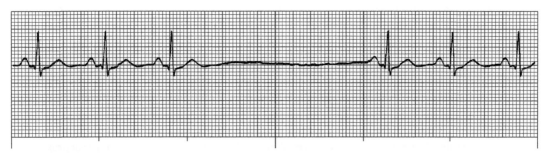

FIGURE 11-23 Sinus rhythm at a rate of 24 to 81 beats/min with an episode of sinus arrest. *From Aehlert B: ECGs made easy, ed 4, St Louis, 2011, Mosby, Inc., an imprint of Elsevier, Inc.*

Periods of sinus arrest lasting as long as 9 seconds have been reported during sleep in young, healthy subjects with apparently normal cardiac function. For these individuals additional dysrhythmias did not occur as a result. For the 13.5 million patients with cardiac disease in the United States, nocturnal asystolic events can set the stage for often life-threatening ventricular arrhythmias.[7]

ATRIAL RHYTHMS

Premature Atrial Contraction

- Rate: Usually normal, but depends on the underlying rhythm
- Rhythm: Regular with premature beats
- P waves: Premature; differ from sinus P waves; may be lost in preceding T wave; upright in modified lead II; one precedes each QRS complex
- PR interval: May be normal or prolonged
- QRS duration: Usually 0.1 seconds or less, unless abnormally conducted
- Conduction: Each P produces a QRS; each premature beat is followed by a *compensatory pause*

The impulse arises as an ectopic atrial focus (outside the SA node) resulting in P waves that appear abnormal (Figure 11-24). The impulse reaches the AV node and conducts through the ventricles in a normal fashion. The patient may be completely unaware of the premature atrial contraction (PAC), or it may be perceived as a "skipped" beat.

Atrial Tachycardia

- Rate: 100-250 bpm
- Rhythm: P-P interval regular; R-R interval regular
- P waves: Atrial waves differ from sinus waves
- PR interval: May be shorter or longer than normal
- QRS duration: Usually 0.1 seconds or less, unless abnormally conducted
- Conduction: A QRS complex follows each P wave

Atrial tachycardia is one of the supraventricular tachycardias—tachycardias that originate above the ventricles. Rhythms and beats that originate above the ventricles have a normal or "narrow" QRS, whereas ventricular rhythms and beats have an abnormally wide QRS complex. Atrial tachycardia occurs when one or more cells or areas of tissue within the atria become irritable and an ectopic focus or foci are responsible for the cardiac rhythm.

Paroxysmal atrial tachycardia appears and ends suddenly. Because of the fast rate, the P wave may be superimposed on the preceding T wave, resulting in a notched appearance, or the P wave may be completely unidentifiable and buried in the T wave. In the latter case, the T waves will be taller than those that occur before or after the period during which atrial tachycardia is present.

In Figure 11-25, the atrial tachycardia abruptly ends as it converts to normal sinus rhythm. Note the

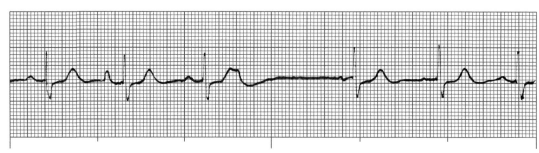

FIGURE 11-24 Sinus rhythm with a nonconducted (blocked) premature atrial contraction. *From Aehlert B: ECGs made easy, ed 4, St Louis, 2011, Mosby, Inc., an imprint of Elsevier, Inc.*

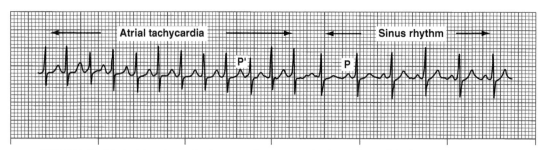

FIGURE 11-25 Atrial tachycardia (a type of supraventricular tachycardia) that ends spontaneously with the abrupt resumption of sinus rhythm. The P waves of the tachycardia (rate: approximately 150 beats/min) are superimposed on the preceding waves. *From Aehlert B: ECGs made easy, ed 4, St Louis, 2011, Mosby, Inc., an imprint of Elsevier, Inc.*

height of the T wave during atrial tachycardia as compared with the T wave during sinus rhythm.

Multiformed Atrial Rhythm

- Rate: Usually 60-100 bpm; if greater than 100 bpm, the rhythm is called *multifocal atrial tachycardia*
- Rhythm: May be irregular as site of conduction shifts from SA node to ectopic atrial locations and AV junction
- P waves: Size, shape, and direction may change from beat to beat
- PR interval: Varies
- QRS duration: Usually 0.1 seconds or less, unless abnormally conducted
- Conduction: A QRS complex follows each P wave

Previously known as *wandering atrial pacemaker*, multiformed atrial rhythm occurs when the dominant pacemaker shifts from the SA node, atria, and AV junction. Identification requires that at least three variations of P wave size, shape, or direction be present (Figure 11-26). Any time the site responsible for origination of the impulse to pace the heart changes, the P wave will also change. The P-P, R-R, and PR intervals will be irregular because of the different sites of impulse formation.[10]

Atrial Flutter

- Rate: Atrial rate 250-450 bpm (flutter waves); ventricular rate variable
- Rhythm: Atrial regular; ventricular regular or irregular
- P waves: No identifiable P waves; sawtoothed "flutter" waves replace them
- PR interval: Not measurable
- QRS duration: Usually 0.1 seconds or less, unless abnormally conducted
- Conduction: Typically either a 2:1, 3:1, or 4:1 flutter wave/QRS relationship

Atrial flutter is easily recognized because two or more sawtooth-shaped flutter waves occur before each QRS (Figure 11-27). Although transitional periods can occur, usually either two, three, or four flutter waves consistently precede each QRS. This is classified as a ratio of 2:1, 3:1, or 4:1 atrial flutter. This is not considered life threatening; however, consult a physician if the patient is symptomatic or does not have a documented history of atrial flutter.

Because blood pools within the atria during atrial flutter, which can lead to the formation of clots, the physician should be contacted in the event of new-onset atrial flutter or if sustained atrial flutter ends during testing in the sleep laboratory.

Atrial Fibrillation

- Rate: Atrial rate 400-600 bpm fibrillation waves; ventricular rate variable
- Rhythm: Chaotic atrial activity; ventricular rhythm usually irregularly irregular
- P waves: No identifiable P waves; fibrillatory waves present; erratic; wavy baseline
- PR interval: Not measurable
- QRS duration: Usually 0.1 seconds or less, unless abnormally conducted
- Conduction: The AV node blocks most impulses

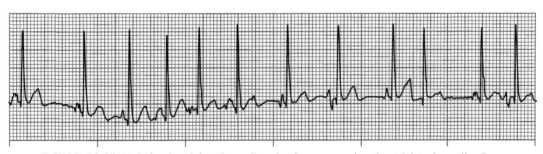

FIGURE 11-26 Multifocal atrial tachycardia, also known as *chaotic atrial tachycardia. From Aehlert B: ECGs made easy, ed 4, St Louis, 2011, Mosby, Inc., an imprint of Elsevier, Inc.*

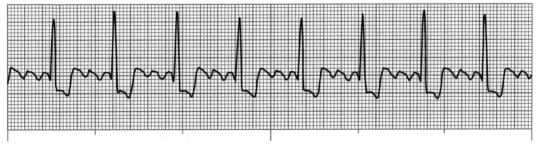

FIGURE 11-27 Atrial flutter. *From Aehlert B: ECGs made easy, ed 4, St Louis, 2011, Mosby, Inc., an imprint of Elsevier, Inc.*

During atrial fibrillation there is no coordinated activation process in the atria (Figure 11-28); the atria are quivering. Although usually benign, the physician should be contacted if the patient becomes symptomatic or no documentation of a history of atrial fibrillation is present. Because pooling of blood within the atria and the formation of blood clots are associated with both new-onset and offset of atrial fibrillation, the physician should be contacted for either.

A clear relationship exists between obstructive sleep apnea (OSA) and atrial fibrillation. It has been reported that 32% of general cardiac patients have OSA, which should not be surprising; however, within the subset of these patients who have atrial fibrillation, 49% are positive for the disorder.[11]

For patients with both atrial fibrillation and OSA, treatment of the atrial fibrillation is not very effective unless the OSA is first treated and the patient is compliant with the prescribed therapy. When patients with documented OSA who were not receiving effective PAP therapy were cardioverted for atrial fibrillation, there was a 12-month recurrence rate of 82%. OSA patients receiving effective PAP had only a 42% recurrence rate.[7]

JUNCTIONAL RHYTHMS

Junctional rhythms originate in the AV node and occur because of failure or disruption in conduction that normally arises from the SA node. The SA node fires an electrical impulse that proceeds in a forward, or **antegrade**, fashion toward the AV node. The impulse travels through the AV node and proceeds to the ventricles. If, however, conduction from the SA node fails and the impulse responsible for AV contraction is initiated at the AV node, the impulse will proceed backward through the atria and forward to the ventricles. These backward flowing, or **retrograde**, impulses result in an inverted P wave. Sometimes the inverted P wave appears before the QRS complex, sometimes after the QRS complex, and sometimes not at all because it occurs during ventricular contraction and is buried within the QRS complex (Figure 11-29).

Junctional rhythms and events are not considered life threatening, so contacting the attending physician and documenting their presence is adequate. Premature junctional contractions are considered benign, which negates the need to contact the physician when they alone occur.

Premature Junctional Complex

- Rate: Usually normal but depends on underlying rhythm
- Rhythm: Regular with premature beats
- P waves: May occur before, during, or after the QRS; if visible will be inverted in modified lead II
- PR interval: If a P wave occurs before the QRS, usually 0.12 seconds or less; otherwise no PR interval
- QRS duration: Usually 0.1 seconds or less, unless aberrantly conducted or an intraventricular delay exists
- Conduction: Retrograde for event

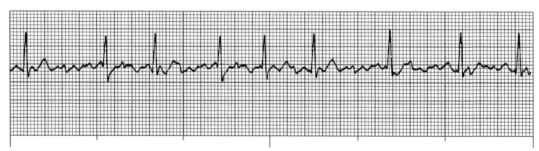

FIGURE 11-28 Atrial fibrillation with a ventricular response of 67 to 120 beats/min.

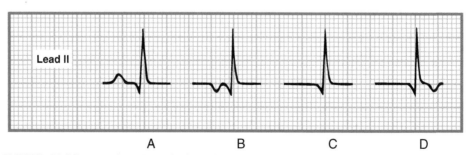

FIGURE 11-29 A, With a sinus rhythm, the P wave is positive (upright) in lead II because the wave of depolarization is moved toward the positive electrode. The P wave associated with a junctional beat (in lead II) may be **B,** inverted (retrograde) and appear before the QRS; **C,** be hidden by the QRS, or **D,** appear after the QRS. *From Aehlert B: ECGs made easy, ed 4, St Louis, 2011, Mosby, Inc., an imprint of Elsevier, Inc.*

A premature junctional complex (PJC) or contraction occurs when an irritable focus within the AV junction fires before the next normal impulse is conducted at the SA node. The retrograde travel of this event disrupts the normal conduction cycle and causes an inverted P wave that can occur before, during, or after the QRS complex. They are not, in and of themselves, worrisome. The recoding technologist should document identification of the abnormality within his or her notes.

Junctional complexes can come early or they can come late. If they are early, the event is a PJC. If the complex is late, it is a junctional escape beat and represents initiation of the cardiac cycle by the AV junction caused by failure of the SA node.[10]

The early beat in Figure 11-30 has an inverted P wave followed by compensatory pause. The P wave of a PJC is earlier than expected for the underlying rhythm, and can be before the QRS, buried within the QRS, or after the QRS. If seen, it will be inverted.

Junctional Escape Beats

- Rate: Usually normal but depends on underlying rhythm
- Rhythm: Regular with *late* beats
- P waves: May occur before, during, or after the QRS; if visible, will be inverted in modified lead II
- PR interval: If a P wave occurs before the QRS, usually 0.12 seconds or less; otherwise no PR interval

- QRS duration: Usually 0.1 seconds or less, unless aberrantly conducted or an intraventricular delay exists
- Conduction: Retrograde for event

A junctional escape beat is generated when an abnormally long amount of time has elapsed since the previous beat. The cardiac impulse does not originate above the AV junction, so it takes over as the cardiac pacemaker. Because the AV junction is waiting for the impulse from above, a junctional escape beat is always late as compared with the underlying rhythm. In Figure 11-31, a sinus arrest lasts approximately 1.4 seconds before an impulse is generated by the AV junction to pace the cardiac cycle.

Junctional Escape Rhythm

- Rate: 40-60 bpm
- Rhythm: Very regular
- P waves: May occur before, during, or after the QRS; if visible will be inverted in modified lead II
- PR interval: If a P wave occurs before the QRS, usually 0.12 seconds or less; otherwise no PR interval
- QRS duration: Usually 0.1 seconds or less, unless aberrantly conducted or an intraventricular delay exists
- Conduction: Retrograde

The junctional rhythm, also referred to as the *junctional escape rhythm,* is several junctional escape beats in a row. In Figure 11-32 there is a total absence of normal P waves; the P waves that can be

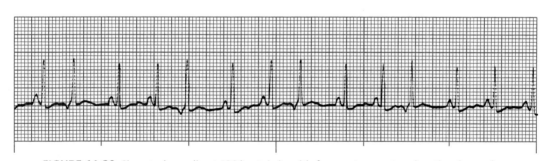

FIGURE 11-30 Sinus tachycardia at 136 beats/min with frequent premature junctional complex. *From Aehlert B: ECGs made easy, ed 4, St Louis, 2011, Mosby, Inc., an imprint of Elsevier, Inc.*

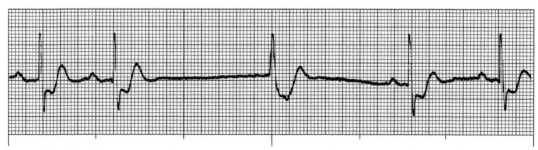

FIGURE 11-31 Sinus rhythm at 71 beats/min with a prolonged PR interval (0.24 sec), an episode of sinus arrest, a junctional escape beat, and ST-segment depression. *From Aehlert B: ECGs made easy, ed 4, St Louis, 2011, Mosby, Inc., an imprint of Elsevier, Inc.*

seen are inverted. The AV junction has taken over as the heart's pacemaker at the intrinsic rate of 40-60 bpm expected for tissue of this area. The technologist should contact the attending physician and document identification of the abnormal rhythm.

At the onset of this rhythm, one should expect to identify a late junctional escape beat followed by the junctional escape rhythm. A pause is normal before all escape beats and all escape rhythms have a rate consistent with the intrinsic rate of the tissue generating them. When a junctional rhythm occurs at a rate less than 40 bpm, it is termed *junctional bradycardia*.[10]

Accelerated Junctional Rhythm

- Rate: 61-100 bpm
- Rhythm: Very regular
- P waves: May occur before, during, or after the QRS; if visible, will be inverted in modified lead II
- PR interval: If a P wave occurs before the QRS, usually 0.12 seconds or less; otherwise no PR interval

- QRS duration: Usually 0.1 seconds or less, unless aberrantly conducted or an intraventricular delay exists
- Conduction: Retrograde

In Figure 11-33 all P waves are inverted and the rate is faster than the inherent rate for this area of tissue. This can be attributed to increased sympathetic nervous system activation, hypoxia, or an active myocardial infarction. As with the junctional escape rhythm, this is not a primary phenomenon and only needs to be brought to the attention of the attending physician. It is likely due to enhanced automaticity of the bundle of His.[10]

Junctional Tachycardia

- Rate: 101-180 bpm
- Rhythm: Very regular
- P waves: May occur before, during, or after the QRS; if visible, will be inverted in modified lead II
- PR interval: If a P wave occurs before the QRS, usually 0.12 seconds or less; otherwise no PR interval

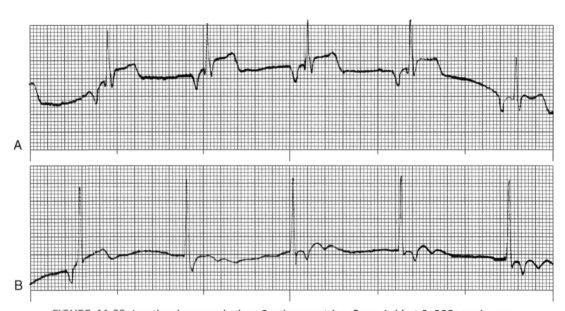

FIGURE 11-32 Junctional escape rhythm. Continuous strips. *From Aehlert B:* ECGs made easy, *ed 4, St Louis, 2011, Mosby, Inc., an imprint of Elsevier, Inc.*

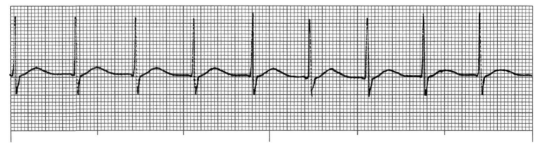

FIGURE 11-33 Accelerated junctional rhythm at 93 beats/min. *From Aehlert B:* ECGs made easy, *ed 4, St Louis, 2011, Mosby, Inc., an imprint of Elsevier, Inc.*

- QRS duration: Usually 0.1 seconds or less, unless aberrantly conducted or an intraventricular delay exists
- Conduction: Retrograde

The junctional tachycardia in Figure 11-34 has a rate of 120 bpm. Note the P waves that consistently fall after the QRS complex. As with all junctional rhythms and complexes, the P wave can occur before, during, or after the QRS. When it falls during the QRS, it is buried by the voltage of the complex and cannot be seen. Junctional tachycardia is an ectopic rhythm that originates in the pacemaker cells found in the bundle of His. When three or more PJCs occur in a row at a rate greater than 100 bpm, a junctional tachycardia exists.

Paroxysmal junctional tachycardia usually starts suddenly with a PJC and ends abruptly. Nonparoxysmal junctional tachycardia usually starts as accelerated junctional rhythm from which the rate gradually increases.[10]

VENTRICULAR RHYTHMS

Excitation originating below the bifurcation of the bundle of His is responsible for ventricular rhythms. Ventricular rhythms are easy to identify because of the frequent lack of a P wave, and a wide and often bizarre QRS complex. The ventricles are the heart's least efficient pacemaker and have an intrinsic rate of 20-40 bpm. The ventricles may assume charge as the pacer if the SA node fails to discharge, if it is blocked as it exits the SA node, if SA node discharge is slower than 40 bpm, or if an irritable focus within either ventricle produces an early beat or rapid rhythm.[10]

Ventricular dysrhythmias have been associated with sleep-disordered breathing, particularly during severe oxyhemoglobin desaturation and in patients with coronary heart disease. Fortunately, these rhythms are virtually eliminated by treatment of the breathing disorder.[7]

Premature Ventricular Complexes (Contractions)

A premature ventricular complex (PVC) represents premature depolarization caused by an irritable focus that arises from within the ventricles. These early beats disrupt the regular cardiac rhythm and are easily distinguished by their wide, bizarre QRS. The vast majority of uniform and unifocal PVCs (Figure 11-35) are benign, but as their frequency increases, they become more worrisome because the heart may become hypoxic. When PVCs are multiform (multifocal), and arise from more than one area within the ventricles (Figure 11-36), or when they fall on the T wave, known as R-on-T PVCs, the physician should be contacted (Figure 11-37).

As with all premature contractions, a compensatory pause follows PVCs. When two PVCs occur in a row, they are referred to as *paired PVCs* or *PVC couplets.* An interpolated PVC does not interfere with the normal cardiac cycle and does not have a full compensatory

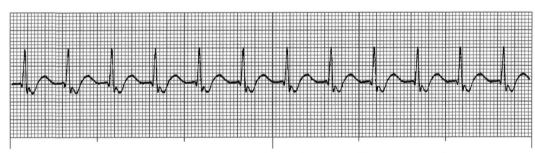

FIGURE 11-34 Junctional tachycardia at 120 beats/min. *From Aehlert B: ECGs made easy, ed 4, St Louis, 2011, Mosby, Inc., an imprint of Elsevier, Inc.*

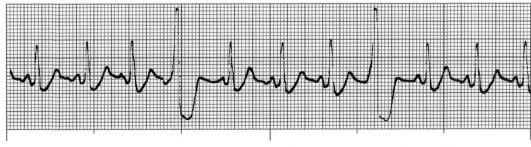

FIGURE 11-35 Sinus tachycardia with frequent uniform premature ventricular complexes. *From Aehlert B: ECGs made easy, ed 4, St Louis, 2011, Mosby, Inc., an imprint of Elsevier, Inc.*

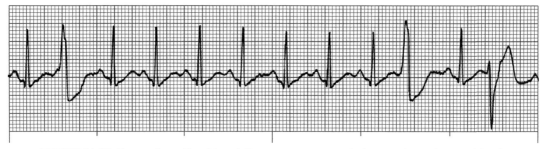

FIGURE 11-36 Sinus tachycardia with multiform premature ventricular complexes. *From Aehlert B: ECGs made easy, ed 4, St Louis, 2011, Mosby, Inc., an imprint of Elsevier, Inc.*

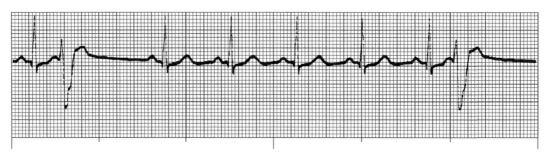

FIGURE 11-37 Sinus rhythm with two R-on-T premature ventricular complexes. *From Aehlert B: ECGs made easy, ed 4, St Louis, 2011, Mosby, Inc., an imprint of Elsevier, Inc.*

pause. When every other beat is a PVC, this is described as *bigeminal PVCs* or *ventricular bigeminy* (Figure 11-38). Trigeminal PVCs, or ventricular trigeminy, describes a rhythm for which every third beat is a PVC, and quadrigeminal PVCs (ventricular quadrigeminy) refers to a PVC that occurs on every fourth beat.[10]

Common causes of PVCs include hypoxia; stress; anxiety; exercise; acid-base imbalance; stimulants, including tobacco and caffeine; increased sympathetic tone; myocardial ischemia; electrolyte imbalance; congestive heart failure; acute coronary syndromes; digitalis toxicity; and various prescription, over-the-counter, and illicit drugs.[10] Given the patient population studied in the sleep laboratory, it is no surprise that PVCs are frequently encountered during the course of testing.

Premature Ventricular Complexes

- Rate: Usually normal, but depends on underlying rhythm
- Rhythm: Essentially regular with premature beats; if the PVC is interpolated, the rhythm will be regular
- P waves: Usually absent or, with retrograde conduction to the atria, may appear after the QRS
- PR interval: None; ectopic beat originates in the ventricle
- QRS duration: Greater than 0.12 seconds, wide, bizarre; T wave usually in opposite direction of the QRS
- Conduction: Ectopic ventricular focus, or foci; retrograde conduction to the atria possible

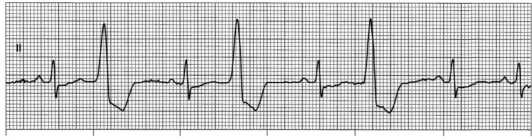

FIGURE 11-38 Ventricular bigeminy. *From Aehlert B: ECGs made easy, ed 4, St Louis, 2011, Mosby, Inc., an imprint of Elsevier, Inc.*

Unifocal Premature Ventricular Complexes

Unifocal PVCs are two or more PVCs with the same appearance that arise from a single irritable focus within a ventricle.

Multifocal Premature Ventricular Complexes

Multifocal PVCs are irritable foci arising from more than one area of the ventricles that have different morphologic characteristics. They manifest as two or more PVCs that differ in morphologic characteristics, amplitude, duration, or polarity.

R-on-T Premature Ventricular Complexes

R-on-T PVCs are serious events that occur when the R wave of a PVC falls on the T wave of the preceding beat (see Figure 11-37). Because the T wave occurs during the relative refractory stage of depolarization, the ventricles are sensitive to any electrical stimulation. It is possible for R-on-T PVCs to cause conversion to a life-threatening dysrhythmia such as ventricular fibrillation (V-fib) or ventricular tachycardia. The attending physician should be contacted when these events are identified.

Ventricular Bigeminy

Ventricular bigeminy exists when every other beat is a PVC. This becomes concerning if it does not resolve in a short period or if the patient is symptomatic. The physician should be contacted if PVCs are multifocal, or if the patient becomes symptomatic.

Ventricular Trigeminy

As with ventricular bigeminy, contact the physician if the PVCs during an episode of ventricular trigeminy (Figure 11-39) are multifocal or if the patient becomes symptomatic. The physician should also be contacted when ventricular escape beats, as discussed in the following section, are noted. All ventricular complexes should be noted in the recording technologist's notes and the sleep study report.

Ventricular Escape Beats

- Rate: Usually normal but depends on underlying rhythm
- Rhythm: Essentially regular with late beats; the ventricular escape beat occurs after an expected sinus beat
- P waves: Usually absent or with retrograde conduction to the atria may appear after the QRS
- PR interval: None with ventricular escape beat; ectopic beat originates in the ventricle
- QRS duration: Greater than 0.12 seconds, wide, bizarre; T wave frequently in opposite direction of the QRS
- Conduction: Ectopic ventricular focus fires in the absence of conduction from the atria; delayed beat

A ventricular escape beat occurs following the pause, during which it is waiting for the supraventricular pacer to fire. The escape beat is late compared with the underlying rhythm as seen in Figure 11-40 following nonconducted PACs. As a protective mechanism, a ventricular escape beat prevents more extreme slowing of the heart or even asystole. All escape beats are late and if the impulse must continue pacing the heart, the escape rhythm will have a rate consistent with the intrinsic rhythm of the tissue within the given area of the heart.

Junctional escape beats can progress to a junctional escape rhythm with a rate of 40 to 60 bpm. When three or more ventricular escape beats occur in a row, the resultant ventricular escape, or idioventricular rhythm (IVR) will have the intrinsic rate of the ventricles, which is 20 to 40 bpm.[10] At minimum, the physician should be contacted any time a ventricular rhythm is noted, and specific ventricular rhythms warrant contacting emergency medical services (EMS) immediately.

Idioventricular Rhythm

- Rate: 20-40 bpm
- Rhythm: Essentially regular
- P waves: Usually absent or with retrograde conduction to the atria may appear after the QRS
- PR interval: None

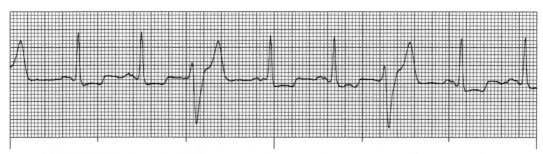

FIGURE 11-39 Ventricular trigeminy. *From Aehlert B: ECGs made easy, ed 4, St Louis, 2011, Mosby, Inc., an imprint of Elsevier, Inc.*

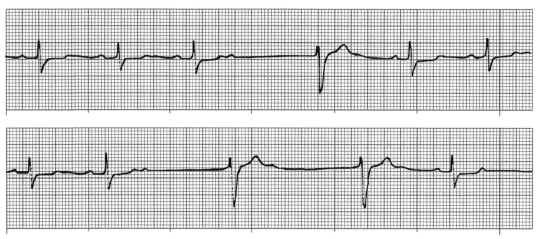

FIGURE 11-40 Sinus rhythm with a prolonged PR interval, ST segment depression. Note the ventricular escape beats following nonconducted premature atrial complexes.

- QRS duration: Greater than 0.12 seconds; T wave frequently in opposite direction of the QRS
- Conduction: Three or more ventricular escape beats in a row

Accelerated Idioventricular Rhythm

- Rate: 41-100 bpm
- Rhythm: Essentially regular
- P waves: Usually absent or with retrograde conduction to the atria may appear after the QRS
- PR interval: None
- QRS duration: Greater than 0.12 seconds; T wave frequently in opposite direction of the QRS
- Conduction: Three or more ventricular escape beats in a row at a rate of 41-100 bpm

Some ventricular rhythms are considered fairly benign in the critical care setting, as they occur normally following events such as myocardial infarction. In the sleep testing environment, however, some of these rhythms, which likely cannot support life in the long term, are viewed quite differently. As an example, at the unlikely onset of either IVR (as seen in Figure 11-41) or accelerated IVR (as seen in Figure 11-42), the technologist should summon EMS and contact the attending physician immediately to ensure patient safety.

Monomorphic Ventricular Tachycardia

- Rate: 101-250 bpm
- Rhythm: Essentially regular
- P waves: May be present or absent; if present they will have no relationship to ventricular rhythm or rate
- PR interval: None
- QRS duration: Greater than 0.12 seconds; often difficult to differentiate
- Conduction: Three or more PVCs in a row; wide, bizarre QRS complexes

Polymorphic Ventricular Tachycardia

- Rate: 150-300 bpm
- Rhythm: May be regular or irregular
- P waves: None
- PR interval: None

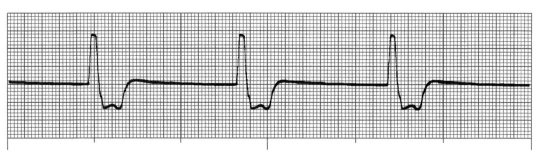

FIGURE 11-41 Idioventricular rhythm at 35 beats/min. *From Aehlert B: ECGs made easy, ed 4, St Louis, 2011, Mosby, Inc., an imprint of Elsevier, Inc.*

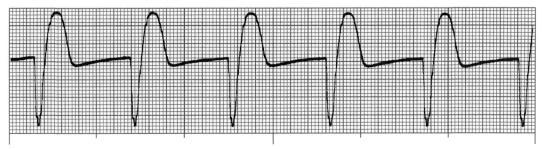

FIGURE 11-42 Accelerated idioventricular rhythm at 56 beats/min. *From Aehlert B: ECGs made easy, ed 4, St Louis, 2011, Mosby, Inc., an imprint of Elsevier, Inc.*

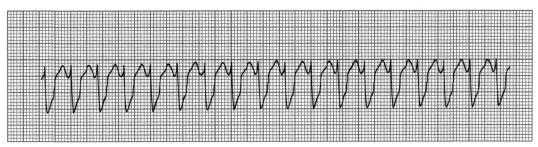

FIGURE 11-43 Ventricular tachycardia. *From Wilkins RL, et al: Clinical assessment in respiratory care, ed 6, St Louis, 2010, Mosby.*

- QRS duration: Greater than 0.12 seconds; often difficult to differentiate
- Conduction: Three or more PVCs in a row; wide, bizarre QRS complexes that vary in shape and amplitude

Three or more PVCs in a row defines a run of ventricular tachycardia (Figure 11-43), which is frequently seen during sleep testing of patients with OSA. When ventricular tachycardia is sustained for greater than 30 seconds, or according to facility policy, assess patient responsiveness, contact EMS and begin cardiopulmonary resuscitation (CPR) as warranted, and notify the attending physician as soon as practical. The life-threatening dysrhythmia can be subclassified as monomorphic (Figure 11-44) or polymorphic (Figure 11-45), but this differentiation is only helpful in recognizing differences in appearance; the technologist response does not differ.

! Polymorphic ventricular tachycardia is a medical emergency and should be dealt with as such by (1) assessing the patient for responsiveness, pulse, and breathing; (2) activating the emergency response system; and (3) initiating CPR with automatic external defibrillator (AED) use. If the patient can be aroused, the tracing is most likely artifactual.

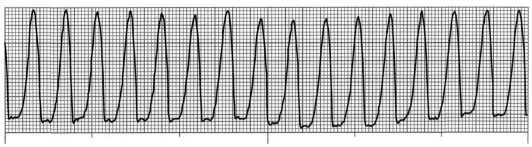

FIGURE 11-44 Monomorphic ventricular tachycardia. *From Aehlert B: ECGs made easy, ed 4, St Louis, 2011, Mosby, Inc., an imprint of Elsevier, Inc.*

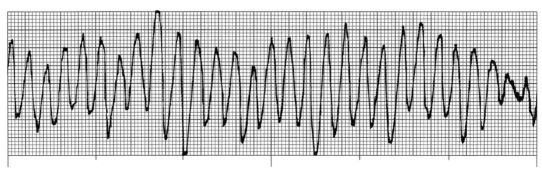

FIGURE 11-45 Polymorphic ventricular tachycardia. *From Aehlert B:* ECGs made easy, *ed 4, St Louis, 2011, Mosby, Inc., an imprint of Elsevier, Inc.*

Ventricular Fibrillation

- Rate: Unable to measure; no discernible waves or complexes
- Rhythm: Chaotic; rapid; no pattern or regularity
- P waves: Not discernible
- PR interval: Not discernible
- QRS duration: Not discernible
- Conduction: The ventricles are quivering; visually classified as coarse or fine; no PQRST

When the ventricles are fibrillating (Figure 11-46), very little if any blood is being pumped through the circulatory system. For this life-threatening dysrhythmia, the technologist should assess patient responsiveness, contact EMS and begin CPR as warranted, and notify the attending physician as soon as practical. If an AED is available, it should be used along with CPR until EMS arrives to take over. The technologist must always assess the patient and never rely solely on the monitor to evaluate a rhythm for which intervention is required. However, to ensure that the rhythm leads to patient assessment and necessary interventions, the technologist must first identify the rhythm as abnormal.

V-fib is classified into two main forms. Fine V-fib (Figure 11-47) can look like a disconnected electrode or electrode board. Coarse V-fib as seen in Figure 11-48, however, is what is typically thought of as V-fib. The response is the same, and the deadly nature of this rhythm is consistent regardless of the classification. Nothing can replace quick technologist response toward assessing the patient, starting CPR, and attaching and using the automated external defibrillator.

> **!** V-fib is a medical emergency and should be dealt with as such by (1) assessing the patient for responsiveness, pulse, and breathing; (2) activating the emergency response system; and (3) initiating CPR with AED. If the patient can be aroused, the tracing is most likely artifactual.

Asystole (Cardiac Standstill)

- Rate: Unable to measure; no discernible QRS but atrial activity may be seen (P wave asystole)
- Rhythm: Ventricular not discernible; atrial may be discernible
- P waves: Usually not discernible
- PR interval: Not measurable

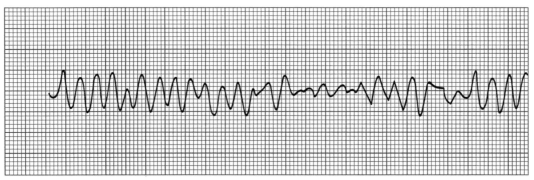

FIGURE 11-46 Ventricular fibrillation. *From Wilkins RL, et al:* Clinical assessment in respiratory care, *ed 6, St Louis, 2010, Mosby.*

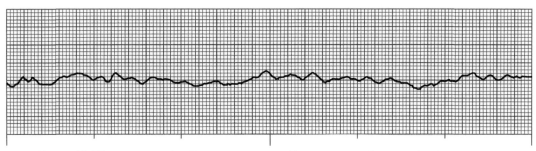

Figure 11-47 Fine ventricular fibrillation. *From Aehlert B: ECGs made easy, ed 4, St Louis, 2011, Mosby, Inc., an imprint of Elsevier, Inc.*

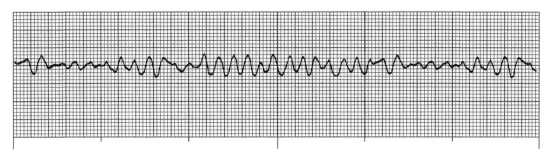

FIGURE 11-48 Coarse ventricular fibrillation. *From Aehlert B: ECGs made easy, ed 4, St Louis, 2011, Mosby, Inc., an imprint of Elsevier, Inc.*

- QRS duration: Absent
- Conduction: No conduction through the heart; pulseless electrical activity may be seen from SA node

Asystole (Figure 11-49) is an absence of electrical and mechanical activity of the heart. If identified on the polysomnogram and the patient can be aroused or a pulse can be palpated, it is most likely artifact from a disconnected electrode. Anytime a life-threatening or potentially life-threatening dysrhythmia is suspected based on pattern recognition of recorded data, the patient should be physically assessed prior to responding with heroic efforts. The technologist must always treat the patient, not the monitor. If asystole is confirmed by patient assessment, EMS should be contacted, CPR should be initiated, and the attending physician contacted as soon as practical.

A phenomenon known as *P wave asystole* or *pulseless electrical activity* (Figure 11-50) occurs when the SA node continues to fire an impulse, but the heart muscle does not capture it. Despite electrical activity on the monitor, the heart is in standstill.

 If on assessment the patient is pulseless and nonresponsive, activate the emergency response system, begin CPR, continue CPR until EMS personnel arrive to take over, and notify the attending physician.

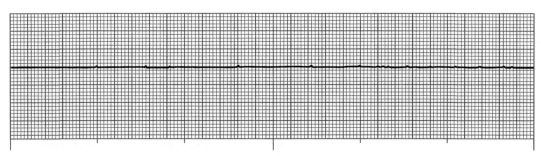

FIGURE 11-49 Asystole. *From Aehlert B: ECGs made easy, ed 4, St Louis, 2011, Mosby, Inc., an imprint of Elsevier, Inc.*

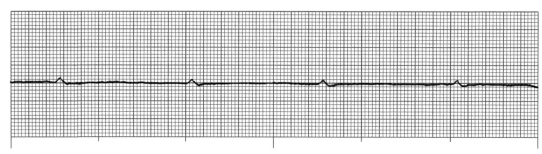

FIGURE 11-50 "P wave" asystole (also known as *ventricular standstill*). *From Aehlert B:* ECGs made easy, *ed 4, St Louis, 2011, Mosby, Inc., an imprint of Elsevier, Inc.*

In the sleep testing center, it is not uncommon for an episode of sinus arrest to last upward of 6 seconds in patients with severe sleep-disordered breathing. This is *not* asystole and does not warrant contacting emergency personnel. However, both sinus pause and sinus arrest should be reported to the physician and documented, and the technologist should continue monitoring the patient's ECG for additional dysrhythmias. If sinus arrest occurs with frequency and is associated with sleep-disordered breathing, application of continuous PAP may be indicated, according to facility policy.

Atrioventricular Blocks

Many people have difficulty with the concept of AV blocks, also known as *heart blocks*. They are very simple to remember if divided into "predictable" and "unpredictable." The predictable blocks are not very worrisome and the unpredictable ones can, in some cases, be cause for great concern. Some heart blocks are, in fact, a complete block in electrical conduction between the atria and ventricles; however, some AV blocks are simply a delay in conduction or an intermittent disruption of the impulse responsible for the cardiac cycle.

First-Degree Atrioventricular Block
- Rate: Usually normal but depends on the underlying rhythm

- Rhythm: Regular
- P waves: Upright in modified lead II; one precedes each QRS complex; normal shape and size
- PR interval: Prolonged (>0.2 seconds) and constant
- QRS duration: Usually 0.1 seconds or less, unless an intraventricular conduction delay exists
- Conduction: A QRS complex follows each P wave

First-degree AV block (Figure 11-51 and comparison Figure 11-52) usually occurs above the bundle of His and is identified by a prolonged PR interval. The normal PR interval is less than 0.2 seconds. The long PR interval is constant, predictable, and benign in that it simply represents a slowing of the atrial impulse through the intranodal pathways. The technologist should document first-degree AV block and continue to monitor the patient's ECG throughout the sleep study.

Second-Degree Atrioventricular Block

Second-degree AV block is segmented into types I and II. One is predictable and the other is unpredictable.

Second-Degree AV Block Type I
- Rate: Atrial rate is greater than the ventricular rate
- Rhythm: Atrial regular (Ps plot through time); ventricular irregular
- P waves: Normal shape and size; some Ps are not followed by a QRS (more P waves than QRS complexes)

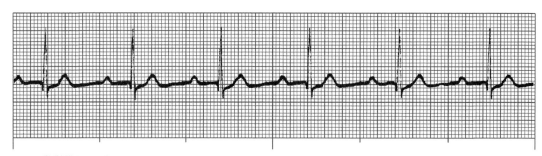

FIGURE 11-51 Consistently prolonged PR interval in first-degree atrioventricular block. *From Aehlert B:* ECGs made easy, *ed 4, St Louis, 2011, Mosby, Inc., an imprint of Elsevier, Inc.*

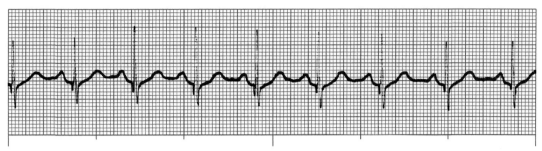

FIGURE 11-52 Normal sinus rhythm with PR interval lasting 0.12-0.20 seconds. *From Aehlert B: ECGs made easy, ed 4, St Louis, 2011, Mosby, Inc., an imprint of Elsevier, Inc.*

- PR interval: Progressively lengthens with each cycle until a QRS is "dropped" (difference may be slight from beat to beat); the PR interval after the nonconducted beat is shorter than others
- QRS duration: Usually 0.1 seconds or less, but is periodically missing
- Conduction: Some P waves are not followed by a QRS complex

Second-degree AV block type I (Wenckebach, Mobitz type I) is identified by a progressive lengthening of the PR interval until a P wave signal fails to continue on to the ventricles; an entire QRST is "dropped" (Figure 11-53). It is posited that this is a dysfunction of the AV node. The occurrence of second-degree AV block type I during sleep testing should be documented to ensure the physician is later aware of it. It is predictable and therefore considered more benign than second-degree AV block type II.

Second-Degree AV Block Type II (Mobitz Type II)
- Rate: Atrial rate is greater than the ventricular rate; ventricular rate is often slow
- Rhythm: Atrial regular (Ps plot through time); ventricular irregular
- P waves: Normal shape and size; some Ps are not followed by a QRS (more P waves than QRS complexes)

- PR interval: Within normal limits or slightly prolonged, but constant for conducted beats; the PR interval after the nonconducted beat may be shortened
- QRS duration: Usually greater than 0.1 seconds, but is periodically missing after P waves
- Conduction: Some P waves are not followed by a QRS complex; the QRS is randomly dropped

Second-degree AV block type II (Figure 11-54) originates below the bundle of His and is identified by a suddenly blocked P wave. There is no progression as seen with type I; an entire QRST is simply dropped without warning. This dysrhythmia warrants close monitoring because it can quickly progress to complete heart block. Second-degree AV block type II should be documented and reported to the attending physician by the recording technologist.

Third-Degree AV Block (Complete Heart Block)
- Rate: Atrial greater than ventricular, ventricular rate is determined by origin of escape rhythm
- Rhythm: Atrial regular; ventricular regular, but no relationship between the two
- P waves: Normal shape and size; some Ps are not followed by a QRS (more P waves than QRS complexes)
- PR interval: No true PR interval; atria and ventricles beat independently of one another

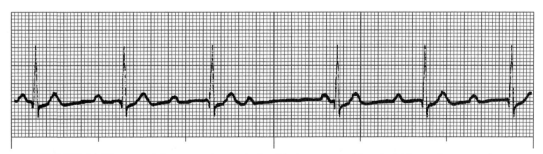

FIGURE 11-53 Second-degree atrioventricular block. *From Aehlert B: ECGs made easy, ed 4, St Louis, 2011, Mosby, Inc., an imprint of Elsevier, Inc.*

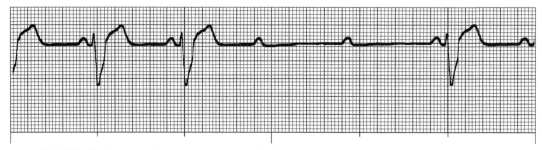

FIGURE 11-54 Second-degree atrioventricular block type II at 20 to 60 beats/min, ST-segment elevation. *From Aehlert B: ECGs made easy, ed 4, St Louis, 2011, Mosby, Inc., an imprint of Elsevier, Inc.*

- QRS duration: Narrow or wide depending on escape pacer location and condition of intraventricular conduction system
- Conduction: All atrial impulses are blocked. No connection between atria and ventricles

Third-degree AV block is the most severe of the heart blocks. With third-degree block (Figures 11-55 and 11-56), there is no relationship to atrial activity and ventricular activity; the P waves have no relationship with the QRS complexes. The signal from the atria does not travel to the ventricles because the pathway is completely blocked. The atrial rate is that of the atrial pacemaker, normally the SA node. The ventricular rate is much slower and based on the origin of the escape rhythm.

> **!** Third-degree AV block is a medical emergency. If the QRS is normal width, contact the attending physician for direction, document, and continue to monitor. If the QRS is wide, contact the emergency response team, assess the patient for responsiveness, prepare the equipment needed to perform CPR, notify the attending physician, and closely monitor the patient and his or her cardiac rhythm. Initiate CPR if warranted based on assessment of the patient.

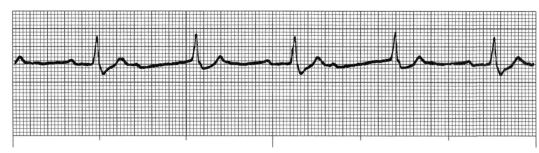

FIGURE 11-55 Third-degree atrioventricular (AV) block with a junctional escape pacemaker (QRS 0.08-0.10 seconds). For third-degree AV block with a narrow QRS width, the physician should be contacted for direction. *From Aehlert B: ECGs made easy, ed 4, St Louis, 2011, Mosby, Inc., an imprint of Elsevier, Inc.*

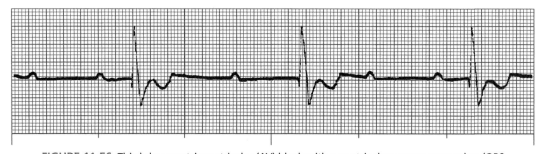

FIGURE 11-56 Third-degree atrioventricular (AV) block with a ventricular escape pacemaker (QRS 0.12-0.14 seconds). Third-degree AV block with a wide QRS warrants contacting the emergency response team, patient assessment, and initiation of cardiopulmonary resuscitation as indicated. *From Aehlert B: ECGs made easy, ed 4, St Louis, 2011, Mosby, Inc., an imprint of Elsevier, Inc.*

CHAPTER SUMMARY

- The anatomy and physiologic characteristics of the cardiopulmonary system are foundational for understanding normal function and the effect abnormalities have on both sleep-related and daytime quality of life.
- Knowledge of the mechanics of breathing and normal cardiac function is necessary toward recognizing the effect normal and abnormal cardiopulmonary function has on sleep.
- The regulation of ventilation is a complex process further complicated by lung disease and sleep-disordered breathing.
- Individuals with obstructive forms of lung disease have difficulty exhaling; those with restrictive lung disease have a hard time getting air into the lungs.
- Recognition of, and response to, abnormalities in cardiac and respiratory function during sleep require the basic skills necessary to assess ventilation, diffusion, perfusion, and gas exchange.
- Recognizing changes to blood gas data improves the technologist's ability to care for the patient and enhances understanding of the complex function of body systems.
- Ventilation and blood gas values change during NREM sleep and REM sleep as compared with waking values.
- Therapeutic intervention must be tailored to, and will be affected by, the patient's cardiopulmonary status.
- Differentiating technologist response to various cardiac dysrhythmias requires the ability to identify the electrocardiographic abnormality and separate it from artifactual data. The technologist must also assess the patient to judge whether the event is life threatening and warrants emergency response, is only significant enough to contact the attending physician, or is benign and requires no more than documentation.

References

1. DesJardins TR: *Cardiopulmonary anatomy and physiology: essentials for respiratory care,* ed 5, Clifton Park, NY, 2008, Thompson Delmar.
2. Shapiro BA, Kacmarek RM, Cane RD, et al: *Clinical application of respiratory care,* ed 4, St. Louis, 1991, Mosby Year Book.
3. Beachey W: *Respiratory care anatomy and physiology: foundations for clinical practice,* ed 2, St. Louis, 2007, Mosby/Elsevier.
4. Wilkins RL, Stoller JK, Kacmarek RM: *Egans's fundamentals of respiratory care,* ed 9, St. Louis, 2009, Elsevier/Mosby.
5. Geers C, Gros G: Carbon dioxide transport and carbonic anhydrase in blood and muscle, *Phys Rev* 80(2), 681-715 (website). http://physrev.physiology.org/content/80/2/681.full.pdf+html.
6. Nattie E, Li A: Central chemoreception is a complex system function that involves multiple, *J Appl Phys* 106:1464-1466. doi: 10.1152/japplphysiol.00112.2008.
7. Kryger M, Roth T, Dement W: *Principles and practice of sleep medicine,* ed 5, Philadelphia, 2011, Elsevier/Saunders.
8. Iber C, Ancoli-Israel S, Chesson A, et al., for the American Academy of Sleep Medicine: *The AASM manual for the scoring of sleep and associated events: rules, terminology and technical specifications,* ed 1, Westchester, Ill., 2007, American Academy of Sleep Medicine.
9. Potter PA, Perry AG, Stockert P, et al: *Basic nursing,* ed 7, St. Louis, 2011, Mosby/Elsevier.
10. Aehlert B: *ECGs made easy,* ed 4, Maryland heights, Mo., 2011, Mosby/Elsevier.
11. Gami AS, Pressman G, Caples SM, et al: Association of Atrial Fibrillation and Obstructive Sleep Apnea, *Circulation* 110: 364-367, 2004.

REVIEW QUESTIONS

1. The bronchial tree represents the:
   a. Major blood vessels
   b. Heart anatomy
   c. Airways
   d. Muscles

2. End tidal carbon dioxide values can be measured using:
   a. Capnography
   b. Oximetry
   c. Plethysmography
   d. Esophageal probe

3. The content of gas remaining in the lungs at the end of normal expiration is:
   a. VC
   b. FRC
   c. ERV
   d. V_T

4. The maximum amount of gas the lungs can contain is:
   a. Total residual volume
   b. Total lung capacity
   c. Tidal volume
   d. Total lung volume

5. The manubrium is a portion of the:
   a. Xiphoid process
   b. Intercostal muscles
   c. Sternum
   d. Sternocleidomastoids

6. Peripheral chemoreceptors are extremely sensitive to changes in:
   a. HCO_3^-
   b. Carbon dioxide
   c. H_2CO_3
   d. Oxygen

7. Hypoxemia occurs as a result of:
   a. Increased carbon dioxide
   b. Decreased oxygen levels
   c. Changes in the pH
   d. Malfunction of the brainstem

8. The pacemaker of the heart is the:
   a. SA node
   b. Tricuspid valve
   c. AV node
   d. SV node

9. The T wave of the cardiac rhythm represents:
   a. Ventricular repolarization
   b. Atrial depolarization
   c. Ventricular depolarization
   d. Atrial repolarization

10. Ventricular tachycardia has:
    a. A heart rate less than 140 bpm
    b. Normal QRS complexes
    c. A rhythmic cardiac rate
    d. Normal P waves

Chapter 12

Noninvasive Monitoring of Gas Exchange During Testing

Buddy Marshall

CHAPTER OUTLINE

LEARNING OBJECTIVES

After reading this chapter, you will be able to:
  1. Explain the role of noninvasive monitoring in sleep disorders testing.
  2. Differentiate between measures of oxygenation and ventilation.
  3. Explain the basic principles of pulse oximeter function.
  4. List reasons why oximetry data are necessary during sleep testing.
  5. Explain the effects of sampling rate, response time, and device memory on acquired data.
  6. Value monitoring CO_2 during sleep disorders testing and treatment.
  7. List physiologic issues that will increase the $P(a\text{-}et)CO_2$ gradient.
  8. Recognize how monitoring CO_2 data may increase patient safety and outcomes.
  9. Differentiate SaO_2, SpO_2, PaO_2, and O_2Hb.
  10. Summarize precautions associated with the use of an oximeter.
  11. Identify factors that may limit the accuracy of oximetric data.
  12. Interface ancillary equipment to a data acquisition system.
  13. Describe limitations of noninvasive CO_2 monitoring methods.
  14. List causes of erroneous results for each noninvasively measured variable.
  15. Explain normal differences in CO_2 values during wake, non–rapid eye movement sleep, and rapid eye movement sleep.
  16. List the basic principles involved in end-tidal CO_2 monitoring.
  17. Choose the sensor site for monitoring pulse oximetry, end-tidal CO_2, and transcutaneous CO_2.
  18. List the basic principles involved in transcutaneous CO_2 monitoring.
  19. Determine sleep-testing patients who will benefit most from CO_2 monitoring.

KEY TERMS

acid-base balance
alveolar-capillary membrane
anemic hypoxia
arterial blood gas (ABG) analysis
averaging (response) time
bicarbonate (HCO_3^-)
capnography
capnometry
carbon dioxide (CO_2)
carbon monoxide (CO)
chronic CO_2 retention
chronic obstructive pulmonary disease (COPD)
circulatory hypoxia
cooximetry
end-tidal carbon dioxide (E_TCO_2)
external respiration
hemoglobin (Hb)
hemoglobinopathies
histotoxic hypoxia
hypercarbia

hyperventilation
hypoxemia
hypoxia
hypoxic hypoxia
infrared spectroscopy
memory capacity
nasal cannula
noninvasive positive pressure
oxygen (O_2)
oxyhemoglobin
oxyhemoglobin (O_2Hb) dissociation curve
oxyhemoglobin (O_2Hb) saturation
P(a-et)CO_2 gradient
palpating
partial pressure of arterial oxygen (PaO_2)
partial pressure of carbon dioxide ($PaCO_2$)
perfusion
pH
photoplethysmography

positive airway pressure (PAP)
pulse oximeter
respiration
restrictive lung disorder
saturation of arterial blood with oxygen (SaO_2)
saturation of peripheral oxygen (SpO_2)
sidestream E_TCO_2 monitoring
signal aliasing
spectrophotometry
standard precautions
time-based capnography
tracheostomy tube
transcutaneous
transcutaneous carbon dioxide ($tcCO_2$)
transcutaneous oxygen (tcO_2)
vasoconstriction
ventilation
ventilation-to-perfusion (V/Q) mismatch

Noninvasive monitoring of gas exchange involves obtaining blood oxygen or **carbon dioxide (CO_2)** values without puncturing the skin or otherwise invading the body. The most common methods of obtaining these data in the sleep testing facility include pulse oximetry for an approximation of **oxyhemoglobin (O_2Hb) saturation** and either end-tidal carbon dioxide (E_TCO_2) or **transcutaneous carbon dioxide ($tcCO_2$)** monitoring. Each monitoring device has both limitations and advantages for use, as compared with the gold standard measures for CO_2 and **oxygen (O_2)**, and when compared with one another. Proper use, and the various options, limitations, and advantages, of noninvasive monitors are more thoroughly covered in later sections of this chapter.

OVERVIEW OF GAS EXCHANGE

Oxygenation values, such as O_2Hb saturation obtained by pulse oximetry and the partial pressure of O_2 obtained by **arterial blood gas (ABG) analysis**, represent the amount of O_2 being carried by the circulating blood. Ideally, circulating blood will carry adequate amounts of O_2 to the tissue for **internal respiration**, the process of gas diffusion between arterial blood and tissue at the cellular level. **Diffusion** is the movement of molecules, driven by a pressure gradient, across a semipermeable membrane. During

this process in the body, O_2 from within the blood moves across the cellular membrane, and CO_2 moves from inside the cell to be transported back to the lungs for removal. Within the lungs, gases diffuse across the **alveolar-capillary membrane**, where pulmonary capillaries and alveoli interface, in a process known as **external respiration**. Here, freshly inhaled air containing 20.95% O_2 moves into the alveoli where it diffuses across the alveolar-capillary membrane into the blood. At the same time CO_2 diffuses from within the blood, across the alveolar-capillary membrane into the alveoli, and is exhaled for removal from the body. Although the term *respiration* is commonly used to denote breathing, **respiration** actually occurs only at the cellular level; it occurs at the membrane of and within cells composing tissues of the body and within the lungs at the alveolar-capillary membrane.

Ventilation is the gross movement of air into and out of the lungs, otherwise described as the process of moving gases between the external environment and the alveoli.[1] Exchange of gases between the external environment and the cells of the body relies on several factors, which will be further explained. To thoroughly understand how gas exchange is monitored, along with the devices used for this purpose, a rudimentary understanding of both oxygenation and ventilation is essential.

HYPOXIA

Hypoxia Classification

When the O_2 content of inspired air is low, O_2 delivery to the blood and tissue is proportionately affected. Inadequate tissue oxygenation is referred to as **hypoxia**, whereas low amounts of O_2 in the blood is **hypoxemia**. When tissue oxygenation is diminished because of inadequate amounts of O_2 in inspired air, the condition is referred to as **hypoxic hypoxia**. Once O_2 diffuses into the bloodstream, it either attaches to **hemoglobin (Hb)** to form O_2Hb or dissolves into the blood plasma.

The majority of O_2 being transported by the bloodstream is carried to the tissue in the form of O_2Hb.[1] When the amount of circulating Hb is low, Hb are abnormal and unable to bind with O_2, or normal Hb have already been saturated with another substance such as **carbon monoxide (CO)**, inadequate O_2 is delivered to the cells of the body.

CO is a colorless, odorless, and tasteless gas that is toxic to humans and animals when encountered in higher concentrations. Any time an individual is exposed to CO, whether from inhaling tobacco smoke, vehicle exhaust fumes, smoke from a fire, or any other source, the CO readily saturates Hb. This is because the affinity of CO for Hb is approximately 210 times the affinity of O_2 for Hb.[1]

When Hb impairment is responsible for the blood's reduced O_2 carrying capacity, the condition is referred to as **anemic hypoxia**. Similarly, when cardiac output is slowed for any reason, O_2 delivery is correspondingly reduced and will likely be unable to keep up with tissue demand. When blood flow is stagnant and does not deliver adequate O_2 to the body, the condition is referred to as **circulatory hypoxia**.

When the tissues become toxic as a result of exposure to certain poisons such as cyanide, the cells are rendered unable to use the O_2 being delivered by the blood. In this scenario, all measures of blood oxygenation yield results indicative of better **oxygenation status** than the patient's clinical presentation, because blood oxygenation is presumably normal. Sufficient amounts of O_2 exist in the circulating blood that the tissues simply cannot use. It is unlikely that this condition, known as **histotoxic hypoxia**, will be encountered in the sleep center; however, it clearly makes the point that simply having O_2 in the bloodstream does not, in and of itself, indicate that the patient's body is being adequately oxygenated. The clinician must always consider multiple factors, including the patient's subjective complaints, his or her work of breathing, and other data obtained through visual assessment prior to making a determination about oxygenation status.

Causes of Hypoxia

Ventilation must be adequate to both move fresh air into the lungs and for exhalation of CO_2, a waste product of cellular respiration. Lung tissue must also be functional for effective external respiration. Anything that impedes the flow of gas to the alveoli, the ability of the lungs to empty, or a gas's ability to diffuse into or out of the blood will inhibit this process.

Lung disease that causes narrowing or blockage of airways, destruction or impairment of lung tissue at the alveolar level, or coating or thickening of the alveolar-capillary membrane, affects both the ability of O_2 to move into the bloodstream and the removal of CO_2. These issues are common for patients who have difficulty exhaling because of a **chronic obstructive pulmonary disease (COPD)**, a group of lung diseases that include chronic bronchitis, bronchiectasis, chronic asthma, and emphysema. Similarly, individuals with obesity hypoventilation, kyphosis, or other **restrictive lung disorder,** have limited lung volumes, which can result in increased blood and tissue CO_2 or decreased blood and tissue O_2.

MONITORING OXYGENATION AND VENTILATION

Oxygenation is most commonly measured by arterial puncture and blood gas analysis, or noninvasively by pulse oximetry. Less commonly, it is monitored via a **transcutaneous** sensor that warms the skin and dilates the capillary bed. The **partial pressure of arterial oxygen (PaO_2)** obtained by arterial puncture and ABG analysis and **transcutaneous oxygen tension ($tcPO_2$)** are measures of the amount of O_2 dissolved in the blood. The **saturation of peripheral oxygen (SpO_2)** is a measure of the percentage of saturated Hb (presumably with O_2), as obtained by pulse oximetry.

The **pulse oximeter** is a non-invasive monitor for estimating the saturation of hemoglobin, presumably with oxygen. Since the pulse oximeter cannot differentiate what is bound to Hb, these data will be erroneous when Hb is saturated with something other than O_2; however, because the majority of O_2 is carried in the blood bound to Hb, the SpO_2 is a very good representation of blood oxygenation under normal conditions. To avoid confusion, the O_2 saturation value obtained by ABG analysis (**saturation of arterial blood with oxygen [SaO_2]**) is a calculated value; it is not a direct measurement of Hb saturation. Oxygenation status along with the approximate relationship between PaO_2 and SpO_2 values, assuming normal physiologic conditions and absence of abnormal Hb, is illustrated in Table 12-1.

Monitoring Carbon Dioxide

Although ventilation is important for the exchange of O_2, changes to ventilation are best represented by

TABLE 12-1

Oxygenation Status Classification: Blood Gas Analysis and Oximetry Values

PaO$_2$	SpO$_2$	Oxygenation Status
80-100 mm Hg	95%-100%	Normal
60-80 mm Hg	90%-95%	Mild hypoxemia
40-60 mm Hg	70%-90%	Moderate hypoxemia
< 40 mm Hg	< 70%	Severe hypoxemia

changes in CO$_2$ levels because ventilation has a very fast, direct effect on blood CO$_2$. The **partial pressure of carbon dioxide (PaCO$_2$)**, which is obtained along with PaO$_2$ as a component of ABG analysis, is the most common way these values are measured. Because of its quick response to changes in breathing, blood CO$_2$ is monitored as a reflection of the adequacy of ventilation.

During periods of **hypoventilation**, the CO$_2$ in the blood rises because it is not being adequately exhaled. When the CO$_2$ rises above its upper normal limit of 45 mm Hg, this is referred to as hypercapnia or **hypercarbia**. Periods of **hyperventilation** result from "blowing off" too much CO$_2$ and the value is reduced below the normal lower limit of 35 mm Hg.

Although ABG analysis is considered the gold standard for assessing both ventilation and oxygenation, arterial puncture can be extremely painful and personnel qualified to perform the procedure may not be available during sleep testing.

Surrogate measures of CO$_2$ are noninvasive and can be implemented in the sleep laboratory with little, if any, disruption to testing. These include the monitoring of either tcPCO$_2$, a process similar to measuring tcPO$_2$ as mentioned previously, and **end-tidal carbon dioxide (E$_T$CO$_2$)**. E$_T$CO$_2$ values are obtained by sampling exhaled gas at the point of end exhalation during the breathing cycle. The results have a fairly linear relationship to PaCO$_2$ values in the absence of respiratory disease. This form of monitoring is suitable for providing a trend measure of ventilation during polysomnography (PSG), although data validity is reduced following application of O$_2$ or **positive airway pressure (PAP)**, and in the presence of respiratory disease.

PAP is the application of pressure above atmospheric to serve as a pneumatic splint for airway patency. Transcutaneous monitoring of CO$_2$ has been employed less often in the sleep laboratory, but deserves reconsideration because of advances in technology during the past couple of decades. It is not affected by initiation of therapeutic interventions such as PAP or supplemental O$_2$. The value and limitations of various methods of monitoring gas exchange are considered in later sections of this chapter.

OXYGENATION AND ACID-BASE BALANCE OVERVIEW

To fully understand the effects of ventilation, and subsequent changes to blood CO$_2$ values, one must possess a functional understanding of **acid-base balance**. Simply knowing to what extent a patient's CO$_2$ value changes as the result of sleep-disordered breathing, or the result of a therapeutic intervention, is not enough. The technologist needs to understand the physiology as a result of these changes. In Chapter 11, ABGs and acid-base balance were introduced. Here, the focus is on the general effects the respiratory system and the metabolic system have on acid-base balance and the practical application of this information.

Arterial Values of Blood Gases

Although not a part of acid-base balance or interpretation, the PaO$_2$ is a parameter from an ABG report that provides a direct measurement of how much O$_2$ is dissolved in the blood. It is considered the gold standard for determining oxygenation status, classified as *normal (80-100 mm Hg), mild hypoxemia (60-80 mm Hg), moderate hypoxemia (40-60 mm Hg),* or *severe hypoxemia (< 40 mm Hg)*. Once oxygenation status is determined, the PaO$_2$ can be put aside. Unfortunately, the SaO$_2$ value obtained by ABG analysis is calculated rather than directly measured. It is not the same measure as SpO$_2$ obtained by oximetry or the SaO$_2$ sometimes reported when **cooximetry** is performed, which is actually a true O$_2$Hb.

Cooximetry is an additional test run in conjunction with ABG analysis that provides a direct measurement of O$_2$Hb saturation, abnormal hemoglobins (carboxyhemoglobin [COHb], methemoglobin [metHb], and fetal Hb), and total hemoglobin (Hb$_{tot}$). The validity of the calculated SaO$_2$ found on an ABG report is based on the assumption that the pH PaCO$_2$, body temperature, Hb, and other parameters are normal. When any of these are abnormal, the value will be erroneous. The technologist must assess oxygenation carefully and understand the value and limitations of the various measures for this purpose. See Table 12-2 for normal ABG values.

TABLE 12-2

Normal Ranges of Arterial Blood Gas Values

Blood Gas Parameter	Arterial Value
pH	7.35-7.45
PaCO$_2$	35-45 mm Hg
HCO$_3$$^-$*	22-26 mEq/L
PaO$_2$	80-100 mm Hg

*Some authorities report the normal HCO$_3$$^-$ range as 22-28 mEq/L.

Assessment of pH Values

The **pH** of the human body must be maintained within a very narrow range to support life. Normal values fall within the range of 7.35 to 7.45 and even a slight change can become life threatening.[2] When the blood pH value falls below approximately 6.8 or exceeds approximately 7.8, cellular metabolism begins to cease and death ensues. Even when a non-lethal acid-base imbalance exists, normal function becomes impaired. It is imperative that the pH remain within normal limits for normal cellular function to be maintained. In general, pH is maintained through balance between the respiratory system and the metabolic system. The metabolic component of acid-base balance is assessed based on the **bicarbonate (HCO$_3^-$)** value, normally 22-26 mEq/L, from a blood gas analysis report.

Changes to HCO$_3^-$ represent changes in the renal system and are used to evaluate overall metabolic function for acid-base balance interpretation. The respiratory component of acid-base balance is the PaCO$_2$, which is maintained between 35 and 45 mm Hg during normal breathing. Hypoventilation results in a value greater than 45 mm Hg and hyperventilation results in a value less than 35 mm Hg. Homeostasis between the metabolic system and respiratory system is responsible for acid-base balance within the body as measured on the pH scale.

If either the HCO$_3^-$ shifts in response to metabolic system changes or the PaCO$_2$ shifts in response to respiratory system changes, homeostasis will be lost and the pH value will change. For simplicity, the PaCO$_2$ can be thought of as the "acid" in the mixture and the HCO$_3^-$ as the "base" or alkaline component within the circulating blood. Balance between the acid and the base is responsible for the pH value. Acidity resides on the lower end of the numerical pH scale, with alkalinity represented by a higher number. Numerically, HCO$_3^-$ tracks with pH; when the bicarbonate increases it causes an upward shift in the pH. Likewise, when it decreases the pH shifts downward. Because CO$_2$ increases the acidity of the mixture, when CO$_2$ increases the pH becomes more acidic and drops to a lower number. This also means that a lower CO$_2$ value will result in a more alkaline mixture and a higher pH.

Regardless of whether CO$_2$ is being measured noninvasively, or by arterial puncture and blood gas analysis, the clinician must recognize that it has an immediate, inverse effect on the pH of the blood. Given that pH balance must be maintained for normal physiologic function, the necessity of monitoring CO$_2$ by some method during sleep testing should be apparent. This is especially the case when augmenting spontaneous ventilation using the various modalities of PAP or applying and titrating supplemental O$_2$.

Although few facilities perform ABG analysis during sleep testing, the technologist must possess the basic skills necessary to interpret these results. This will lead to a better understanding of the effect CO$_2$ values obtained noninvasively have on human physiology. Additionally, the technologist must be able to interpret ABG results when available in the medical record, especially when the patient has end-stage COPD and chronic retention of CO$_2$ in the blood. The flow charts illustrated later in this chapter provide a step-by-step approach for easy interpretation of acid-base balance and ABG interpretation.

PULSE OXIMETRY

Pulse oximetry, often referred to as the "fifth vital sign," is a simple, noninvasive technique used to monitor tissue oxygenation in a wide variety of settings.[3] For the purposes of this chapter, the use of oximetry is presented as an integral component of PSG and as a stand-alone screening tool for triaging patients with sleep-disordered breathing. Data are obtained by pulse oximetry via a probe placed on each side of a vascular bed, typically the finger or ear. The resultant data represent the percentage of saturated Hb, presumably with O$_2$. Refer to Figure 12-1 for a schematic diagram of a typical pulse oximeter and sensor.

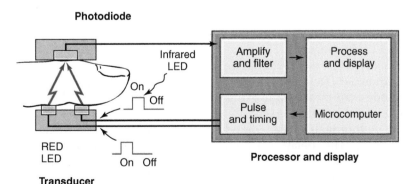

FIGURE 12-1 Schematic block diagram of a pulse oximeter. *Modified from Gardner RM: J Cardiovasc Nurs 1:79, 1987.*

The term used to identify these data is *saturation of peripheral O_2* because the measurement is obtained during pulsations at the peripheral capillary level. This is also sometimes referred to as O_2Hb saturation obtained from pulsatile data or by pulse oximetry. Although both are measures of oxygenation, a distinction should be made between SpO_2 and the SaO_2 as derived by either blood gas analysis or directly measured by hemoximetry (cooximetry) of an arterial blood sample. These values have significant differences and should not be confused.

ORIGINS OF PULSE OXIMETRY

The origins of pulse oximetry date back to the early 1930s when German investigators were researching light transmission through the skin. In 1939, German researchers reported the use of an "ear O_2 meter," but there was not great interest in this new technology until World War II with the emerging need to evaluate oxygenation of pilots at high altitudes.

In the early 1940s, a British researcher, Glen Millikan, developed a lightweight ear O_2 meter for use in aviation monitoring, for which he coined the term *oximeter.* Millikan's oximeter, mainly used in physiology, aviation, and experimental studies, was modified throughout the 1940s and 1950s and was eventually manufactured by the Waters Company.

In the 1970s, Hewlett Packard marketed a system for use in the clinical setting; however, because of its weight of approximately 35 pounds, price of about $10,000, and bulky earpiece, there were practical limitations to use. In 1972, the modern oximeter was developed by a Japanese bioengineer, Takuo Aoyagi, while he was working on developing a noninvasive cardiac output measurement.

The first reliable and affordable oximeter that was commercially available for clinical use was introduced by Nellcor in 1980. Throughout the 1980s, Nellcor, Ohmeda, and Novametrix continued to make improvements that resulted in decreased size, lower cost, and the development of probes for use at multiple anatomical sites.[4,5] Today's oximeters are small, lightweight, affordable, and can run on battery for extended periods. Many digital acquisition systems used for sleep testing can be purchased complete with an internal oximeter to avoid potential issues related to interfacing an ancillary device. At times, however, use of an external device can be advantageous. The decision to use an internal or external oximeter should be made based on the specific needs of the testing facility. Figures 12-2 and 12-3 provide examples of some oximeter probe types currently available for use.

Reusable sensors must be thoroughly cleaned and disinfected between patients. The delay between physiologic changes in oxygenation status and changes to the value obtained by pulse oximetry is directly affected by how far blood leaving the cardiopulmonary

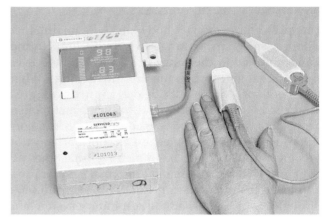

FIGURE 12-2 Reusable adult-size clip-type pulse oximeter sensor. *From Elkin MK, et al: Nursing interventions and clinical skills, ed 4, St Louis, 2008, Elsevier.*

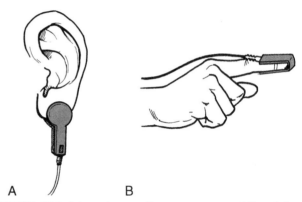

FIGURE 12-3 Pulse oximeter clip-type ear sensor (*A*) and finger sensor (*B*). *From Linton AD:* Introduction to medical-surgical nursing, *ed 5, St Louis, 2012, Elsevier.*

system must travel to the recording site. When selecting sensor type, keep in mind that there will be a longer delay between sleep-disordered breathing events and the associated O_2Hb desaturation when the sensor is located farther away from the central organs.

THEORY OF OPERATION

Pulse oximeters use the principles of **spectrophotometry** and **photoplethysmography** to estimate the percentage of saturated Hb in the blood. According to the principles of spectrophotometry, every substance has its own pattern of light absorption, and this pattern varies predictably with the amount of the substance that is present. Photoplethysmography uses light to detect the minute volume changes between the baseline component and pulsatile component of blood flow through the tissue bed. These represent the venous and capillary blood flow, and the arterial blood flow through the tissue, respectively.[6]

The pulse oximeter uses two wavelengths of light: red and infrared. The sensor consists of a light-emitting diode (LED) that emits alternating pulses of red and infrared light. On the other side of the sensor, which is

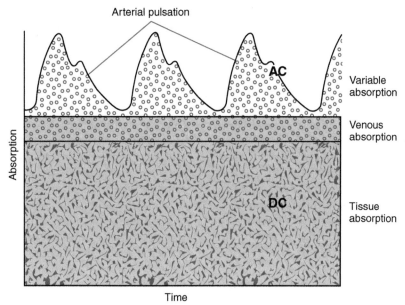

FIGURE 12-4 Measurement principle of standard pulse oximetry. *From Ruppel GL:* Manual of pulmonary function testing, *ed 9, St Louis, 2009, Elsevier.*

placed on the opposite side of the vascular bed, a photodiode measures the intensity of the transmitted light. By comparing the light absorbance during the pulsatile component with the baseline value at each wavelength, a pulse-added measure independent of incident light is obtained. The oximeter's microprocessor then calculates the SpO_2 as the ratio of the pulse-added absorbance measured at the two different wavelengths.[6] Figure 12-4 provides a graphical representation of tissue, venous, and arterial pulsatile absorption.

Transmitted light (at wavelengths of 660 and 940 nm) consists of two components. A large, fixed component, the DC component, represents light passing through tissue and venous blood without being absorbed. A smaller portion is pulsatile in nature and changes absorption as blood pulses through the arterioles; this is represented as the AC component. The pulse oximeter divides the AC signal by the DC signal at each wavelength, effectively canceling the DC component. The ratio of the AC signals at the two wavelengths is then a function of the relative absorptions of O_2Hb and reduced Hb. Modern pulse oximeters include sophisticated digital filters to better distinguish the AC and DC components of the signal.

CONTRAINDICATIONS, PRECAUTIONS, AND INFECTION CONTROL

According to the American Association of Respiratory Care position paper, *Clinical Practice Guideline: Pulse Oximetry* (Box 12-1), the only relative contraindication to pulse oximetry is the presence of an ongoing need for measurement of pH, $PaCO_2$, Hb_{tot}, and abnormal hemoglobins.[7] Fortunately, these considerations are not relevant to the majority of patients undergoing

---

BOX 12-1

Pulse Oximetry: American Association for Respiratory Care Clinical Practice Guidelines—Summary of Sleep Testing–Related Considerations

INDICATIONS

- To monitor the adequacy of O_2Hb saturation
- To quantify the O_2Hb saturation response to therapeutic intervention
- To comply with mandated regulations
- To abide by recommended standards of practice

RELATIVE CONTRAINDICATIONS

- The ongoing need for actual measurement of arterial pH, $PaCO_2$, total Hb, or abnormal Hb

PRECAUTIONS

- Device limitations causing false-negative results for hypoxemia, normoxemia, or hyperoxemia may lead to inappropriate treatment of the patient.
- Accuracy of SpO_2 vales may be affected by nail polish, skin pigmentation, motion, low perfusion, and abnormal Hb, among other factors.

ASSESSMENT OF NEED

- Pulse oximetry is appropriate for continuous or prolonged monitoring of O_2Hb saturation.
- Pulse oximetry may be adequate when assessment of acid-base balance or PaO_2 is not required.

Hb, Hemoglobin; *O_2Hb,* oxyhemoglobin; *$PaCO_2$,* partial pressure of carbon dioxide; *SpO_2,* saturation of peripheral oxygen. Data from *Respir Care* 37(8):891-897, 1992.

a polysomnographic evaluation. Of these, changes to blood CO_2 during sleep, and during the application and titration of PAP modalities and supplemental O_2, are of most concern in the sleep-testing patient population. CO_2 can be monitored noninvasively with relative ease and is further discussed later in this chapter. In a time when the number of people with latex allergies continues to climb, the material from which the sensor is constructed may be another relative contraindication to oximetry. Some prior-generation, reusable sensors may contain latex, although no currently available models are known to contain it. If a question exists regarding the material used to construct a particular oximeter sensor, the manufacturer should be consulted prior to use.

Precautions

Some additional precautions should be considered when monitoring patients using pulse oximetry. The oximeter sensor LED produces heat, although the amount of heat is typically nominal. With prolonged use, however, care should be taken that skin at the probe site is not burned and that the sensor does not cause a pressure sore. A sensor that has been applied too tightly has the potential to cause pressure injury, including tissue necrosis, at the site of placement. Information provided by the manufacturer in reference to the particular oximeter and sensor should be consulted for recommendations regarding how long a sensor may be left in one place.

A good practice during PSG, regardless of whether the manufacturer-recommended time has elapsed, is to change the site of the probe whenever technologist intervention is required at the bedside. PAP initiation and patient restroom breaks provide perfect opportunities to change the sensor site. It is also recommended that the technologist question the patient regarding sensor-site comfort, as early as the beginning of testing. Although uncommon, the patient with low sleep efficiency during PSG will occasionally comment that the sensor was uncomfortable all night when questioned about the poor night's sleep on the morning following testing.

Routine Safety Practice

Routine safety practices should be followed when using any electrical device, particularly in the provision of patient care. At minimum, the device, power cord, and input cable should be physically assessed for damage prior to each use. If the manufacturer originally provided the device with a three-prong grounded electrical plug, it should never be bypassed and the outlet being used should be tested for a patent ground connection at a regular interval. In addition, as with all electronic medical devices, an oximeter should be regularly tested for excessive electrical leakage current and the power cord should never be altered. One specific consideration to electrical safety

should be noted in regard to the sensor. Regardless of connection compatibility, probes not specifically intended for a given oximeter should never be used. Electrical shock and burns may result from the substitution of incompatible probes between equipment.[7]

Infection control

Infection control precautions, also known as **standard precautions,** should be used during all patient contact and should be applied to all patients in all situations. Gloves, or another appropriate barrier, should be donned when exposure to any bodily fluid, secretion, or excretion other than sweat is anticipated. Although it is unlikely that such exposure would occur during this procedure, standard precautions are always to be followed when the technologist is involved in direct-patient contact. Typically, a few preventative measures practiced diligently will be sufficient to avoid cross-contamination between equipment and patients. Some important considerations related to the performance of pulse oximetry monitoring are outlined in Box 12-2.

The oximeter sensor should be thoroughly cleaned and disinfected after each patient use when a reusable probe is employed. Disposable probes should not be

---

BOX 12-2
Important Considerations for Performing Pulse Oximetry

- Follow the manufacturer's recommendations to ensure data accuracy and patient safety.
- Use only a sensor specifically intended for the recording device.
- Set the response averaging time to 3 seconds or less.
- Ensure sensor is the correct size and style according to patient and recording site.
- Remove nail polish and nail coverings when a finger probe is used.
- Question the patient regarding sensor site comfort prior to lights out.
- Confirm adequacy of pulse signal before accepting oximetry data.
- Check site to confirm sensor is not placed too tightly or too loosely.
- Recognize that the delay between physiologic change and SpO_2 data is directly proportionate to sensor site distance from the cardiopulmonary system.
- Inspect sensor site and change location periodically.
- Validate SpO_2 values against arterial blood gas measures when possible.
- Confirm patient comfort during each subsequent bedside intervention.
- Clean and disinfect a reusable sensor, cable, and the instrument case between uses.
- *Do not* initiate emergency response based on oximetry data alone; assess patient.

SpO_2, saturation of peripheral oxygen.

used between patients; they are intended for single-patient use only. Additionally, the extension cable and the oximeter itself should be cleaned between uses unless they are not accessible to the patient. The manufacturer's operation manual may provide cleaning and disinfection recommendations for a given device; however, standard practice for low-level disinfection of oximeter sensors involves use of 70% isopropyl alcohol, whereas disinfecting the device itself can be accomplished by wiping it down with a 10% household bleach solution or a high-grade disinfectant intended for use on surfaces in healthcare facilities.

LIMITATIONS TO TESTING AND THE RELIABILITY OF RESULTS

Many factors can affect the accuracy of oximetry data, which may, in some cases, influence clinical decision making.[8-10] Because the recording technologist is present during data acquisition, it is important that he or she recognize discrepant data and at minimum report it to the interpreting clinician. Ideally, the technologist will be able to intervene and correct the issue during acquisition when data are not as expected. Any time questionable data exists, the occurrence should be thoroughly documented, along with how the technologist attempted to correct the problem.

Oxyhemoglobin Dissociation Curve

The relationship between the PaO_2 and the SpO_2, as well as the effects of the **oxyhemoglobin dissociation**

curve on this relationship as influenced by the partial pressure of arterial CO_2, acid-base balance, and other factors must be well understood by the sleep technologist (Figure 12-5). Otherwise, physiologically relevant SpO_2 data may be erroneously thought to be artifactual. Because the majority of O_2 transported to the cell is carried through the bloodstream attached to Hb, any abnormality in this carrying capacity will result in decreased tissue oxygenation. Pulse oximeters estimate the percentage of Hb that is saturated; pulse oximeters cannot determine what the Hb is saturated with.

If the patient has abnormally elevated levels of metHb or COHb, the SpO_2 value obtained by pulse oximetry may be normal or elevated when the actual O_2Hb is relatively low, resulting in clinical tissue hypoxia. Likewise, when the amount of Hb in the bloodstream is low, the oximeter simply measures the saturation of the Hb that is present. If the amount of Hb cannot adequately carry O_2 to the tissue, the patient may present with clinical hypoxia (anemic hypoxia) despite having a normal percent saturation as obtained by pulse oximetry. Less commonly seen, **hemoglobinopathies** like sickle cell anemia cause a decrease in the overall O_2 carrying capacity of the blood. In contrast to these situations, pulse oximetry data in the presence of a hemoglobinopathy accurately reflect the patient's hypoxic state.

Although less common in the sleep center than in the acute care setting, diminished peripheral **perfusion** as the result of peripheral vascular disease,

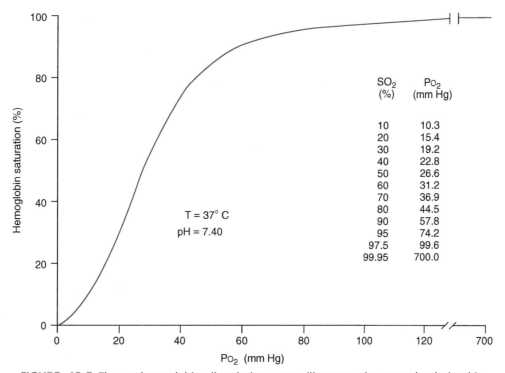

FIGURE 12-5 The oxyhemoglobin dissociation curve illustrates the normal relationship between the partial pressure of arterial blood (PaO_2) and oxyhemoglobin saturation (O_2Hb) as measured by cooximetry. *From Lane EE, Walker JF: Clinical arterial blood gas analysis, St Louis, 1987, Mosby.*

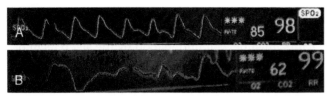

FIGURE 12-6 Normal plethysmographic waveform (A) and abnormal, unreliable plethysmographic waveform (B). *From Sandberg WS, et al: The MGH textbook of anesthetic equipment, ed 1, Philadelphia, 2011, Elsevier-Saunders.*

hypoxemia, hypotension, cold extremities, peripheral **vasoconstriction,** or a reduction in the diameter of blood vessels, from any other cause, can make obtaining valid oximetry data difficult. The term perfusion means to supply with blood, or the process of delivering blood to a capillary bed in the tissue. Insufficient pulsatile data can impair the oximeter's ability to differentiate arterial from background signal sources, and produce an erroneous reading on the display or a complete loss of the signal. For the patient with diminished peripheral perfusion, the technologist should choose the best perfused (warmest) site for probe placement and verify the oximetry data against a clinical assessment of the patient and ABG results, if available.

Examining by touch, or **palpating** the patient's pulse to ensure the oximeter waveform represents pulsatile data, is a good indication of signal adequacy. Figure 12-6 is an example of an acceptable and a variable plethysmographic waveform that can be used to assess whether the oximeter is sensing sufficient pulsatile data. Because the ear is closer in proximity to the central organs, it may provide a better-perfused site for probe placement than a digit.

Another related condition exists when the SpO_2 falls to less than 70%. When the O_2 content of blood falls, the body responds with peripheral vasoconstriction in an effort to shunt blood toward the central organs. Lack of perfusion to the extremities makes it difficult to obtain a pulsatile signal, resulting in data of questionable validity in a reading of less than 70%. In fact, most clinicians consider SpO_2 readings less than 80% unreliable.[6]

Additional Considerations for Pulse Oximetry Monitoring

Nail coverings and nail polish should be removed prior to using a digit as the oximeter probe site during polysomnographic testing. Although it has been reported that some colors of nail polish affect the accuracy of pulse oximetry less than others, removal is always recommended for this all-night, elective procedure.

Consideration should also be given to clinical issues that could potentiate increased motion artifact. During preparation for testing, the technologist should assess the patient for movement disorders, such as those that cause tremors, and choose a probe site to best minimize motion artifact.

Technical and Environmental Considerations

Many technical factors exist that may influence the accuracy of data obtained by pulse oximetry. Most notably, improper placement of the sensor will result in the inaccurate measurement of O_2-saturated Hb, or the introduction of excessive motion artifact into the recording. Improper attachment to the skin can lead to erroneous data if ambient light is allowed to reach the photodiode of the sensor.

As previously mentioned, the sensor should be placed so that the transducer and photodiode lie directly across a vascular bed from one another. Traditional sites for sensor placement include the nail bed, ear lobe, toe, and nasal bridge. The side of the foot is commonly used for sensor placement on neonates.

A sensor for forehead placement using reflectance technology was introduced to the market in recent years, although due to the expense, this technology may be more feasible in the critical care setting where patients with diminished peripheral perfusion require long-term monitoring. Reflective sensors detect light reflected from the bone underlying a vascular bed. Table 12-3 provides a listing of some factors responsible for erroneous data.

TABLE 12-3

Factors Resulting in Erroneous Oximetry Values

Factor	Effect on SpO_2%
Nail polish (particularly black and blue)	Falsely high
Dark skin pigmentation	Falsely high
Presence of COHb	Falsely high
High metHb	Falsely low if > 85% Falsely high if < 85%
Presence of fetal Hb	None
Anemia (low Hb/hematocrit)	None or low
Ambient light	Varies
Movement	Unpredictable; spurious
Poor perfusion (vasoconstriction)	Poor signal; varies
Hypothermia (vasoconstriction)	Poor signal; varies
Hypotension (vasoconstriction)	Poor signal; varies

COHb, Carboxyhemoglobin; *Hb,* hemoglobin; *metHB,* methemoglobin.

Software Limiting Factors for Oximetry

Limiting factors that result from the technology employed by a particular brand of oximeter, or even a specific software revision, include **memory capacity**, **sampling rate**, **averaging time (response time)**, and data output capabilities.[11] A good technologist will become familiar with the operating manual of each oximeter in his or her facility, including those both used in conjunction with PSG or as a stand-alone recorder.

The sampling rate refers to the number of data points stored to memory during a defined period, usually 1 second. Averaging time is a moving window within which data points collected during a defined period are averaged for a reported value. As an example, a given oximeter may obtain 30 samples per second although values on the display, and those sent to the output, are only updated once each second. The value that is displayed in this scenario is the average of 90 values measured during the past 3 seconds. This is described as a 3-second response time, which is actually a 3-second moving window. The next time the oximeter updates its value, the window will move 1 second and the new window of data consisting of the 90 values collected during the course of the past 3 seconds will be averaged and displayed.

Memory capacity refers to the ability of an oximeter to store data for download to a software program or recorder at a future time. Limitations to this process may include inadequate storage space for the desired length of recording and the frequency of samples stored within the memory of the oximeter. Insufficient frequency of samples stored in memory will result in a drop off, or distortion, of resolution on the downloaded tracing or the numerical data obtained. Digital data is at best a close approximation of the original signal. **Signal aliasing** occurs when digitized data are distorted because of inadequate sampling rate.

The terms response time, averaging time, and recording settings have been used interchangeably to mean the same thing. Response time is a product of the sampling rate and the proprietary algorithms used by the manufacturer of a pulse oximeter. Depending on the model in question, this value may be represented as fast, normal, or slow, as a number of seconds (e.g., 3 seconds; 6 seconds; 12 seconds), or a range of seconds (e.g., 2-4 seconds; 4-6 seconds; 6-8 seconds). The slower the setting (longer amount of time) the more artifact will be averaged out of the displayed value of the recording. This can be helpful in settings such as critical care or a neonatal intensive care unit where oximetry may be used only as a trending device. This will, however, reduce both the absolute value of the O_2Hb desaturation nadir and the relative change of individual desaturations.[11] .

Figure 12-7 provides an example of the effect of various averaging time settings on O_2Hb saturation values simultaneously recorded from the same patient. Three oximeters were set at different averaging time settings (3, 6, and 12 seconds). The O_2Hb desaturation events were the result of sleep-disordered breathing. Note the difference in the relative change in saturation, along with the absolute saturation values, at the various settings caused by signal aliasing

Optimizing Oximetry During Polysomnography

Because pulse oximetry is used as an integral part of a polysomnographic evaluation, it is important to use

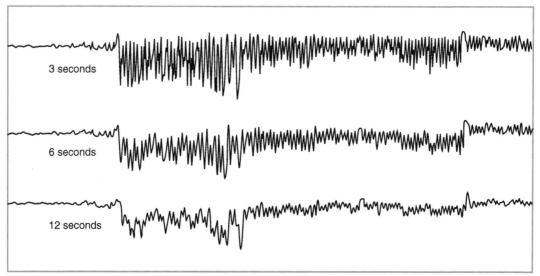

FIGURE 12-7 One patient's data obtained simultaneously by three separate oximeters set at different averaging time settings (3, 6, and 12 seconds).

the fastest (lowest number of seconds) response time setting available to ensure data are not lost because of excessive averaging. In fact, the American Academy of Sleep Medicine (AASM) *Manual for the Scoring of Sleep and Associated Events,* first published in 2007 and updated in 2012, requires that a maximum signal averaging time of 3 seconds be used when recording oximetry in conjunction with PSG for scoring of respiratory events.[12]

When evaluating pulse oximeters for use in PSG, the data output capabilities should be considered as well as available response time settings. As discussed in detail later in this chapter, most oximeters capable of being interfaced with a PSG acquisition system provide a 0-1 volt (V) direct current (DC) signal for this purpose. Some newer pulse oximeters only provide a digital output signal and no longer provide the analog output necessary to interface the device to most acquisition systems and strip chart recorders.

Regardless of the amount of planning that goes into a sleep-testing facility, technical issues are inevitable and the recording technologist must become proficient at troubleshooting equipment problems as they arise. Troubleshooting the device when results are not as expected may be less difficult once a few basic questions, as outlined in Box 12-3, are answered. Despite simplification of acquisition systems during the past years, most consist of various pieces of equipment and sensors interfaced to a primary recorder. In most centers, a stand-alone pulse oximeter is connected to the acquisition system by way of a separate interface cable as described in the following section.

RECORDING OXIMETRY DATA

The importance of the operation manuals for the oximeter and the acquisition system cannot be overemphasized in regard to the next three sections. These manuals provide instructions for interfacing devices and transferring data, input and output connections, device-specific settings, and calibration procedures. A limited number of acquisition systems are equipped with an internal, original equipment manufacturer (OEM), oximeter board. The equipment operations manual provides detailed instructions for the device, but it is only necessary for the technologist to know how to calibrate the device to confirm data accuracy. It is also important, however, that the technologist know the manufacturer and device characteristics, such as response time setting, when using an acquisition system with an OEM oximeter board. Settings on some of these systems are preset, whereas settings on others are user-definable. This information should be available in the operating manual that came with the acquisition system.

BOX 12-3
Considerations for Basic Equipment Troubleshooting

I. Are data between the oximeter and acquisition system consistent?
   a. If yes, refer to II.
   b. If no:
      1. Ensure that the oximeter's output voltage is set correctly if user-definable.
      2. Generate a calibration signal from the oximeter and verify accuracy on the recorder.
      3. Check all connections between the oximeter output and acquisition system input.
      4. Ensure that the acquisition system is properly calibrated (or correct montage and calibration files are in use).
      5. Replace interface cable.
      6. Consider replacing oximeter (output may be faulty).
II. Do the plethysmographic waveform and other proprietary signal quality indicators appear adequate?
   a. If yes, refer to III.
   b. If no:
      1. Visually assess the patient.
      2. Check probe placement.
      3. Assess perfusion to probe site.
      4. Consider alternate probe site.
      5. Consider replacing probe or input cable.
      6. Consider replacing oximeter.
III. Additional ways to verify function when values remain in question:
   1. Compare palpated heart rate to rate measured by the oximeter.
   2. Compare values to that of another oximeter when practical.
   3. Compare oximetry results to arterial blood gas data with cooximetry when practical.

Generally, the process of interfacing a stand-alone oximeter with an acquisition system only requires connecting a two-conductor cable between the devices to transfer analog data in the form of a 0-1 V, DC signal for each parameter being transferred. Most oximeters are capable of, at minimum, an output for both heart rate and SpO_2.

OXIMETRY CALIBRATION

Calibration of the oximeter with the acquisition system is a simple procedure. However, it is imperative that one knows the characteristics of the specific devices in use. Most oximeters generate calibration signals of 0 V and 1 V, which represent 0% and 100% SpO_2, respectively. Some of these devices allow the user to select an additional 0.5 V signal, which represents 50%. With these devices, one must decide whether to set up the acquisition system to record

SpO_2 in the range of either 0 to 100% or 50% to 100%. If the range of 0 to 100% is chosen, a calibration voltage of 0 V followed by 1 V should be generated to confirm accuracy of the recording channel. If 50-100% is selected, calibration signals of 0.5 V and 1 V are used to test the span of the acquisition system channel.

An alternate method provided by the manufacturers is to allow the user to select the SpO_2 span represented by a 0-1 V signal via software settings. With these devices the acquisition system settings are the key. On the oximeter, the 0-1 V signal is set to represent either 50% to 100% or 0 to 100%. Using these values, the acquisition system is then set to 0 V = 50% or 0 V = 0%, and 1 V = 100% to determine the recording range.

SELECTING THE APPROPRIATE OXIMETER FOR BOTH IN-LAB AND OUT-OF-LAB TESTING

It is important to use the fastest response time setting available to ensure data are not lost because of excessive averaging when pulse oximetry is used as a part of a polysomnographic evaluation. When evaluating equipment for purchase, it is imperative that the end user determines whether settings are user definable, consistently default to acceptable values, and are of sufficient range for their designated purpose. When purchasing an acquisition system with an integrated oximeter, the buyer must ensure that settings are not predefined and fixed at undesirable values.

The current Centers for Medicare and Medicaid Services (CMS) policy on supplemental O_2 requiring cumulative saturation values ≤ 88% for ≥ 5 minutes when taken in sleep, make it difficult to qualify patients with short-lived, repetitive O_2Hb desaturation events.[13]

In fact, in an effort to obtain the required documentation to qualify the patient for O_2 under these guidelines, when a stand-alone oximeter is interfaced to the acquisition system during overnight PSG, it can be downloaded the following morning.

Oximetry alone is not considered an adequate diagnostic tool in sleep medicine. Although it can be useful in identifying potential disorders in sleep, it cannot differentiate sleep disorders or identify confounding disorders. Clearly, it is an integral component of a comprehensive polysomnographic evaluation.

Both the CMS guidelines and the AASM recommendations require an associated O_2Hb desaturation to score a hypopnea.[12,14] When SpO_2 values are excessively manipulated by an oximeter's software, relative desaturations may not be significant enough to score hypopneas. In lieu of CMS guidelines for O_2 qualification, consideration should be given to whether a particular device has sufficient memory and that data are easily transferred in the event it needs to be downloaded in the morning following sleep testing. Because most acquisition systems rely on an analog

signal from the stand-alone oximeter, the ability to interface the two devices must also be confirmed.

Despite its limitations as a stand-alone diagnostic device, oximetry is a valuable tool for managing patients before and after comprehensive sleep testing as long as all limitations are considered. Prior to testing it can be an effective means of triaging patients when the wait time for an in-laboratory sleep study is excessive. It can also be very useful to the clinician when evaluating the efficacy of treatment with PAP or supplemental O_2 therapy following evaluation, testing, and titration. When used to assess the patient at home, recorder settings and memory capacity must be sufficient to avoid signal aliasing.

MONITORING VENTILATION DURING SLEEP

As previously described, blood CO_2 levels provide the most accurate representation of the adequacy of ventilation. This can be measured by ABG analysis or by a surrogate, noninvasive method. To document and score hypoventilation for adult subjects, 2012 AASM guidelines require an increase in $PaCO_2$ ≥10 mmHg during sleep to a value exceeding 50 mmHg for ≥ 10 minutes, or an increase to a value >55 mmHg for ≥10 minutes as measured by ABG analysis, E_TCO_2 monitoring, or $tcCO_2$ monitoring.[12] For pediatric subjects, E_TCO_2 and $tcCO_2$ monitoring are primarily utilized.[12] These noninvasive measures can be reliable for documenting trends of increasing or decreasing CO_2 levels regardless of the cause.

IMPACT OF HYPOVENTILATION DURING SLEEP

Individuals who are healthy, those with cardiorespiratory disease, and those with sleep-disordered breathing all hypoventilate during sleep; everyone has elevated blood CO_2 levels during sleep as compared with their baseline values while awake. Normal adults without sleep-disordered breathing or respiratory disease experience an increase in $PaCO_2$ of 2-8 mm Hg during NREM sleep, and 5-10 mm Hg during REM sleep as compared with baseline. These expected changes have little effect on physiologic function; however, in the presence of underlying medical disease or sleep-disordered breathing, patients may hypoventilate severely enough to affect the body's pH. When $PaCO_2$ is either elevated or decreased enough to shift blood pH to dangerously acidic or alkaline levels, respectively, metabolic function will be compromised. Often, an acid-base imbalance is accompanied by hypoxemia, which further complicates the issue of diminished metabolic function.

Because in most cases it is impractical to perform arterial puncture for blood gas analysis during sleep, changes to CO_2 values most often go unmonitored during PSG. Even in facilities where prestudy arterial blood samples are drawn to obtain baseline blood gas values, repeat testing during sleep is rarely performed. A handful of sleep laboratories do, to their credit, obtain a repeat blood gas sample immediately after awakening the patient. These laboratories typically repeat testing following therapeutic intervention when baseline ABGs yield an elevated $PaCO_2$. The threshold for repeat testing is typically greater than a value between 45 and 50 mm Hg, as determined by the attending physician based on the individual patient history and current clinical scenario. When a surrogate measure is obtained, comparable values are used, ideally as validated against blood gas data across various patient groups.

Failure to monitor CO_2 during sleep testing, particularly that of the patient with an elevated baseline value can result in suboptimal, even disastrous consequences. When there is no way of knowing the effect PAP has on the patient's acid-base balance it is difficult to make intelligent titration decisions toward optimal outcomes, including how her first impression of therapy will influence long-term compliance. This is particularly true in regard to both titrating **noninvasive positive pressure** to improve ventilation and the application of supplemental O_2.

Ideally, a CO_2 value will be obtained at baseline prior to therapeutic intervention and at the optimally titrated continuous positive airway pressure (CPAP) or bilevel PAP. In fact, a significant increase following CPAP titration warrants a bilevel PAP titration for improved ventilation. For individuals with a history that is compelling for **chronic CO_2 retention**, a baseline value should also be obtained prior to supplemental O_2 application and titration. Chronic CO_2 retention is characterized by chronically elevated CO_2. A blunted carboxic drive, and failure to identify this condition, can lead to worsening hypoventilation and deterioration of the patient's condition, including respiratory arrest if supplemental O_2 satisfies the hypoxic drive on which his breathing relies.[15]

When O_2 is administered to a patient from within this population, subsequent testing needs to be performed to determine that CO_2 retention is not exacerbated. Alternatively, the ordering practitioner may provide a maximum SpO_2 value, for instance 88% to 90%, in an effort to minimize the likelihood that supplemental O_2 will "knock out" the hypoxic drive. Whether baseline data are obtained by ABG analysis or a surrogate measure, CO_2 should be evaluated against the same measure 20 or more minutes following O_2 administration and adjustment.

END-TIDAL CARBON DIOXIDE MONITORING

E_TCO_2, also known as **capnometry**, has a rich history in the pediatric sleep-testing facility. In addition to

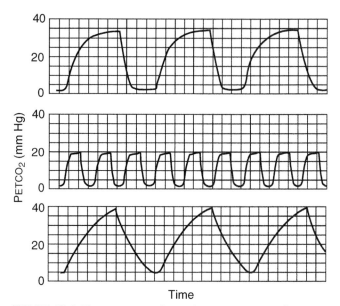

FIGURE 12-8 Three capnography tracing patterns: normal pattern, hyperventilation, and ventilation-perfusion mismatching. *From Ruppel GL: Manual of pulmonary function testing, ed 9, St Louis, 2009, Elsevier.*

numerical E_TCO_2 values obtained by capnometry, the graphical display of the flow curve from which values are measured, known as **capnography**, is typically displayed and recorded as part of the polysomnogram (Figure 12-8).

Evaluation of the amplitude and morphology of the capnograph over time can provide valuable information about the patient's breathing pattern, underlying respiratory disease, and sleep-disordered breathing events. With the limited effect pediatric sleep-disordered breathing often has on oxyhemoglobin saturation and the speed with which pediatric patients typically recover, increases in the E_TCO_2 signal provide an additional means of identifying hypoventilation. Similarly, a complete loss of data is a reliable indicator of apnea.

When ventilation is disrupted for any reason, it can be identified by capnometry long before the onset of an O_2Hb desaturation because of the time it takes for blood to flow to the site of the pulse oximeter sensor. The delay between an increase in E_TCO_2 and decrease in SpO_2 is lengthened even further when the patient is receiving supplemental O_2 because O_2Hb saturation may be maintained despite hypoventilation.[16]

According to the AASM, capnography can be used as an alternative measure for scoring apneas, to meet the secondary criterion of a respiratory event–related arousal, and to document the required increase associated with hypoventilation of pediatric subjects.[12] Because E_TCO_2 is oversensitive as a measure of airflow, it should only be used as a backup to AASM-recommended sensors for this purpose.[17] Clearly, value exists for the use of E_TCO_2 in the pediatric sleep laboratory as an alternative measure for respiratory event scoring, identification of breathing trends, hypoventilation, and more.

MONITORING CO_2 IN THE ADULT POPULATION

The expired CO_2 of three patients is plotted over time in Figure 12-8. In each example, expiration is marked by a rapid increase in CO_2 to a peak, representing the partial pressure of exhaled CO_2, followed by a return to baseline during inspiration. The top graph depicts a normal respiratory pattern with E_TCO_2 near 40 mm Hg and a relatively flat alveolar phase. Rapid respiratory rate and low E_TCO_2 (20 mm Hg) indicative of hyperventilation, with a normal expiratory waveform can be seen in the middle example. In the bottom tracing, the abnormal expired CO_2 waveform morphology is representative of a ventilation-perfusion mismatch. This pattern might be seen while recording data of a patient with severe COPD, among other disorders.

Monitoring CO_2 in exhaled gas has been employed less often in the adult sleep laboratory, although most technologists report reliable trending values during the diagnostic phase of study for both adult and pediatric patients. In fact, according to a 2006 study reported in *Sleep* both E_TCO_2 and transcutaneous CO_2 measures are noninvasive, validated, quantitative, indirect predictors of arterial CO_2 level, and both have been widely adopted for use during pediatric and adult PSG.[19] Unfortunately, the data can only be used to satisfy the scoring criteria for hypoventilation on adult studies. This is likely due to the failure of adult sleep testing facilities to embrace the technology and the subsequent lack of consensus during development of the AASM scoring manual.

When increased flow is present as the result of PAP application, and possibly supplemental O_2 administration, waveforms are dampened and recorded values often unreliable. This may account, in part, why end-tidal sampling has not been embraced in adult testing facilities or incorporated into adult respiratory event scoring criteria. Although E_TCO_2 can accurately predict the partial pressure of alveolar CO_2 under many circumstances, the accuracy is diminished when an alveolar-perfusion mismatch or other cardiovascular or pulmonary disease is present.[20,21] Despite these limitations, the technology can still provide good trend data even though the difference between the partial pressure of arterial CO_2 and E_TCO_2, for which the acronym **P(a-et)CO_2 gradient** is used, increases as compared with that for patients with normal pulmonary function.

THEORY OF OPERATION

Through direct measurement of exhaled gas values obtained through end-tidal sampling of exhaled gas, an E_TCO_2 monitor approximates the partial pressure of CO_2 in arterial blood. Infrared CO_2 analyzers use a gas's known absorption of infrared radiation to determine its concentration in a sample through a process known as *spectroscopy*. **Infrared spectroscopy** is based on the principle that molecules containing more than one element absorb infrared light in a characteristic manner.[22]

Other more advanced technologies exist that can measure CO_2 along with various other gases in a single aspirated sample of gas; however, because these are not used in the typical bedside E_TCO_2 monitor, only infrared spectroscopy is introduced in this chapter. The analyzer can determine how much of a gas is present by measuring the infrared radiation that is not absorbed, because certain gases, include CO and CO_2, absorb infrared radiation.

Mainstream and sidestream testing are the two primary methods of end-tidal monitoring of gas exchange. Mainstream devices are used when a closed-system breathing circuit is in use along with an endotracheal or **tracheostomy tube**. A tracheostomy tube is an artificial airway that is surgically placed into the trachea and bypasses the upper airway. For spontaneously breathing individuals, including those receiving noninvasive PAP therapy, a sidestream device is employed.

A traditional infrared absorption analyzer contains two infrared sources from which the beams they emit pass through parallel cells. One cell contains a reference gas; the other contains the gas sample to be analyzed. A rotating blade segments the beams rhythmically. When both the reference and sample cells contain the same amounts of gas, identical amounts of radiation reach each half of the detector cell. When a gas sample is introduced, it absorbs some infrared radiation. Different amounts of radiation reach the two halves of the detector cell, causing the diaphragm separating the compartments of the detector to oscillate. This oscillation is transformed into a signal proportional to the difference in gas concentrations.[23] Both CO and CO_2 can be simultaneously measured when four beams are used. A modern double-beam infrared absorption analyzer is depicted by schematic in Figure 12-9.

When the sample is contaminated by the presence of another gas or water vapor, absorption of infrared radiation increases and erroneously high values will be obtained. Components exist within the analyzer to minimize water vapor and filter other gases from the sample in an effort to maintain reliable results. There is also an external water filter intended to prevent liquid from entering the sampling chamber. It is imperative that the external water filter be changed when saturated with water or secretions, and that large amounts of condensation be removed from the tubing throughout testing. Some devices incorporate a water trap that is useful for long-term monitoring. If present, it should be emptied frequently.

Sidestream E_TCO_2 Monitors

Sidestream E_TCO_2 monitoring involves aspiration of gas into the sampling chamber at the point of end

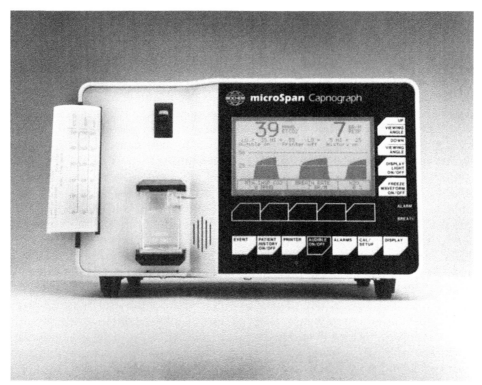

FIGURE 12-9 A microprocessor-controlled infrared carbon dioxide monitor. *Courtesy BCI, Inc., a Smiths Medical company.*

exhalation through a small tube. Typically, gas is sampled from the nares through a special **nasal cannula** very similar to the larger bore version used for supplemental O_2 delivery. A nasal cannula is a device consisting of two small tubes that fit in the nares and connect to a single larger tube.

Exhaled gas can also be effectively obtained for sampling from the distal end of a tracheostomy tube or through a nasal cannula or other tube positioned in front of the mouth. Tracheostomy bypasses the resistance of the upper airway, reducing or eliminating airflow at the mouth and nares. Because the gas being sampled at end exhalation contains little, if any, dead space (V_D) gas from the conducting airways, its content will be closer to the partial pressure of alveolar CO_2 (P_ACO_2) than the partial pressure of arterial CO_2. This is the primary reason for the 4-mm Hg to 6-mm Hg difference in values between end-tidal and arterial sampling in healthy individuals.

Displaying E_TCO_2 Data

Single-breath and **time-based capnography** are ways of displaying data. Time-based capnography used in PSG provides a numerical value of the maximum pressure of exhaled CO_2 for each breath, and displays either a breath-by-breath waveform or breathing trend over time; along with the patient's respiratory rate.[24] Single-breath capnometry has little application in the sleep testing environment.

For both methods of sidestream monitoring it is imperative that a good signal with adequate plateau is obtained during exhalation. Otherwise, the PCO_2 can be severely underestimated.

A vigilant technologist must regularly clear secretions, moisture, and organic material from the sampling tubing, and ensure its proper placement. The filter can also become saturated with moisture or other material and must be evaluated along with the tubing any time there is signal dampening, disruption, or loss. In Figure 12-10, the infrared CO_2 monitor allows presentation of E_TCO_2 values, respiratory rate,

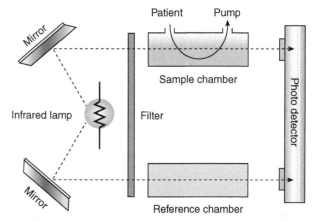

FIGURE 12-10 A simple schematic of a double-beam infrared capnometer. *From Kacmarek RM, et al: Egan's fundamentals of respiratory care, ed 10, St Louis, 2013, Elsevier.*

and CO_2 waveforms on the LCD screen. This particular capnograph includes a printer and alarms, along with a water trap to remove condensation from the sample line. In addition to the integrated strip-chart recorder, an analog output can be interfaced with the acquisition system for recording CO_2 data along with other physiological variables.

Figure 12-9, shown previously, represents a simple schematic of a double-beam infrared capnometer. A filtered infrared light source passes through a sample chamber, after which a lens focuses the remaining, unabsorbed radiation onto an electric photodetector. Because CO_2 absorbs infrared radiation, the greater the concentration of CO_2 in the sample, the less infrared light arrives at the detector; thus, variations in the concentration of CO_2 alter the electrical output of the detector. The signal is then used to either display the numerical CO_2 concentration (capnometer) or to generate a real-time graphic display (capnogram).

The tracing in Figure 12-11 is a normal capnogram. On the left side of the recording, the time base has been lengthened (reduced paper speed) so that compressed data from five tidal breaths can be assessed. The frequency of breathing is regular and CO_2 values are consistent over time. The phases on the single-breath capnogram on the right are as (1) beginning exhalation during which gas from the conducting airways (V_D ventilation) is expelled; (2) active exhalation made up of a mixture of V_D ventilation and alveolar ventilation; (3) the alveolar plateau, a measurement of the alveolar partial pressure of CO_2; and (4) active inhalation. End exhalation, during which gas is sampled, is denoted by the broken line.

ADVANTAGES AND LIMITATIONS OF TECHNOLOGY

E_TCO_2 monitoring is used extensively for monitoring children in the sleep laboratory, and less frequently as a parameter of adult PSG. When the patient is being ventilated using a closed circuit via a tracheostomy tube or endotracheal tube, E_TCO_2 can be measured directly; however, because sidestream sampling is most often performed using a nasal cannula with spontaneously breathing patients in the sleep laboratory, the signal will not always be reliable. When mask CPAP or bilevel PAP is applied, and possibly even low-flow O_2 supplementation, the increased flow within the open circuit tends to dilute the gas sampled at end exhalation. For this reason the numerical value, and sometimes the displayed waveform, can be distorted by therapeutic intervention.

Mouth breathing can also be problematic, but placing the sampling cannula in the air stream in front of the mouth or the use of a multisite sampling tube may provide a satisfactory solution to this issue. Distortion of the E_TCO_2 waveform caused by expiratory flow limitation, severe airway obstruction, and mouth breathing can influence the accuracy of values. Additionally, any time there is an increased **ventilation-to-perfusion (V/Q) mismatch** as characteristically seen with severe COPD the $P(a\text{-}et)CO_2$ will be greater than the normal 4-6 mm Hg. A V/Q mismatch occurs in this patient population when blood passes through the pulmonary circulation without exchanging gases with the alveoli. This variation must be considered, along with the fact that trend values can be less accurate when monitoring patients with COPD.

Some modern E_TCO_2 monitors like the one in Figure 12-12 are available with integrated pulse oximetry and provide an estimation of both ventilation and oxygenation. When simultaneous E_TCO_2 and SpO_2 values are desired during sleep testing, they can be measured and displayed on a single device, interfaced with the data acquisition system. Although both noninvasive measures have inherent limitations, they provide excellent trend data.

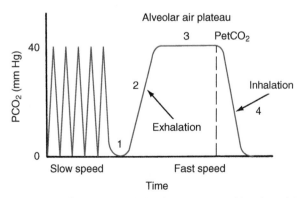

FIGURE 12-11 A capnogram from a normal, healthy, resting subject breathing room air. *From Cairo JM: Pilbeam's mechanical ventilation: physiological and clinical applications, ed 5, St Louis, 2012, Elsevier.*

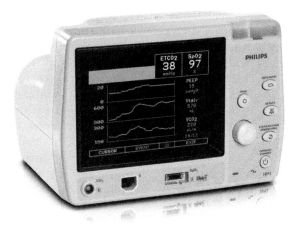

FIGURE 12-12 A capnometer with integrated pulse oximetry. *From Cairo JM:* Pilbeam's mechanical ventilation: physiological and clinical applications, *ed 5, St Louis, 2012, Elsevier.*

COMPARISON OF OBTAINED VALUES

Most studies comparing noninvasive measures of CO_2 to $PaCO_2$ as measured by ABG analysis have been performed in critical care units or during surgery under anesthesia, rather than in the sleep testing environment. In general, these studies show good correlation between arterial, end-tidal, and transcutaneous CO_2 values. However, E_TCO_2 monitoring tends to underestimate CO_2 values obtained from arterial blood, most notably in hypercapnic subjects and those with respiratory disease.[15]

Under normal circumstances the difference between the $P(a\text{-}et)CO_2$ gradient is 4-6 mm Hg in adults; the E_TCO_2 is 4-6 mm Hg lower than the $PaCO_2$ during normal tidal breathing. The $P(a\text{-}et)CO_2$ gradient is an index of alveolar V_D, and will therefore increase in the presence of lung disease or anything else that adds to alveolar V_D such as low cardiac output, hypovolemia, and pulmonary embolism. In the patient population studied in the outpatient sleep-testing facility it is unlikely that severe examples of these latter conditions will be seen. Although technologists should recognize this limitation of testing, the majority of patients for whom the $P(a\text{-}et)CO_2$ will be more than 4-6 mm Hg will be those with congestive heart failure, emphysema, or another chronic lung disease.

Although rarely an issue in the sleep laboratory, E_TCO_2 is not considered a good tool when precise CO_2 monitoring is required.[25] In the sleep laboratory relative changes typically suffice. Even with the difference in absolute values, monitoring of CO_2 by any means that provides trend data will be beneficial to patient outcomes as long as data are reliable during PAP titration, particularly noninvasive positive pressure ventilation (NPPV). Unfortunately, the reliability of E_TCO_2 is diminished in the presence of increased flow associated with PAP and O_2 administration, which makes it less valuable during titration studies. Figure 12-13 is a hypnogram displaying trend capnography data. Figures 12-14 through 12-17 are polysomnogram tracings that include examples of capnography in various scenarios.

A capnography educational site that is regularly updated and maintained by Harvard professor Bhavani-Shankar Kodali, MD, is located at www.capnography.com. This site provides many useful graphics and information about capnography, although not specific to polysomnographic technology.

(Text continued on page 300)

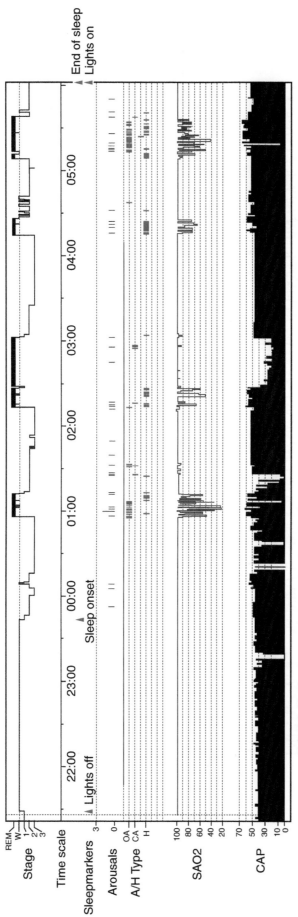

FIGURE 12-13 Clusters of elevated carbon dioxide values aligned with obstructive apneas and oxyhemoglobin desaturations are seen on this hypnogram from a 4-year-old girl. *From Beck SE, Marcus CL: Pediatric polysomnography,* Sleep Med Clin *4:393-406, 2009.*

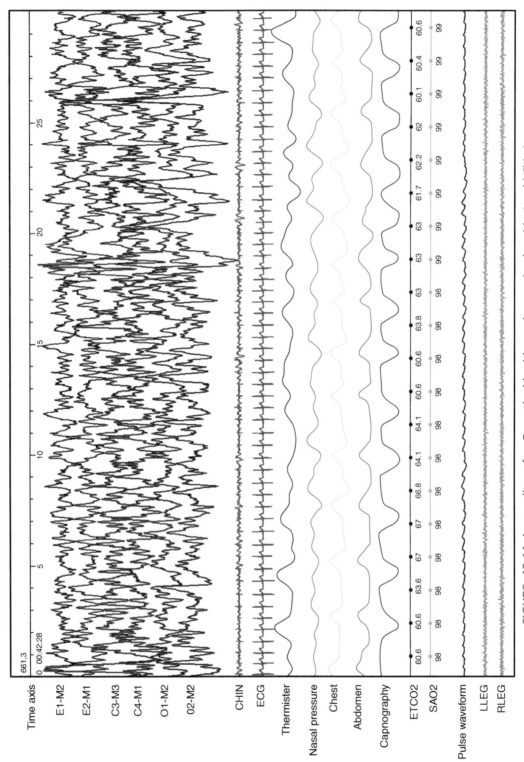

FIGURE 12-14 A recording of a 7-month-old with Arnold-Chiari malformation and central hypoventilation. Note the excellent carbon dioxide waveform and expiratory plateau. *From Beck SE, Marcus CL: Pediatric polysomnography, Sleep Med Clin 4: 393-406, 2009.*

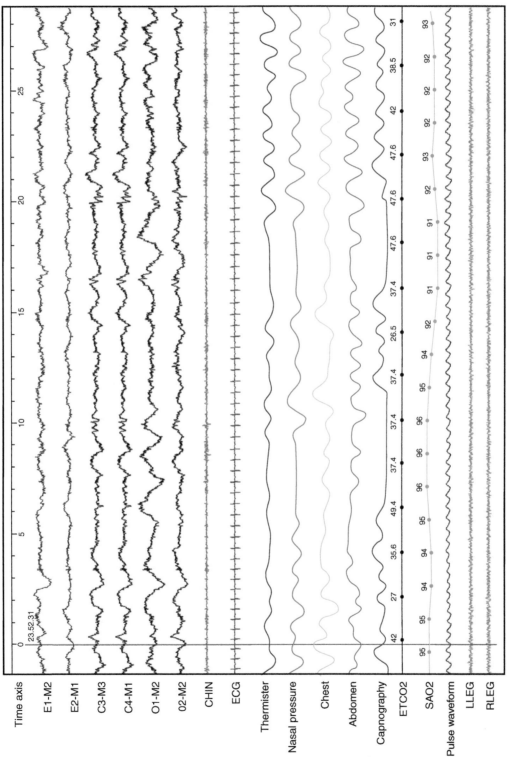

FIGURE 12-15 A recording from a 4-month-old infant with obstructive sleep apnea. Note the short obstructive apneas, associated with paradoxical chest and abdominal wall motion and desaturation, but no arousal. *From Beck SE, Marcus CL: Pediatric polysomnography, Sleep Med Clin 4:393-406, 2009.*

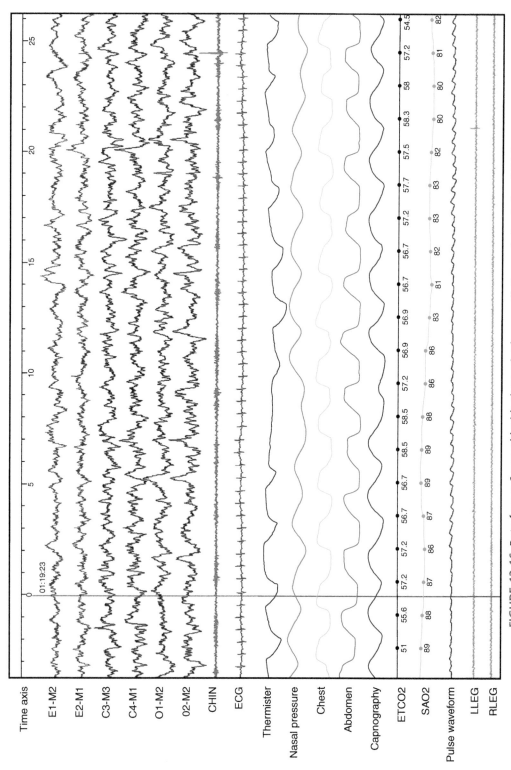

FIGURE 12-16 Data from a 6-year-old with obstructive hypoventilation and elevated end-tidal carbon dioxide with prolonged desaturation. *From Beck SE, Marcus CL: Pediatric polysomnography, Sleep Med Clin 4:393-406, 2009.*

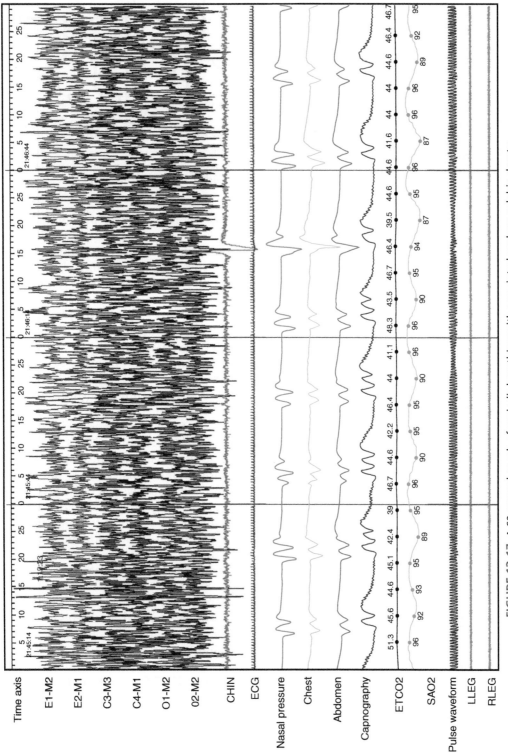

FIGURE 12-17 A 60-second epoch of periodic breathing with associated oxyhemoglobin desaturations and fairly stable end-tidal carbon dioxide values recorded from a 4-month-old infant. *From Beck SE, Marcus CL: Pediatric polysomnography, Sleep Med Clin 4:393-406, 2009.*

CONTRAINDICATIONS, PRECAUTIONS, AND INFECTION CONTROL

Although not a precaution or contraindication, the technologist must carefully evaluate data obtained by sampling of end-tidal gas. Because the sample must be aspirated from exhaled gas and drawn through tubing to be measured in the sampling chamber of a nearby analyzer, a delay exists between the signals displayed on the capnogram as compared with the patient's actual breathing cycle. When being recorded along with other parameters of a polysomnogram, it can be difficult to determine which respiratory waveform on the sleep study corresponds to a particular breath recorded by capnography.

The gas sampling tubing and moisture filter that make up the circuit of an E_TCO_2 monitor are disposable, single-patient-use items that are discarded between patient uses. Because exhaled gas is aspirated into the tubing with each patient breath, water vapor, secretions, and possibly solid organic material can be drawn into the tubing. Condensation and secretions can both occlude the tubing and saturate the moisture filter that resides between the tubing and sampling device. When either or both have become occluded, the tubing can be either carefully blown out with compressed air, or replaced; however, the moisture filter must be replaced when saturated. Partial occlusion of the sampling circuit results in a dampened waveform and erroneous values. Accurate results can be obtained only when a good alveolar plateau is present; data should be suspect any time the plateau is distorted.

No absolute contraindications exist to monitoring E_TCO_2. A relative contraindication to E_TCO_2 monitoring occurs when there is a continuous need for monitoring of $PaCO_2$ and pH. This absolute necessity should not be present during typical outpatient sleep disorders testing.

TRANSCUTANEOUS MONITORING OF OXYGEN AND CARBON DIOXIDE

Transcutaneous monitoring approximates PaO_2 and $PaCO_2$ values by dilating the capillary bed with heat, and measuring capillary blood O_2 and CO_2 values through the skin. Monitoring CO_2 through human skin was first mentioned by Severinghouse in 1960.[26] However, the first commercially available **transcutaneous carbon dioxide (tcCO2)** sensor was not introduced until approximately twenty years later.[26] The first **transcutaneous oxygen (tcO2)** sensor, however, was used in 1967 when the polarographic O_2 electrode was modified for transcutaneous use.[27] A heating element was incorporated into transcutaneous monitoring sensors later, which yielded values that more closely represent those obtained from arterial blood (Figure 12-18).

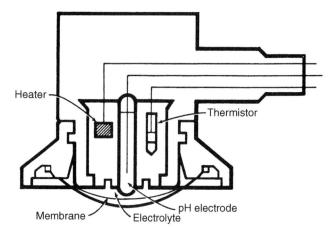

FIGURE 12-18 Graphic of a transcutaneous carbon dioxide electrode. *From Cairo JM, Pilbeam SP:* Mosby's respiratory care equipment, *ed 9, St Louis, 2011, Elsevier.*

Initially, sensors were predominately used in the intensive care nursery initially. Sensors required frequent membrane changes, and monitor calibration was required multiple times daily using gases of a known low and high value. Replacing the sensor membrane was a tedious, delicate, and often time-consuming process that could challenge even the most patient practitioner. Additionally, the sensors had to be moved to a new site as frequently as every 2 hours. Depending on the integrity of the patient's skin, repositioning of the sensor would be required even more frequently to avoid burns, blisters, and skin breakdown.

Some sleep laboratories adopted this technology early on, but as the business of sleep medicine grew, most adult testing facilities discontinued recording the parameter because of labor intensity, patient discomfort, and inconsistency of results in this patient population. Early sensors provided more reliable and consistent values along with pediatric PSG and more facilities testing these patients continued using the technology.

During the past two decades, particularly the last 10 years, improvements to technology have made $tcCO_2$ monitoring in the sleep laboratory more practical. Most notably, accurate values can now be obtained with less heating of the sensor site, resulting in less discomfort and less potential for damage to the skin. Modern devices require warming of the monitoring site to only 42° C for adults and 41° C for neonates, as compared with temperatures as high as 45° C that were necessary in the past.

Manufacturers claim that the sensor can remain in one location for as long as 8 or 12 hours, although the technologist should establish a routine to move it for comfort every few hours as practical. Repositioning the sensor each time the patient needs a restroom break, and during other patient-technologist interactions, is typically more than adequate.

Modern, small, lightweight sensors can be effectively applied to various locations of the body, including the thorax, abdomen, forearm, and for increased patient comfort the earlobe where it can generally be left in place the longest. Additionally, both $tcCO_2$ and tcO_2 can be monitored using one dual-sensor probe, although tcO_2 is not a value typically monitored during sleep testing.

Many of the studies comparing $tcCO_2$ with arterial CO_2 measured by blood gas analysis have been performed using samples obtained during surgery because of the practical limitations of maintaining indwelling arterial lines or obtaining serial blood gas results by arterial puncture in other patient populations. Comparison studies using pediatric, adult, and geriatric subjects have continuously and reliably shown agreement between these non-invasively obtained data and arterial CO_2.[28-32]

ADVANTAGES AND LIMITATIONS OF TECHNOLOGY

Transcutaneous monitoring is another noninvasive method of indirectly obtaining CO_2 values, and can also provide an estimation of the PaO_2. During sleep testing, CO_2 values measured noninvasively using transcutaneous technology are extremely valuable because they provide information about how therapeutic modalities, sleep-disordered breathing, and underlying medical disorders augment the patient's ventilation.

Unlike pulse oximetry and E_TCO_2 monitoring, which rely on spectrophotometric analysis, $tcPCO_2$ and $tcPO_2$ are measured at the surface of the skin using modified blood gas electrodes. The optimal location for sensor placement is an area of high capillary density and minimal skin thickness. The ear lobe, forearm, chest, and abdomen are often used. The obvious advantage of transcutaneous monitoring as compared with serial blood gas testing is that there is typically no need to draw arterial blood for analysis. Another significant advantage of transcutaneous sampling during sleep testing is the ability to monitor and obtain reliable results during PAP or supplemental O_2 administration and titration, during which the increased flow typically dilutes end-tidal samples. This is likely the single most important advantage of this technology as compared with end-tidal monitoring.

Given the evolution of the field and patient population, more advanced cases of sleep-disordered breathing and other medical issues requiring nocturnal ventilation are being seen in many sleep laboratories. The treatment goal for the majority of these patients is improved control of ventilation. Likewise, supplemental O_2 is titrated either in concert with the various modalities of PAP, or as stand-alone therapy. Careful addition of supplemental O_2 can typically be accomplished safely by a knowledgeable technologist; however, when a patient with severe CO_2 retention is hypersensitive to even a small dose of supplemental O_2, hypercapnia can significantly worsen.

Even application of continuous PAP will occasionally cause an increase in arterial CO_2, particularly for patients with respiratory disease with or without known chronic CO_2 retention. Unless CO_2 is being monitored by some means in the sleep laboratory, the technologist has no way of knowing the exact effect of therapeutic modalities on physiology. In some cases the technologist is not even aware of a patient's CO_2 retention status.

During the past two decades there have been numerous advances in transcutaneous monitoring technology. Among the most notable includes the ease with which newer models are used in general, less frequent need for and simpler membrane changes, safety and comfort in regard to lower sensor temperature and smaller sensor size, and improved accuracy of results. New technology has also been developed for simultaneous monitoring and display of $tcCO_2$ and SpO_2 data that are recorded using a single sensor. This sensor, ideal for the sleep laboratory, has been shown to provide accurate results for both parameters on critically ill patients and patients with sleep apnea using an electrode temperature of $42°$ C.[33]

One potential disadvantage of transcutaneous monitoring pertains to the need for the recording site to be warmed by the sensor in order to enhance capillary vasodilation for increased accuracy. In the sleep laboratory, with sufficient planning for patient monitoring, this should not be problematic. When the site is changed in the middle of therapeutic titration, however, reliable data may not be immediately available. This issue is found throughout the literature with the optimal warm-up time ranging from 12 to 30 minutes. Apparently the technological advances that require less heat have also sped the warming process. In recent literature, short times (e.g., 12 minutes) were offered, whereas the lengthier times before values could be trusted were found in older studies.

COMPARISON OF OBTAINED VALUES

The diffusion capacity of CO_2 is greater than that of O_2, which makes transcutaneous monitoring of CO_2 much more reliable than transcutaneous monitoring of O_2. Major concern is lessened because the CO_2 value provides additional information and tcO_2 adds little when SpO_2 is already being monitored during sleep testing. According to available studies, transcutaneous monitoring of CO_2 has a smaller bias compared with $PaCO_2$ than that of the $PaCO_2$ and E_TCO_2. Alternately, however, $tcCO_2$ tends to slightly overestimate the $PaCO_2$.[18] Fortunately, most commercial manufacturers of transcutaneous monitors incorporate correction factors into the software to remove any discrepancy between $PaCO_2$ and E_TCO_2.[22] These devices will not only provide valid trend data, they will also provide reliable absolute values when compared with the $PaCO_2$ from ABG analysis.

Because E_TCO_2 data are affected by the presence of increased flow, $tcCO_2$ provides the most reliable data for determining the effects of therapy on ventilation throughout the course of a sleep study. It can also provide valid results during sleep testing on patients for whom E_TCO_2 may not be reliable, such as those with hypercapnia caused by alveolar hypoventilation, chronic airflow obstruction, or morbid obesity, with or without sleep apnea.[34]

SpO_2 values are relied on for monitoring oxygenation and O_2Hb desaturations during a sleep study, for scoring of sleep-disordered breathing events, and to qualify the patient for home use of supplemental O_2. For this reason, tcO_2 is a parameter of little value during a typical sleep study. When dual-monitoring capability is an option, a device that records both $tcCO_2$ and SpO_2 holds the most utility in the sleep-testing facility.

CONTRAINDICATIONS, PRECAUTIONS, AND INFECTION CONTROL

There are no known absolute contraindications to transcutaneous monitoring of O_2 or CO_2. Transcutaneous monitoring guidelines that may be applicable to sleep testing for neonatal and pediatric patients are summarized in Box 12-4. A potential relative contraindication to end-tidal monitoring exists when there is a need for continuous pH and $PaCO_2$ monitoring. Also, because the sensor site is heated, the technologist must be careful not to allow the probe to remain in one place too long in an effort to avoid damage to the skin. When choosing a location for sensor placement, the integrity of the skin should be thoroughly assessed. Likewise, each time the technologist enters the room, he or she should verify that there are no burns and that no evidence of skin breakdown exists. These simple precautions should avoid thermal injury issues when using modern recording technology.

Maintenance of infection control should present few, if any, problems as long as skin integrity is frequently assessed. The sensor, cable, and even the recorder should be cleaned and disinfected between each patient. Many manufacturers recommend that the sensor membrane be replaced prior to use on each patient.

ANALYSIS OF ACID-BASE BALANCE OF ARTERIAL BLOOD GAS RESULTS

Assess the pH and follow the steps in Figures 12-19 and 12-20:

If pH is within the normal range of 7.35-7.45, follow the steps outlined in Figure 12-19.

If pH is either above 7.45 (alkaline) or below 7.35 (acidic) follow the steps in Figure 12-20.

See Table 12-4 for acid-base balance quick reference.

BOX 12-4

Summary of American Association for Respiratory Care Clinical Practice Guidelines Transcutaneous Blood Gas Monitoring for Neonatal and Pediatric Patients

INDICATIONS

- Monitoring the adequacy of arterial oxygenation and ventilation
- The need to quantify the response to diagnostic and therapeutic interventions (e.g., administering enriched oxygen mixtures, application of PEEP)

CONTRAINDICATIONS AND COMPLICATIONS

Transcutaneous monitoring may be relatively contraindicated in patients with poor skin integrity or adhesive allergy.

MONITORING

The following should be recorded when monitoring transcutaneous measurements:

- Clinical appearance of the patient, including subjective assessment of perfusion, pallor, and skin temperature
- Date and time of the measurement
- Patient position
- Respiratory rate
- Physical activity level
- Inspired oxygen concentration and the type of oxygen delivery device if supplemental oxygen is being administered
- Mode of ventilator support (i.e., ventilator or CPAP settings)
- Electrode placement site, electrode temperature, and time of placement
- Results of simultaneous measurements of PaO_2, $PaCO_2$, and pH

CPAP, Continuous positive airway pressure; *PaCO₂,* partial pressure of carbon dioxide; *PaO₂,* partial pressure of arterial oxygen; *PEEP,* positive end-expiratory pressure.
From Cairo JM: *Pilbeam's mechanical ventilation: physiological and clinical applications,* ed 5, St Louis, 2012, Elsevier/Mosby.

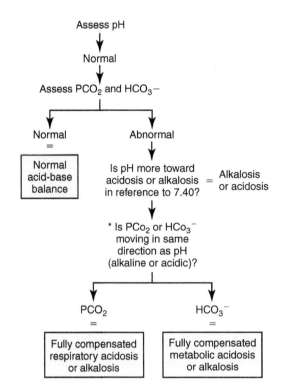

FIGURE 12-19 Acid-base with normal pH.

* The other parameter will be moving in the opposite direction of the pH (acid or alkaline) to compensate

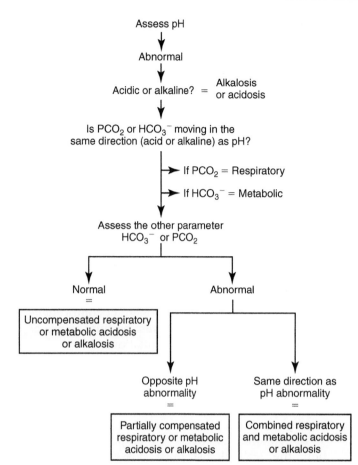

FIGURE 12-20 Acid base with abnormal pH.

TABLE 12-4
Acid-Base Balance Quick Reference

	Acute	Partially Compensated	Fully Compensated
Respiratory Acidosis			
pH	↓	↓	↓N*
PaCO$_2$	↑	↑	↑
HCO$_3^-$	N	↑	↑
Respiratory Alkalosis			
pH	↑	↑	↑N
PaCO$_2$	↓	↓	↓
HCO$_3^-$	N	↓	↓
Metabolic Acidosis			
pH	↓	↓	↓N
PaCO$_2$	N	↓	↓
HCO$_3^-$	↓	↓	↓
Metabolic Alkalosis			
pH	↑	↑	↑N
PaCO$_2$	N	↑	↑
HCO$_3^-$	↑	↑	↑

Continued

TABLE 12-4

Acid-Base Balance Quick Reference—cont'd

	Combined Acidosis[†]	Combined Alkalosis
pH	↓	↓
$PaCO_2$	↑	↓
HCO_3^-	↓	↑

*↑N or ↓N means that the pH has returned to a value within the normal limits of 7.35-7.45 through compensation by the opposing system. It will remain on the low or high side of absolute normal (7.40) because the body cannot overcompensate. When the results are partially compensated, the pH remains outside the normal range but has begun being shifted back toward normal by the effects of the opposing system.

†It would be atypical for an outpatient arriving for a sleep study to have results consistent with a combined acid-base imbalance. However, these values may be in the patient's medical record, especially if she or he was previously hospitalized for critical care.

CHAPTER SUMMARY

- Oximetry is an integral component of comprehensive PSG. The technologist must be fully aware of its various capabilities and limitations.
- A practical understanding of this technology is an essential skill of a qualified sleep technologist.
- As sleep technology evolves, standardization to both policy and available recording products is needed.
- To understand the effects of therapeutic intervention, the technologist must possess a working knowledge of ventilation and oxygenation, and the various ways these parameters are measured.
- Failure to understand the differences between measures of oxygenation can lead to erroneous interpretation of data and assessment of the patient, with possible application or titration of an inappropriate therapeutic modality.
- According to the AASM, oximetry data documenting an accompanying desaturation ≥ 3% are required for the identification and scoring of hypopneas.
- To qualify patients for supplemental O_2 in the home during sleep, CMS requires documentation of cumulative saturation values ≤ 88% for ≥ 5 minutes obtained by pulse oximetry
- To understand the patient's baseline status and effects of treatment modalities, the technologist must be able to assess oxygenation status from various measures and appreciate the effect of CO_2 on acid-base balance.
- When recorder settings are not understood, or are incorrectly applied, misinterpretation of data is possible that may affect clinical decision making.
- Safe and effective use of noninvasive monitors requires knowledge found in the operation manuals for the monitor and data acquisition system. Various ancillary devices can be interfaced with a recorder, via a two-wire conductor, and calibrated to accept a 0-1 V DC signal representative of the recorded measure.

- Oximeter response time and sampling rate must be user definable or appropriate if predefined and fixed.
- Trend CO_2 values are beneficial for determining adequacy of the patient's ventilation when noninvasive measures are reliable as compared with $PaCO_2$. Transcutaneous CO_2 monitoring provides reliable results as compared with $PaCO_2$ once the warm-up period has elapsed.
- E_TCO_2 monitoring is more widely used in PSG than $tcCO_2$ monitoring, likely because of the latter's past need for excessive heating of the sensor site and excessive calibration.
- End-tidal values can be "washed out" as a result of supplemental O_2 or PAP, which limits the value of this technology during the therapeutic phase of testing.
- Monitoring of CO_2 can be very useful during supplemental O_2 titration when the patient has chronic CO_2 retention and when augmenting ventilation with PAP.

References

1. DesJardins TR: *Cardiopulmonary anatomy and physiology: essentials for respiratory care*, ed 5, Clifton Park, NY, 2008, Thompson Delmar.
2. Potter PA, Perry AG, Stockert PA, et al: *Basic nursing*, ed 7, St. Louis, 2011, Elsevier/Mosby.
3. Birnbaum, S: Pulse oximetry: identifying its applications, coding, and reimbursement, *Chest* 135:838-841, 2009.
4. Severinghouse JW, Astrup PB: History of blood gas analysis. VI. Oximetry, *J Clin Monit* 2:270-288, 1986.
5. Severinhouse JW, Honda Y: History of blood gas analysis. VII. Pulse oximetry, *J Clin Monit* 3(2):135-138, Apr 1987.
6. Wilkins RL, Stoller JK, Kacmarek RM: *Egan's fundamentals of respiratory care*, ed 9, St. Louis, 2009, Elsevier/Mosby.
7. AARC clinical practice guideline: pulse oximetry, *Respir Care* 37(8):891-897, 1992.
8. Davila DG, Richards KC, Marshall BL, et al: Oximeter's acquisition parameter influences the profile of respiratory disturbances, *Sleep* 1:91-5, 2003.
9. Zafar S, Krieger AC, Rappaport DM: Choice of oximeter affects apnea-hypopnea index, *Chest* 127:80-88, 2005.
10. Birnbaum S: Pulse oximetry: identifying its applications, coding, and reimbursement, *Chest* 135:838-841, 2009.

11. Davila DG, Richard KC, Marshall BL, et al: Oximeter performance: the influence of acquisition parameters, *Chest* 122:1654-1660, 2002.

12. Berry R, Brooks R, Gamaldo C, et al: *The AASM manual for the scoring of sleep and associated events* V2.0, Darien, Ill., 2012, American Academy of Sleep Medicine.

13. Centers for Medicare and Medicaid Services: Local coverage article for oxygen and oxygen equipment—policy article—effective October 2011 (A22750), DME Region C (website). http://www.cms.gov/medicare-coverage-database/license/cpt-license. Accessed July 3, 2012.

14. Centers for Medicare and Medicaid Services: National coverage determination (NCD) for continuous positive airway pressure (CPAP) therapy for obstructive sleep apnea (OSA) (240.4). http://www.cms.gov/medicare-coverage-database/details/ Accessed on August 3, 2012.

15. Marcus CL, Carroll JL, Bamford O, et al: Supplemental oxygen during sleep in children with sleep-disordered breathing, *Am J Respir Crit Care Med* 152(4 Pt 1):1297-1301, 1995.

16. Green SM: Research advances in procedural sedation and analgesia, *Ann Emerg Med* 49(1):31-36, 2007.

17. Beck SE, Marcus CL: Pediatric polysomnography, *Sleep Med Clin* 4:393–406, 2009.

18. Redline S, Budhraja R, Kapur V, et al: The scoring of respiratory events in sleep: reliability and validity, *J Clin Sleep Med* 3(2): 169-200, 2007.

19. Kirk VG, Batuyong ED, Bohn SG: Transcutaneous carbon dioxide monitoring and capnography during pediatric polysomnography, *Sleep* 29(12):1601-1608, 2006.

20. Breen PH: Arterial blood gas and pH analysis. Clinical approach and interpretation, *Anesthesiol Clin North Am* 19:885-906, 2001.

21. Wahba RWM, Tessler MJ: Misleading end-tidal CO_2 tensions, *Can J Anaesth* 43:862-6,1996.

22. Cairo JM: *Pilbeam's mechanical ventilation: physiological and clinical applications*, ed 5, St. Louis, 2012, Elsevier/Mosby.

23. Ruppel GL: *Manual of pulmonary function testing*, ed 9, St. Louis, 2008, Elsevier/Mosby.

24. Waugh JB, Epps CA: Ventilation for life: efficient ventilation utilizing noninvasive capnography, *AARC Times* 12-16, March 2009.

25. Nosovitch MA, Johnson JO, Tobias JD: Noninvasive intraoperative monitoring of carbon dioxide in children: end-tidal versus transcutaneous techniques, *Pediatr Anaesth* 12:48-52, 2002.

26. Eberhard P: The design, use, and results of transcutaneous carbon dioxide analysis: current and future directions, *Anesth Analg* 105(65):Suppl S48-S52, 2007.

27. Evans NTS, Naylor PFD: The systemic oxygen supply to the surface of human skin, *Respir Physiol* 3:21-37, 1967.

28. Casati A, Squicciarini G, Malagutti G, et al: Transcutaneous monitoring of partial pressure of carbon dioxide in the elderly patient: a prospective, clinical comparison with end-tidal monitoring, *J Clin Anesth* 18:436-440, 2006.

29. Reed C, Martineau R, Miller D, et al: The comparison of transcutaneous, end-tidal, and arterial measurements of carbon dioxide during general anaesthesia, *Can J Anaesth* 39(1):31-36.

30. Oshibuchi M, Cho S, Hara T, et al: A comparison evaluation of transcutaneous and end-tidal measurements of CO_2 in thoracic anesthesia, *Anesth Analg* 97:776-779, 2003.

31. Rohling R, Biro P: Clinical investigation of a new combined pulse oximetry and carbon dioxide tension sensor in adult anesthesia, *J Clin Monit Comput* 15:23-27, 1999.

32. Reid CW, Martinez RJ, Hull DR, et al: A comparison of transcutaneous end-tidal and arterial measurements of carbon dioxide during general anaesthesia, *Can J Anaesth* 39:31-36, 1992.

33. Senn O, Clarebach CF, Kaplan V, et al: Monitoring carbon dioxide tension and arterial oxygen saturation by a single earlobe sensor in patients with critical illness or sleep apnea, *Chest* 128:1291-1296, 2005.

34. O'Donoghue FJ, Catcheside PG, Ellis EE, et al: Sleep hypoventilation in hypercapnic chronic obstructive pulmonary disease: prevalence and associated factors, *Eur Respir J* 21: 977-984, 2003.

REVIEW QUESTIONS

1. In respect to adult sleep testing, which of the following is the most notable improvement to noninvasive monitoring of carbon dioxide during the past 2 decades?
   a. Reduced size of the gas sampling cannula
   b. Lower sensor temperature requirement
   c. Integrated heated-wire circuit technology
   d. Digitization of CO_2 values during testing

2. Which measure of CO_2 is *most* reliable for monitoring throughout both the diagnostic and therapeutic portions of a sleep study?
   a. ABG analysis
   b. COHb testing
   c. $tcCO_2$ monitoring
   d. E_TCO_2 monitoring

3. What is the normal $P(a\text{-}et)CO_2$ gradient for adults?
   a. 0-3 mm Hg
   b. 4-6 mm Hg
   c. 5-10 mm Hg
   d. 7-12 mm Hg

4. For patients with which of the following conditions would an increase in the $P(a\text{-}et)CO_2$ gradient be *most* expected?
   a. Chronic neuromuscular disease
   b. Restrictive thoracic cage disorders
   c. Obstructive pulmonary disease
   d. Obesity hypoventilation syndrome

5. Which monitoring method will produce the most accurate measure of carbon dioxide?
   a. ABG analysis
   b. COHb testing
   c. $tcCO_2$ monitoring
   d. E_TCO_2 monitoring

6. When inspired air contains an insufficient amount of oxygen, the resulting condition is:
   a. Stagnant hypoxia
   b. Histotoxic hypoxia
   c. Anemic hypoxia
   d. Hypoxic hypoxia

7. The affinity of CO for Hb is _____ times the affinity of O_2 for Hb.
   a. 120
   b. 160
   c. 210
   d. 320

8. Following an exposure to CO, its affinity for Hb will result in which of the following?
   a. Normal or elevated SpO_2, normal PaO_2, and reduced tissue oxygenation
   b. Significantly low SpO_2, reduced PaO_2, and normal tissue oxygenation
   c. Normal or elevated SpO_2, reduced PaO_2, and normal tissue oxygenation
   d. Significantly low SpO_2, normal PaO_2, and reduced tissue oxygenation

9. What is the greatest obstacle to routine use of $tcCO_2$ monitoring during sleep testing of adult subjects?
   a. Results lack an adequate relationship with $PaCO_2$ data
   b. The potential for thermal injury and breakdown to the skin
   c. It is impossible to obtain a valid signal on adult subjects
   d. It is not recognized by, nor included in, AASM scoring rules

10. What range of SpO_2 and PaO_2 values represent mild hypoxemia?
    a. 70% to 90%; 40-60 mm Hg
    b. 80% to 90%; 70-80 mm Hg
    c. 90% to 95%; 60-80 mm Hg
    d. 95% to 97%; 80-95 mm Hg

Chapter 13

Diagnosis, Treatment, and Outcome Management of Sleep-Disordered Breathing

Bonnie Robertson

CHAPTER OUTLINE

LEARNING OBJECTIVES

After reading this chapter, you will be able to:
1. Recognize respiratory events contributing to sleep disorders.
2. Titrate continuous positive airway pressure, bilevel positive airway pressure, adaptive servo ventilation, noninvasive positive-pressure ventilation, and supplemental oxygen to achieve optimal outcomes.
3. Follow "best practice" treatment guidelines.
4. Identify alternative therapies for sleep-disordered breathing.
5. Educate patients regarding disease process and therapy recommendations.
6. Follow patients' progress on positive airway pressure therapy and treatment recommendations.
7. Assist patients with positive airway pressure adherence issues.
8. Identify positive airway pressure therapy outcomes.

KEY TERMS

adaptive servo ventilation

adherence

apnea-hypopnea index (AHI)

central apnea

clinical sleep educator

compliance

continuous positive airway pressure (CPAP) emergent

enhanced expiratory rebreathing space (EERS)

mixed apnea

noninvasive positive pressure ventilation (NPPV)

obstructive sleep apnea (OSA)

paradoxical breathing

pressure support (PS)

respiratory inductive plethysmography (RIP)

split-night sleep study

titration

Obstructive sleep apnea (OSA) is the most common diagnosis seen in a sleep-testing center. OSA manifests as intermittent cessations of airflow during sleep with continued efforts to breathe. Population-based studies have documented that possibly up to 25% of the population have at least a mild to moderate degree of sleep-disordered breathing.[1] Because of the high occurrence of the disorder, this group of patients composes the majority of sleep studies performed in sleep testing centers.

Since approximately 1985, continuous positive airway pressure (CPAP) therapy has been the accepted gold standard for the treatment of OSA.[2] The continuous positive pressure acts as a splint to maintain a patent airway during sleep.

Patients who are studied in sleep-testing facilities often undergo a **split-night sleep study**. This type of study involves the use of a diagnostic protocol for the first half of the testing period followed by a therapeutic protocol for the second half of the testing period, if the patient meets predetermined diagnostic factors. This type of testing has increased in popularity during the past 10 years. It has been shown to be an effective pathway to diagnosis and treatment at a significantly reduced expense for the third-party payor as well as the patient, compared with performing two separate nights of sleep testing: one for diagnosis and a second test for the **titration** of positive airway pressure (PAP).

Titration is manual or auto manipulation of the positive airway pressure setting to treat sleep disordered breathing. This strategy, used by some programs since the early 1990s, has been identified as an effective method of reducing patient wait time as the time from referral to study in many prominent facilities grew to 6 months or longer because of public and professional awareness of sleep disorders. Whatever the motivation for conducting split-night procedures, one must recognize that not all patients are good candidates.

More recently, other therapies have emerged for the treatment of more complex patients. These patients may have comorbidities that contribute to an increased difficulty in the establishment of diagnosis and treatment. Central apnea and PAP-emergent central apnea present challenges for the sleep technologist during both diagnostic and therapeutic sleep studies. They also require more advanced technologist skills to recognize and identify the related events.

The sleep technologist must be confident in skills related to diagnostic waveform recognition to make well-informed decisions regarding the application of PAP during a split-night study. Failure to correctly identify, differentiate, and tabulate (i.e., scoring maneuvers) respiratory events can result in nontreatment or inadequate treatment of the patient. The astute learner-technologist will spend many hours of hard work developing the skills necessary for competent respiratory event identification. At times, even knowledgeable, skilled technologists experienced in event recognition and polysomnogram (PSG) scoring may have difficulty differentiating some respiratory event types, among other scoring parameters.

The titration of PAP and other advanced therapy modalities requires tremendous attention to proper event recognition, true understanding of the mechanics of breathing and the effect of therapy application. A competent understanding of treatment options and the decision making related to those options are of the utmost importance. A technologist must understand and comprehend how the devices work and how they affect the sleep architecture, cardiac system, and respiratory status of each patient.

RESPIRATORY EVENT RECOGNITION

The waveforms displayed on the PSG system montage representing breathing are captured by recording sensors and equipment that convert the mechanical activity into an electrical signal, which is digitalized for display. The accepted standardized recording mechanism for respiratory effort used during sleep testing is **respiratory inductive plethysmography (RIP)**. The gold standard for respiratory effort recording requires insertion of an esophageal pressure monitoring probe; however, because this procedure is invasive in nature, most sleep testing centers do not use it as a first-line sensor.[3]

PARADOXICAL BREATHING

The proper application and fit of RIP belts is paramount to accurate recording and recognition of in-sync versus **paradoxical breathing**, or desynchronized breathing pattern. This pattern is illustrated in figure 13-1. In addition, the polarity of the respective respiratory effort recording channel must be properly adjusted during periods of normal breathing. These factors, all controlled by the technologist, result in the recording of accurate information, and thus recognition of waveform patterns by the technologist and the interpreting physician. An obstruction of the upper airway frequently manifests with paradoxical breathing. The thorax collapses during inspiration when the airway is blocked because negative pressure, created as the strong diaphragm muscles pull the abdomen down and out, displaces the chest wall. During exhalation the opposite occurs. Upon resolution of airway obstruction, in-phase thoraco-abdominal movement returns.

CENTRAL APNEA

Central apnea demonstrates little or no effort on either the chest or abdominal respiratory effort channel in addition to little or no airflow. An illustration of how this may appear on a monitor is shown in Figure 13-2. Many patients with cardiovascular disease have central apnea during sleep. The technologist must be able to trust the data when the effort belts do not record movement. Ensuring proper placement and proper size of the belts enhances the accuracy of the RIP recording system. Confirmation that size and placement are appropriate will add value to, and the technologist's trust in, the recorded data.

CHEYNE-STOKES RESPIRATIONS

Patients with cardiovascular disease may have Cheyne-Stokes respirations (CSR) during wake and sleep (Figure 13-3). Studies indicate that 45% of stable, optimally treated patients with congestive heart failure (CHF) have an **apnea-hypopnea index (AHI)** > 26 events per hour of sleep.[4] Furthermore, the treatment of sleep-disordered breathing improves left ventricular systolic function, improving ejection fraction from 25 ± 2.8 to 33.8 ± 2.4 percent ($P < 0.001$).[5]

MIXED APNEA

A patient may demonstrate central and obstructive efforts during a single respiratory event. When these mixed efforts have little or no airflow, the event is known as a **mixed apnea;** it starts as a central apnea with no effort and no airflow, and converts to an obstructive apnea in the latter half of the event as effort resumes (Figure 13-4).

HYPOPNEA

Respiratory events during sleep may also manifest as hypopneas (Figure 13-5). The American Academy of Sleep Medicine (AASM) defines a hypopnea of an adult subject as a respiratory event lasting a minimum of 10 seconds with a $\geq 30\%$ reduction in peak signal excursion as compared with the baseline signal, and associated with at least a 3% oxygen desaturation or an EEG arousal.[6]

COMPLICATED BREATHING PATTERNS

Many patients have complicated breathing patterns because of restriction of the thoracic ribcage in addition to obstruction of the upper airway. Patients with significant obesity have restricted ribcage movement from the weight of the body fat on the chest, resulting in impeded respiratory movement. Patients with neuromuscular disease have an impediment to free breathing through reduced movement of the ribcage and also demonstrate a complexity of breathing problems during a sleep study[7] (Figure 13-6). These patients may require **noninvasive positive-pressure ventilation (NPPV)** as their disease state progresses.[8]

A histogram demonstrates complicated breathing events, including central apneas, mixed apneas, obstructive apneas, central and obstructive hypopneas with severe oxygen desaturations, and extremely disturbed sleep as evidenced by the stage plot.

TITRATION TECHNIQUES

CONTINUOUS POSITIVE AIRWAY PRESSURE

OSA frequently has the identifying characteristics of loud snoring, gasping for air, disrupted sleep, and tiredness during waking hours. In the sleep laboratory setting, PAP is the most common treatment for resolving airway obstruction with CPAP as the therapy of choice for a high percentage of the patients with sleep-disordered breathing. CPAP is easy to administer in the testing environment and titration typically requires a straightforward approach. Once identification of OSA is confirmed during the sleep study, a patient may be placed on CPAP for titration purposes, often allowing diagnosis and treatment in one visit to the sleep center. CPAP creates a splint for the obstructed airway, keeping it open throughout the respiratory cycle (Figure 13-7). In these patients, the airway typically collapses at the end of exhalation, just before negative pressure is exerted against it at beginning inspiration. With the pneumatic splint of CPAP continuously exerting pressure on the walls of

(Text continued on page 316)

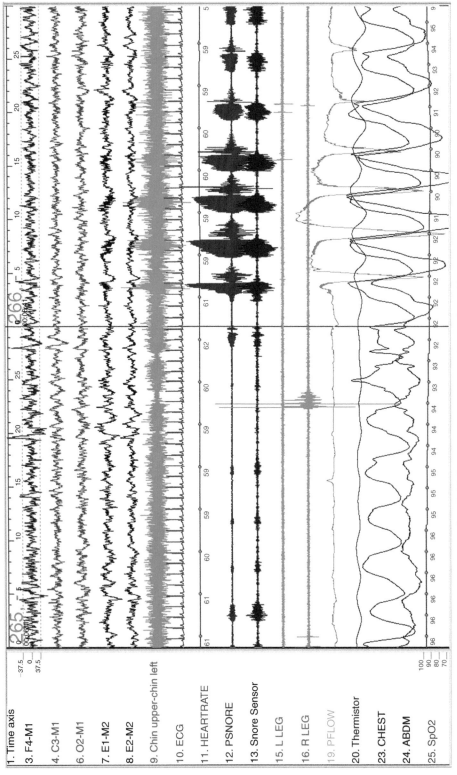

FIGURE 13-1 Obstructive apnea with paradoxical breathing.

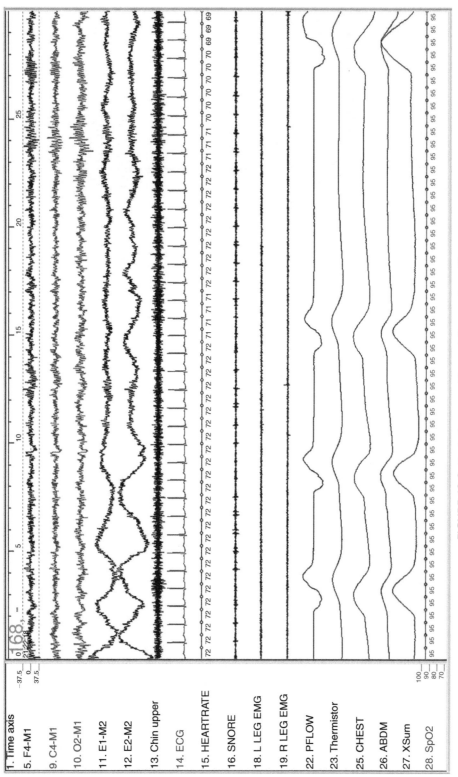

FIGURE 13-2 Central apnea with no airflow and no effort.

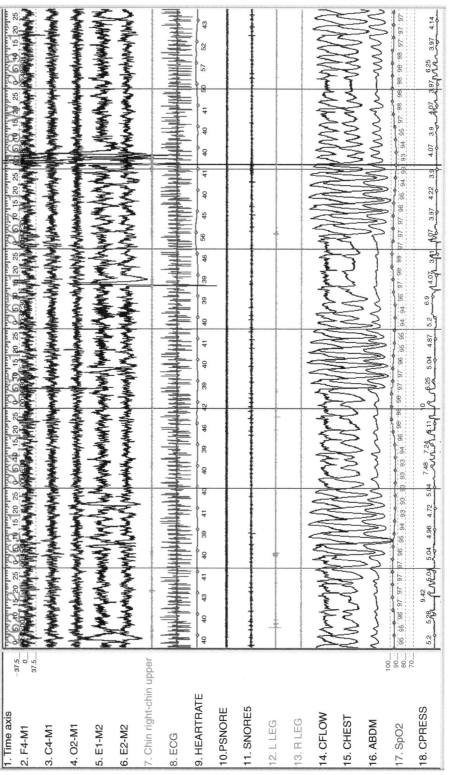

FIGURE 13-3 Cheyne-Stokes respirations with waxing and waning patterning.

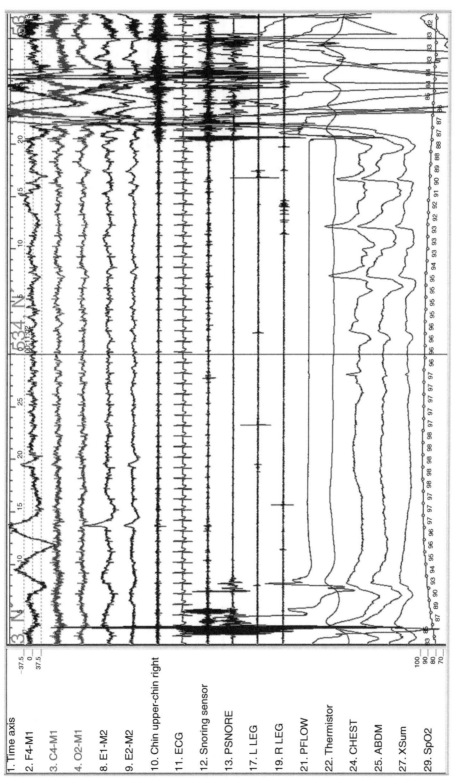

FIGURE 13-4 Mixed apnea.

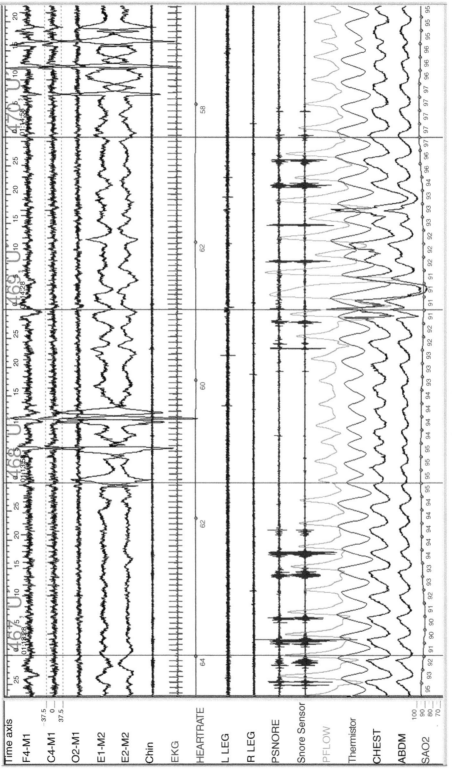

FIGURE 13-5 Hypopnea.

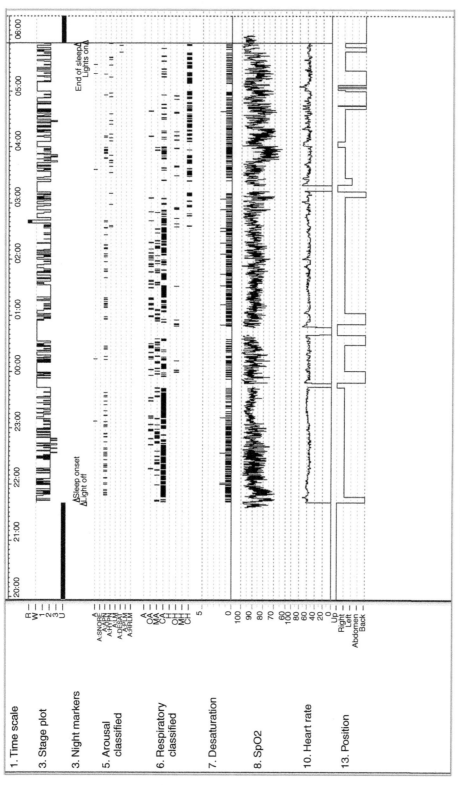

FIGURE 13-6 Histogram of sleep study with complicated breathing.

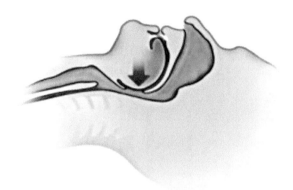

FIGURE 13-7 Partial airway obstruction. *Used with permission from ResMed Corp., San Diego, California. www.resmedialibrary.com.*

the airway, soft tissues in the upper airways will no longer collapse at end exhalation when the correct prescriptive CPAP pressure is determined. End exhalation is the critical point in the respiratory cycle during which pressure must be applied to the airway at a therapeutic level.

Any patient presenting to the sleep laboratory for suspected OSA should receive education regarding his or her breathing disorder, his or her health as it relates to obstructed breathing during sleep, and the necessity of treatment for the disease if the patient is found to have the disorder.[9] The patient's willingness to accept therapy must be reinforced and continually confirmed by the entire sleep team. Beginning with the physician who initially identifies the potential for sleep-disordered breathing, and including each health care member, the importance of therapy must be discussed openly and candidly.

CPAP compliance and **adherence** can be a challenge once the patient begins using therapy at home. In PAP therapy, the term compliance refers to measurement of specific usage determinants. Adherence refers to the extent to which the patient continues the agreed-upon mode of PAP under limited supervision when faced with conflicting demands. Inclusion of family members or supportive friends in the education process can certainly help set the stage for success.

Guidelines for Titrating CPAP

The AASM has published guidelines for the titration of CPAP in the sleep laboratory. These guidelines are an industry standard for CPAP titration protocol development in sleep centers: Clinical Guidelines for the Manual Titration of Positive Airway Pressure in Patients with Obstructive Sleep Apnea.[10]

In addition, the AASM has developed a practice parameter for the use of CPAP and level positive airway pressure (BPAP) therapy: *Practice Parameter for the Use of Continuous and Bilevel Positive Airway Pressure Devices to Treat Adult Patients with Sleep-Related Breathing Disorders.*[2]

These resources are quite helpful for the technologist who is learning techniques for the titration of CPAP. Those who have worked in sleep medicine for many years often refer to titration as an art. Indeed, sleep technologists do hone this skill as they experience different types of patients, different types of problems, and different solutions that work.

During a CPAP titration for OSA, the patient typically exhibits either obstructive apneas or obstructive hypopneas that will respond well to CPAP. A titration can be started at 4-5 cm H_2O to allow the patient to adapt and to provide an opportunity for the patient to reinitiate sleep. Additionally, as little as 5 cm H_2O will result in a patent airway for the occasional, mildly obstructed patient. Beginning with low CPAP settings will prevent over-titration of less severe patients.

As the patient falls asleep, it is common for respiratory events to occur as the chemoreceptors adjust during this transitional phase. If the patient continues to exhibit respiratory events once sleep has resumed, typically a 1 to 2 cm H_2O increase will help open the airway better and thus decrease the number and severity of the respiratory events. If the patient continues to exhibit OSA, the pressure can be increased again in an attempt to alleviate the events. This pathway requires the technologist to be vigilant and to also have a clear recognition of the type of respiratory events the patient is experiencing.

Titration Variations Based on Age

For adults, the AASM suggests an initial titration pressure of 4 cm H_2O with a recommended maximum CPAP setting of 20 cm H_2O.[10] An upward titration in 1 cm H_2O increments following each 5-minute period should be continued until greater than 30 minutes is observed without respiratory defined events. A higher starting pressure may be used if necessary to accommodate breathing requirements of patients with elevated body mass index (BMI) or if the patient is being retitrated on PAP therapy. For patients younger than 12 years of age, the Academy recommends an upward titration in 1 cm H_2O increments following a minimal 5-minute period, if continued sleep-disordered breathing events are observed.

The AASM guidelines provide general recommendations based on consensus of the task force[10]:

- The recommended maximum CPAP should be 15 cm H_2O for patients <12 years of age and 20 cm H_2O for patients ≥12 years of age.
- CPAP should be increased by at least 1 cm H_2O with an interval no shorter than 5 minutes, with the goal of eliminating obstructive respiratory events in all sleep stages and body positions.
- CPAP should be increased if at least one obstructive apnea is observed for patients <12 years of age or if at least two obstructive apneas are observed for patients ≥12 years of age.
- CPAP should be increased if at least one hypopnea is observed for patients <12 years of age or if at least three hypopneas are observed for patients ≥12 years.
- CPAP should be increased if at least three respiratory effort–related arousals (RERAs) are observed for patients <12 years or if at least five RERAs are observed for patients ≥12 years.
- CPAP may be increased if at least 1 minute of loud or unambiguous snoring is observed for patients <12 years or if loud or unambiguous snoring is observed for at least 3 minutes for patients 12 years.

Managing Complications and Side Effects of CPAP Therapy

The technologist monitoring the patient and making PAP titration decisions must have a clear understanding of the hows and whys of CPAP with a specific understanding of the following:

What keeps the airway open?
- Breathing is spontaneous.
- Patient-generated, relatively negative inspiratory airway pressure and positive expiratory airway pressure are present.
- Pressures remain positive and do not return to a zero baseline.
- One level of pressure exists for both the inspiratory and expiratory phase of breathing.

What comfort features are available to add tolerance and adherence to CPAP?
- Ramp-delivered pressure increases, up to that prescribed, over a preset timeframe.
- Airway pressure release ventilation (ResMed EPR, Respironics C-Flex) – pressure drops at beginning exhalation for comfort, and returns to the therapeutic level before end exhalation
  - Also known as *pressure waveform modification*
  - Also known as *pressure-relief CPAP*

What are potential complications and side effects of CPAP?
- Barotrauma (pressure trauma to the chest wall)
- Epistaxis (nose bleed)

- Rhinorrhea (runny nose)
- Nasal bridge sore
- Skin irritation and breakdown
- Nasal drying
- Rhinitis and nasal congestion
- Aerophagia (intake of air into the stomach)
- Central apnea

What is leak and how can it be managed?
Intentional leak—controlled port leak
- Washes out carbon dioxide (CO_2) and prevents rebreathing

Unintentional leak—mouth leak or mask leak
- Mask refit or readjustment should be performed.
- Addition of a chinstrap may help mouth leak.
- Switching to a direct nasal interface may help.
- Switch to an oronasal mask for mouth leak.
- Increased risk of aerophagia, abdominal distention, and vomiting
- Heated humidification reduces nasal resistance.

According to AASM standards, the goal of proper PAP titration is to perform and obtain an optimal titration defined as the pressure needed to respond to all events during REM sleep in the supine position.[2] The technologist must weigh several aspects during the performance of the titration and keep several goals in mind:

- Observe all positions and stages of sleep, as practical for the optimal outcome.
- Apply adequate pressure to resolve disruptive snoring.
- Minimize arousals and cardiovascular effects.
- Avoid excessive pressure, particularly if sleep fragmentation, patient intolerance, or central apneas occur.
- Seek improvement in gas exchange (increased functional residual capacity) and oxygenation, although this is not always possible.

It may not be possible to completely resolve all respiratory events because the negative effect of excessive pressure may outweigh the benefit of reaching "optimal" PAP.

Overtitration of CPAP can result in central apneas called **CPAP emergent** central apneas or complex apnea. Morganthaler and colleagues describe the characteristics of complex sleep apnea as typically emergent during titration of CPAP, not present during the diagnostic PSG, emerging when pressure is applied to alleviate OSA events, and occurring at approximately 30-second intervals.[7] An estimated 15% of patients with sleep-disordered breathing may have this disorder.

The AASM recommends a switch to BPAP with a backup rate to treat CPAP emergent central apneas.[10] A titration protocol must include steps for the technologist to adapt or change the titration technique when noting these types of events. If the use of CPAP does not correct apnea, hypopnea, and snoring, it may also be necessary to switch to BPAP therapy during a fairly routine PAP titration.

SPONTANEOUS BILEVEL POSITIVE AIRWAY PRESSURE (BPAP-S)

Indications for Transition from CPAP

BPAP in the spontaneous mode (BPAP-S) can be beneficial to the patient requiring a high therapeutic pressure, or who has difficulty adjusting to the sensation of pressure because the lower expiratory pressure is often more comfortable (Figure 13-8). The AASM's task force outlined the following general recommendations for BPAP titration studies[10]:

Switch to BPAP-S from CPAP if:
- The patient becomes intolerant of high CPAP settings.
  - Sensation of smothering
  - Swallowing air (aerophagia)
  - Difficulty exhaling
- Obstructive respiratory events persist once a pressure of 15 is achieved.
- CPAP has caused an increase in the partial pressure of carbon dioxide (PCO_2).

Guidelines for Titration of BPAP-S

Refer to the following for spontaneous mode guidelines:
- A pressure is set for inspiration (IPAP).
- A pressure is set for exhalation (EPAP).
- For the treatment of OSA in spontaneously breathing subjects. The greater the IPAP – EPAP difference (Δ), known as **pressure support (PS),** the greater the tidal volume (V_T), for improved ventilation, and oxygenation, and decreased CO_2.
- Minimum Δ 4 cm H_2O
- Maximum Δ 10 cm H_2O
  Once the decision is made to begin BPAP-S:
- The recommended minimum starting pressures are an IPAP of 8 cm H_2O and an EPAP of 4 cm H_2O for adults and pediatrics. Higher starting pressures may be needed when switching from CPAP or following a prior titration.
- Increases in the IPAP setting and/or the EPAP setting will be titrated in a minimum of 5-minute increments according to the respective number of observed respiratory events until the maximum IPAP level of 20 cm H_2O for patients <12 years of age or 30 cm H_2O for patients >12 years of age is reached. It is possible that the titration unit being used for this purpose may have pressure limitations.
- The technologist must know the capabilities of the laboratory-based titration device in use. When pressures higher than typical are required, availability of a device capable of delivering the prescribed therapy must be confirmed with the home PAP device supplier.
- The recommended minimum pressure support (PS) is 4 cm H_2O.

- The recommended maximum PS is 10 cm H_2O using BPAP-S for the treatment of OSA.

Optimally, the final BPAP settings will reduce the respiratory disturbance index (RDI) to less than five per hour during at least fifteen minutes of REM sleep in the supine position.[10]

CENTRAL APNEA, CHEYNE-STOKES RESPIRATIONS, AND CPAP-EMERGENT CENTRAL APNEA

Even the most seasoned technologist may be challenged by the patient with central breathing events during a PAP titration (Figure 13-9). Frequently, central apneas emerging early in a titration during transitional sleep will resolve once the patient's sleep continuity improves. During a PAP titration, time should be allowed for the patient's chemoreceptors to reset and to allow the patient time to adjust to the changes in positive pressure in order to reestablish sleep. Often this readjustment period is all that is needed to resolve some central apnea events.

Technologist review of the raw data from the diagnostic portion of a split night or full night PSG is recommended to determine a plan of action for the patient's titration. Many patients exhibit central apneas during the diagnostic portion of testing. When central events are predominant during diagnostic testing, the initial approach during titration may differ.

Pathology associated with periodic breathing and CSR may involve an exaggerated response to changes in CO_2. Increases in CO_2 elicit a hyperventilation response, whereas decreases in CO_2 may elicit central events in these patients. The goal of titration is to normalize minute ventilation, to minimize the exaggerated response to blood gas changes, and allow the patient's CO_2 level and breathing pattern to stabilize.

BPAP Therapy as Noninvasive Ventilation for Central Apnea

Indications for Use

The first line of therapy for central apnea patients may be BPAP therapy with a back-up rate to supplement spontaneous breathing. To determine the best EPAP setting for a BPAP titration, the physician or the technologist may review previous titration results or compliance data to determine if a low level of CPAP resolved existing obstruction. The review should also determine if an increase in pressure at a specific point in the titration resulted in an increase in central events to determine titration settings for use at the beginning of the BPAP study.

Technologists often find a flowchart helpful when determining next steps. The AASM provides specific guidelines to assist with titrations using BPAP and a back-up rate.[8,10]

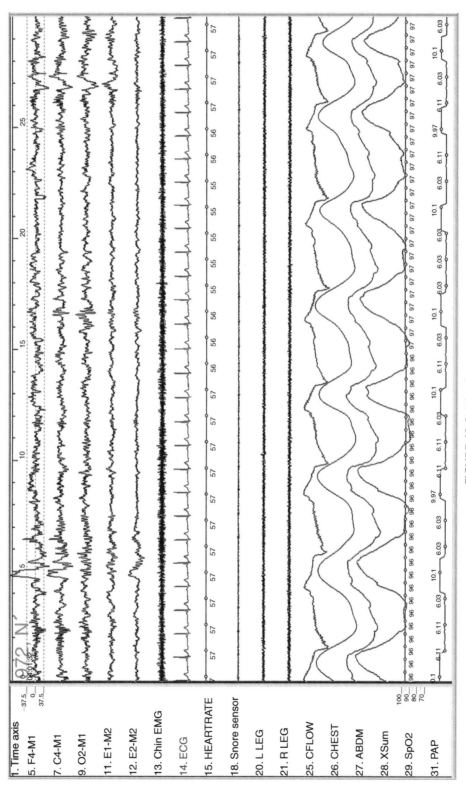

FIGURE 13-8 Bilevel spontaneous.

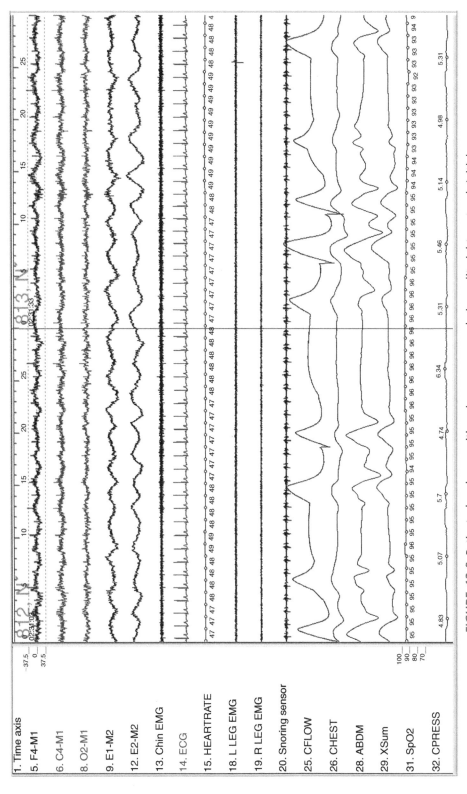

FIGURE 13-9 Patient placed on positive airway pressure during split-night protocol. Initial response: central apneas on 5 cm H_2O.

Guidelines for Titration

For properly setting NPPV, the following guidelines should be met:

- Breaths delivered when the back-up rate cycles the machine to IPAP are synchronized with spontaneous breathing. This is typically the S/T, or spontaneous-timed, mode on the BPAP device.
- The rate is set so timed breaths are delivered in the absence of spontaneous breathing. Often, a setting equal to two breaths below the patient's resting respiratory rate while awake is a good starting point.
- Ventilatory support is provided for all central apnea and complex apnea events.
- Initial IPAP and EPAP settings may be higher for increased BMI, retitration, or air hunger.
- When switching from CPAP, set EPAP at the titrated CPAP level that eliminated obstructive events or slightly lower.
- When switching to NPPV, IPAP set two above and EPAP set two below the effective CPAP setting may prevent over use of EPAP because the mean airway pressure is responsible for airway patency

> **!** IPAP of more than 30 cm H_2O may result in barotrauma; however, most laboratory titration devices cannot deliver more than 25 cm H_2O.

NOTE: The pressure difference between IPAP and EPAP is referred to as pressure support (PS) and has a direct effect on the delivered V_T (Figure 13-10).

The patient interface chosen for NPPV is a critical factor in the success of the therapy. Each breath, whether patient assisted or machine generated, is optimally delivered if the nasal or oronasal device fits well and seals effectively.[11]

Adaptive Servo Ventilation

Indications for Use

Adaptive servo ventilation (ASV) is a mode of ventilation used to treat Cheyne-Stokes breathing, complex sleep apnea, and other central forms of sleep-disordered breathing by dynamically augmenting pressure support, as needed on a breath-by-breath basis, to ensure target minute ventilation is achieved. The need for ASV may be determined by diagnostic testing, or through effective home compliance monitoring that indicates a patient with a high degree of central apnea is unlikely to be responsive to BPAP, even with a back-up rate.

A decision may be made by the attending physician to attempt an ASV trial to control the central apneas. This mode of therapy has been shown to be beneficial for patients with CSR associated with CHF, periodic breathing caused by idiopathic central sleep apnea (CSA), and opioid-induced CSA.[4]

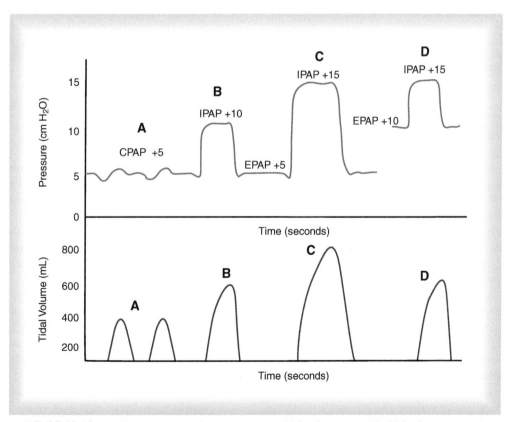

FIGURE 13-10 Continuous positive airway pressure and bilevel support with tidal volume comparisons. *From Kacmarek RM, et al: Egan's fundamentals of respiratory care, ed 10, St Louis, 2013, Elsevier.*

Guidelines for Titration

Servo ventilation uses a minimum end-expiratory pressure to control any component of upper airway obstruction, PS above the set expiratory pressure to augment delivered V_T, and a back-up rate to supplement the patient's own breathing efforts.

The ASV devices on the market at the time of this publication vary in their approach to adaptation. The Philips Respironics BiPAP autoSV Automatic Servo Ventilation device targets the peak flow during a 4-minute moving window and adjusts the delivered PS breath by breath when necessary. In addition, the device automatically calculates a back-up breathing rate based on the patient's spontaneous efforts.

The ResMed VPAP Adapt SV's algorithm continuously calculates target minute ventilation by monitoring the patient's respiratory rate and estimated V_T. The target maintains 90% of the patient's average minute ventilation by gradual variance and adaptation throughout the night. To meet the required minute volume, as determined by averaging data over a 3-minute window, machine-delivered breaths and PS are adjusted within the set range on a breath by breath basis.

Prior to implementing an ASV titration, the technologist must determine initial device settings. The settings may be included in the physician's orders, or the starting parameters may be a technologist decision. If the patient had some degree of obstruction during the diagnostic sleep study and it responded well to a particular CPAP setting, a setting at, or one slightly lower, should be used as the starting end-expiratory pressure for the ASV titration. Typically the default PS and back-up rate settings recommended by the respective manufacturer will prove adequate for adaptation.

Treatment Challenges

The most difficult challenge for the sleep technologist performing an ASV titration is practicing patience during the process, especially if the sleep technologist is accustomed to "fixing" patients and "tweaking" PAP settings to make every physiologic signal "pretty" (Figures 13-11 and 13-12). Titrating the ASV patient requires an uninterrupted sleep opportunity to ensure the adaptation has time to respond. The intricacies of cardiac and neurologic biofeedback associated with CSR, CHF, idiopathic CSA, and opioid-induced CSA require additional time to adapt and respond to the ventilatory support. The technologist's primary focus in regard to pressure changes is to make conservative adjustment to the end-expiratory pressure in response to clearly obstructive events. A physician may decide to use a gentle sleep aid or an antianxiety medication on the night of ASV titration to reduce the patient's tension and help with sleep initiation.

Treatment failure for patients with respiratory instability and resultant central apneas on positive pressure therapy is a challenge for the health care provider. Some patients fail all attempts at treatment, including trials on CPAP, BPAP with and without a back-up breathing rate, and eventually adaptive servo ventilation. Termed *chemo-reflex modulated sleep apnea*, individuals with this response demonstrate a hypocapnic breathing pattern. Recently, the use of **enhanced expiratory rebreathing space (EERS)** has been used to shift the apnea threshold for patients with possible abnormal reflexive chemoreceptors.[12] After determining the baseline arterial carbon dioxide pressure ($PaCO_2$), dead space and a nonvented mask are used to increase the $PaCO_2$ to just above the apnea threshold. Significant progress has been shown toward improving the sleep-disordered breathing of these challenging patients.

NPPV IN COMPLEX RESPIRATORY DISEASES

Sleep disorder centers are seeing an increase in the acuity of patients presenting for diagnosis and treatment. With the wide acceptance of out-of-center testing (home sleep testing), many straightforward OSA patients are being diagnosed in the home and treated with empiric or autotitrating PAP therapy in many areas of the United States. The more complicated, "sicker" patient will continue to be diagnosed and titrated in the sleep laboratory and a well-trained, highly skilled sleep technologist is required to manage the more difficult titrations. The acute OSA patient requires intensive patient education regarding disease management, therapeutic options, treatment in the home setting, and continual management of the disease process.

CHRONIC HYPOVENTILATION SYNDROMES

Patients with a chronic alveolar hypoventilation syndrome need ventilatory assistance during the night, and eventually around the clock, to maintain a $PaCO_2$ level in an acceptable range.[13] These particular patients present with respiratory compromise during the waking hours and, with the physiologic changes that take place during sleep, the compromised $PaCO_2$ state is intensified.

Even healthy individuals experience decreased chemoreceptor sensitivity during sleep, with a change in both oxygen level and CO_2 level. This normal decreased response, combined with additional cardiopulmonary disorders that result in a decrease in arterial oxygen pressure (PaO_2) and an increase in $PaCO_2$, places patients with alveolar hypoventilation at a significantly increased risk of impaired breathing during sleep.

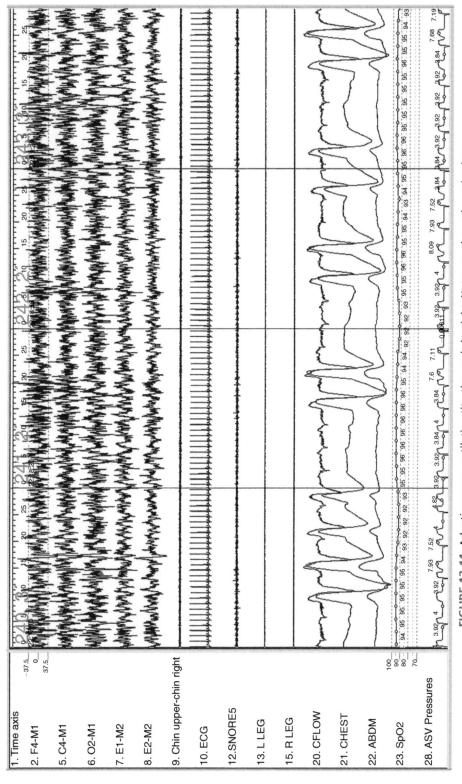

FIGURE 13-11 Adaptive servo ventilation titration early in night. Note complete adaptation has not been achieved, but sleep continuity shows improvement. The patient continues to exhibit significant central events.

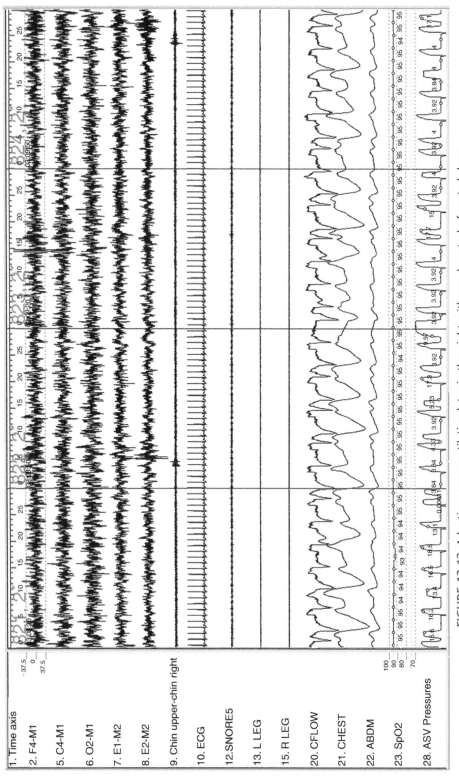

FIGURE 13-12 Adaptive servo ventilation later in the night with good control of central sleep apnea, stable oxygen saturation, and consolidated sleep.

Indications for NPPV

Respiratory insufficiency, or respiratory failure, results from the inability to achieve adequate ventilation necessary to eliminate CO_2, known as hypercapnia, and the inability to provide adequate oxygen to the cells, or tissue hypoxia. By definition, respiratory failure results when the patient is unable to maintain a $PaCO_2$ at or below 45 mm Hg. Respiratory failure is further defined by the inability to maintain the blood pH within the normal limits of 7.35-7.45.

Individuals with chronic respiratory failure experience excessive work of breathing, respiratory muscle fatigue and dysfunction, inadequate alveolar ventilation, and severe hypoxemia. These individuals have experienced a chronically elevated $PaCO_2$ for so long that the metabolic system, particularly the renal system, has retained bicarbonate to normalize the blood pH in the presence of an elevated $PaCO_2$. Patients with chronic respiratory failure and chronically elevated $PaCO_2$ with normal blood pH are hypersensitive to supplemental oxygen. Care should be taken when titrating supplemental oxygen that central and peripheral chemoreceptors are not overwhelmed by a sudden rise in the PaO_2 resulting in cessation of breathing caused by "knocking out" the hypoxic drive mechanism.

Goals of NPPV

The goal of NPPV is to relieve the work of breathing, improve and stabilize gas exchange, improve the duration and quality of sleep, prolong survival, and maximize the quality of life.[14] For many patients, the use of NPPV early in the disease process provides much needed relief in a noninvasive manner and delays the need for invasive ventilation. When invasive ventilation can be delayed, the patient's quality of life is greatly enhanced.

Implement or increase the backup rate in the spontaneous timed (ST) or timed (T) modes:
- When $PaCO_2$ cannot be kept within an acceptable range without excessive IPAP
- When the technologist is concerned that the required IPAP may cause barotrauma (e.g., in the presence of bullous lung disease)
- When the technologist is concerned that the necessary IPAP may cause patient intolerance
- When central apneas emerge in the absence of respiratory alkalosis (patient is normocapnic)
- To decrease excessive spontaneous respiratory rate or work of breathing
- To maintain the $PaCO_2$ between awake values and 10 mm Hg lower for hypercapnic patients, provided that the pH remains at or below 7.49

Guidelines for Titration with NPPV

Spontaneous Timed or Timed Mode

- Set the respiratory rate at the resting wake rate or lower, or at a stable value during sleep.

- Adjust rate *and* IPAP based on blood gases or surrogate measures of oxygenation and ventilation:
  - To reduce elevated spontaneous respiratory rate
  - To reduce the patient's work of breathing
- Adjust EPAP to eliminate upper airway obstruction.
- Adjust IPAP:
  - To augment spontaneous breathing by increasing V_T
  - To decrease the $PaCO_2$
  - To ventilate the patient during central events

Inspiratory to Expiratory Ratio

- The normal inspiratory-to-expiratory time (T_E) ratio is 1:2.
- Patients with chronic obstructive pulmonary disease (COPD) may benefit from a longer inspiratory time (e.g., 1:3).

SPECIAL CONSIDERATIONS FOR THE USE OF NPPV

Chronic Obstructive Pulmonary Disease and Overlap Syndrome

NPPV may be indicated for individuals with COPD or *overlap disorder,* a term used to describe patients with concurrent COPD and OSA, restrictive thoracic disorders, obesity hypoventilation and other forms of hypoventilation, and neuromuscular disorders. Patients with any of these disorders are significantly affected by body position changes during sleep, and by the normal breathing changes that occur during REM sleep.

Patients with COPD prone to overlap syndrome present with the following symptoms:
- Daytime hypercapnia or both daytime and nighttime hypercapnia
- Moderate to severe reduction in the forced expiratory volume in 1 second measure assessed by pulmonary function testing
- Obesity (BMI >30)
- Snoring
- Morning headaches

Chronic Obstructive Pulmonary Disease

- COPD patients often need longer T_E: typically an I:E ratio of 1:3 or 1:4 will be more comfortable.
- If the noninvasive ventilator has the option to adjust inspiratory time (T_I) by percentage of the breathing cycle, use the following rule of thumb: If the normal T_I is 37%, for COPD always use a reduced percentage T_I such as 30% or 25%, because COPD patients benefit from a faster T_I and a longer time for expiration (T_E).
- When inspiratory flow rate (IFR) is adjustable, increase the IFR or peak IFR to deliver a shorter inspiratory time (T_I) and subsequently a longer T_E.

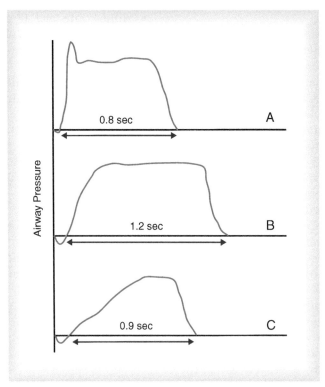

FIGURE 13-13 Rise time and slope. *Modified from Branson RD, Campbell RS, Davis K, et al: Altering flow rate during maximum pressure support ventilation (PSVmax): effect on cardiorespiratory function,* Respir Care 35:1056-1069, 1990. *From Kacmarek RM, et al:* Egan's fundamentals of respiratory care, *ed 10, St Louis, 2013, Elsevier.*

Restrictive Lung Disease

- A longer T_I and shorter T_E (%T_I > 37%; I:E ratio = 1:1.5) will improve lung expansion by more gradually filling areas with increased resistance.
- *Rise time* is the time it takes in seconds for the IPAP max to be delivered.
  - A longer rise time makes the inspiratory phase more sinusoidal and results in a decreased flow rate (Figure 13-13).
  - Adjusting rise time affects patient comfort during breath delivery.
  - Adjusting rise time does not alter the I:E ratio.

Selection of NPPV Device Settings

- I:E ratio: Decrease T_I or increase T_E to allow longer expiratory phase of breathing for COPD patients. *The opposite may improve ventilation with restrictive disorders.*
- Inspiratory flow rate: Decrease to allow ease of filling of airways with increased resistance; results in a longer T_I. *The opposite results in a longer T_E and may improve ventilation with COPD.*
- Rise time: Determines how flow is delivered during the inspiratory phase of breathing and changes the characteristics of the delivered breath. More sinusoidal flow results in improved comfort.

Sleep-testing facilities are beginning to see more patients for NPPV titration for the purpose of use in the home for ventilatory support. BPAP therapy, either in the spontanous mode or using a timed back-up rate,

may be used to augment the spontaneous ventilation of patients with chronic respiratory insufficiency. Monitoring and recording airflow, oxyhemoglobin saturation, V_T, leak, and delivered pressure signals are mandatory in the sleep laboratory setting to determine best settings for home use. In addition, transcutaneous CO_2 monitoring, end-tidal CO_2 monitoring, or arterial blood gas testing must be done to assess ventilation. Without a measure of CO_2, there is no accurate way to assess the patient's response to therapy.

Oxygenation should be monitored continuously while on therapy in the sleep laboratory. Ventilation should be monitored by $PaCO_2$ or a surrogate measure during titration and assessed periodically while on therapy at home. Long-term treatment requires assessment of $PaCO_2$ at least biannually.

The AASM has published guidelines for NPPV in the sleep center.[8] Using these guidelines, a NPPV titration protocol should be developed by each laboratory that includes procedural information to help the technologist in the decision-making process.

GENERAL RECOMMENDATIONS FOR NPPV*

Table 13-1 provides an overview of the anticipated results of adjusting ventilator settings. In general:
1. Increase IPAP or EPAP, or both as indicated, to eliminate apneas, hypopneas, RERAs, and snoring.

---

*Vary according to device.

TABLE 13-1
Expected Results of Changing Noninvasive Ventilator Settings

Setting	Adjustment Anticipated Result
IPAP	
↑	↑ V_T, ↑ minute ventilation, ↓ $PaCO_2$
↓	↓ V_T, ↓ minute ventilation, ↑ $PaCO_2$
EPAP	
↑	↑ FRC, ↑ PaO_2, ↓ V_T If intrinsic PEEP is present, fewer missed trigger attempts and improved patient-ventilator synchrony
↓	FRC, ↓ PaO_2, ↑ V_T ↓ $PaCO_2$ Possible rebreathing of CO_2 if EPAP < 4 cm H_2O
FiO_2	
↑	↑ PaO_2; if bleeding O_2 into circuit, maximum expected FiO_2 is approximately 0.5; increasing O_2 flow >15 L/min may adversely affect triggering
↓	↓ PaO_2
RATE CONTROL*	
↑	↑ minute volume in timed modes, ↓ $PaCO_2$
↓	↓ minute volume in timed modes, ↑ $PaCO_2$

CO_2, Carbon dioxide; *EPAP*, exhalation positive airway pressure; *FiO_2*, fraction of inspired oxygen; *FRC*, functional residual capacity; *IPAP*, inspiration positive airway pressure; *O_2*, oxygen; *PaCO_2*, arterial carbon dioxide pressure; *PaO_2*, arterial oxygen pressure; *PEEP*, positive end-expiratory pressure, *V_T*, tidal volume.
*Rate control is generally set at 8 to 10 as a backup rate and not changed in spontaneous or timed mode.

2. Increase PS to maintain desired V_T.
3. Increase PS if $PaCO_2$ trends 10 mm Hg or more above desired $PaCO_2$.
4. Increase PS if needed to provide respiratory muscle rest.
5. Increase PS if SpO_2 remains below 90% for greater than 5 continuous minutes.

A back-up rate should be used to provide support for all patients with respiratory muscle weakness, low respiratory rates, and central alveolar hypoventilation. Increase to provide an adequate respiratory rate to meet minute ventilation goals. Adjust inspiratory time to meet the patient's needs and typically provide 30% to 40% of the total respiratory cycle time.

Supplemental oxygen can be added to optimize oxyhemoglobin saturation when the SpO_2 remains at less than 90% for greater than 5 minutes after adjustments to the PS and respiratory rate have failed to improve oxygenation.

Continuously assess ventilation by monitoring respiratory rate, V_T, and CO_2. Continually assess oxygenation by SpO_2. Attempt to maintain a stable CO_2 level throughout the sleep cycle.

Conditions Associated with the Use of NPPV

The following is a list of conditions associated with respiratory failure and the use of NPPV:
- Lung disease and end-stage COPD
  - Decreased ventilation and ventilation-to-perfusion mismatch
  - Chronic or sleep-related hypoxemia
  - Chronic or sleep-related respiratory failure
  - Overlap syndrome
- Chronic alveolar hypoventilation syndromes
  - Central respiratory disturbances
  - Restrictive thoracic cage disorders (e.g., kyphoscoliosis)
  - Hypoventilation syndromes (e.g., obesity hypoventilation)
  - Neuromuscular disorders
  - Amyotrophic lateral sclerosis, stroke, Guillain-Barré syndrome, myasthenia gravis, Duchenne muscular dystrophy, etc.

CONTRAINDICATIONS FOR NPPV

- Unstable cardiorespiratory status
- Uncooperative patient
- Patient unable to protect airway because of impaired swallowing or cough
- Recent facial, esophageal, or gastric surgery
- Recent craniofacial trauma or burn
- Anatomic lesions of upper airway
- Excessive aerophagia that may result in vomiting, and aspiration of vomitus

The following conditions are relatively contraindicated for the use of NPPV:
- Extreme anxiety
- Massive obesity
- Copious secretions
- Need for continuous or nearly continuous ventilatory assistance
- Bullous lung disease
- Hyperventilation
- Hypoventilation
- Night-to-night variability of need

OPTIMIZING NPPV

A histogram demonstrating the incorrect use of BPAP on patients with chronic hypoventilation, for example, using a narrow IPAP:EPAP delta window and using high EPAP settings instead of wide bilevel split with a lower EPAP setting can be seen in Figure 13-14. The goal of BPAP is to reduce the chronically elevated $PaCO_2$ by increasing the patient's minute ventilation (V_TRR). A BPAP PS of

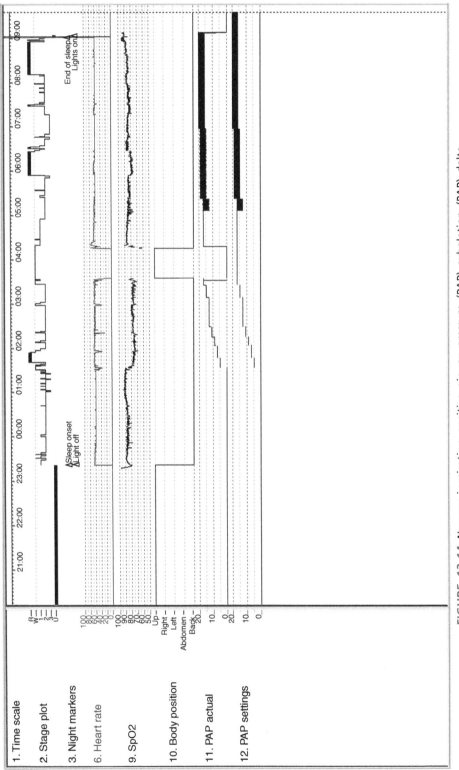

FIGURE 13-14 Narrow inspiration positive airway pressure (PAP)–exhalation (PAP) delta window.

8 cm H_2O or more may be needed to augment the spontaneous V_T. In fact, PS greater than or equal to 10 cm H_2O may be needed to ventilate some patients with significant neuromuscular disease.[8]

Newer devices on the market act primarily as bilevel PS ventilators and actually provide a constant V_T, rate, and minute ventilation. The pressure differential between end-expiratory pressure and required PS adjusts to the patient's breathing to maintain a consistent minute ventilation. Some of these devices also provide a more natural breathing waveform that is comfortable for the patient and is similar to normal breathing. This sinusoidal waveform provides an easier transition between inspiration and expiration than most traditional bilevel devices, which have a square waveform for transition. This can be an important factor for patients who "fight" the device or have difficulty with synchrony.

Improving patient comfort and synchrony with the device is an important factor for long-term adherance to therapy. Pressure relief and rise time settings can be adjusted to optimize synchrony of breathing between the patient and the NPPV device. Mask leak must be within acceptable range to allow the NPPV device to provide adequate ventilation. As always, heated humidity will be a key factor to control complaints of nasal and oral dryness and congestion, as well as daytime runny nose that can occur when the body overcompensates for airway drying at night.

SUPPLEMENTAL OXYGEN

The technologist must be aware of the patient's history and note if there is potential for oxygenation issues during wake and sleep. Having baseline arterial blood gas values available is optimal, but may not occur consistently in true practice. Placing the oximeter probe on the patient prior to the "lights out" maneuver gives the technologist an opportunity to observe the patient's oxygen saturation measured by pulse oximetry (SpO_2) levels during wake.

GUIDELINES FOR USE OF SUPPLEMENTAL OXYGEN

The sleep laboratory should have a supplemental oxygen protocol that addresses the need to apply supplemental oxygen with or without PAP therapy.

The AASM has published guidelines for the use of oxygen in the sleep laboratory setting.[10]

- Supplemental oxygen should be considered if a patient's awake supine SpO_2 on room air is $\leq 88\%$. It may also be added during a PAP titration if the SpO_2 remains $\leq$ at 88% for > 5 minutes in the absence of respiratory events. Supplemental oxygen should be added at 1 L/min for adults and pediatrics and titrated to achieve an SpO_2 between 88% and 94%.
- The oxygen should be titrated in 15-minute intervals to allow for stabilization of blood gases and the resulting SpO_2 indication.
- When applying PAP, supplemental oxygen is connected to the PAP device outlet.
- BPAP may be implemented to assist in the downward titration or weaning of supplemental oxygen.

Considerations for the Use of Supplemental Oxygen

The patient's awake baseline SpO_2 must be considered as many patients with advanced respiratory disease have compensated respiratory acidosis (chronic CO_2 retention) and additional oxygen can be detrimental.[16] Conversely, a severely hypoxic patient may require a higher setting.

In the absence of specific physician orders or a clear facility policy, the technologist must rely on clinical judgment. When the patient with end-stage COPD and chronic CO_2 retention requires supplemental oxygen, it may be prudent to start at less than 1 L/min. For this group of patients it may also be wise to maintain the $SpO_2 \leq 90\%$ as supplemental oxygen is titrated. Because this is normal for most of these patients, increasing the SpO_2 to more than 90% may satisfy the hypoxic drive that is relied on because the carboxic drive has become impaired as a result of high levels of CO_2. If this happens, the respiratory rate and depth will begin decreasing and respiratory arrest may eventually ensue. If a patient with known or suspected CO_2 retention significantly hypoventilates as a response to supplemental oxygen and an increase in SpO_2 to approximately 90%, the O_2 should be withdrawn until breathing is again stimulated by mild to moderate hypoxemia.

NOTE: The PAP device flow may increase because of high leak and affect the inspired oxygen concentration.

A sleep study histogram is beneficial to demonstrate severe hypoxemia during sleep unresponsive to both CPAP and the narrow delta bilevel with supplemental oxygen at 2 liters per minute (Figure 13-15). A wider difference between the EPAP and the IPAP may have helped; however, as the patient still had significant obstructive events even at high CPAP levels, it may be difficult to create a pressure gradient to suffice. This patient had a BMI in the 50s and eventually needed a tracheotomy to treat his sleep disordered breathing.

Figure 13-16 represents the polysomnogram of a severely hypoxic patient with severe OSA. Signficantly

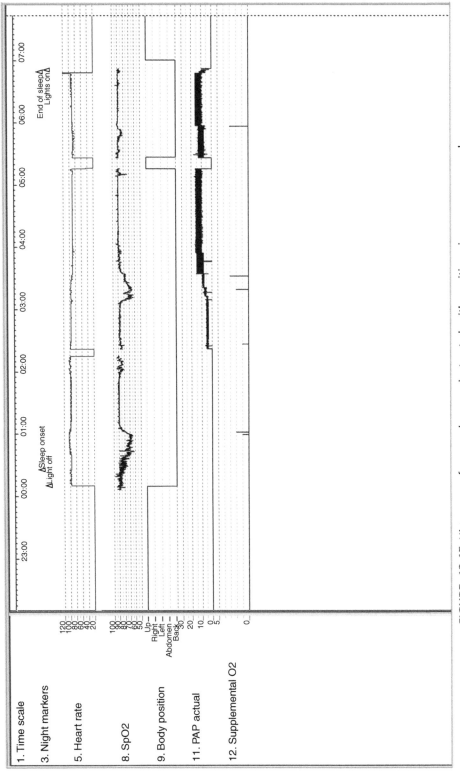

FIGURE 13-15 Histogram of severe hypoxemia treated with positive airway pressure and supplemental oxygen.

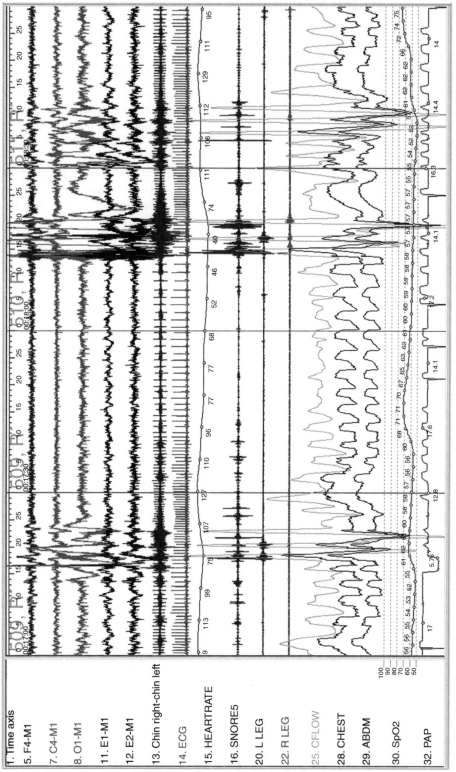

FIGURE 13-16 Severe hypoxemia affects cardiac function.

low SpO$_2$ levels in the 50s and 60s during REM sleep are accompanied by severe bradytachycardia with a variable heart rate between the low 30s to 110 bpm within a very short time frame. The patient's electrocardiogram tracing (modified lead II) has a pattern associated with an atrioventricular block.

ALTERNATIVE TREATMENTS FOR OBSTRUCTIVE SLEEP APNEA

TRACHEOSTOMY

Prior to the emergence of CPAP as an available home therapy, many patients had no option except to undergo a tracheostomy for the treatment of OSA. Indeed, a tracheostomy is an effective cure for OSA and is still used today when a patient cannot tolerate PAP therapy or when the effect of nontreatment is extremely detrimental to the patient's health and well being (Figure 13-17). It is not an easy decision to make and the patient will need education and support to undertake what may be a lifelong lifestyle change.

Advantages

- Provides a patent airway
- Obstruction bypassed
- Upper airway bypassed
- Work of breathing decreased

Disadvantages and Risks

- Long-term risk of tracheal stenosis
- Increased risk of infection
- Secretion management
- Social implications
- Tracheostomy care
- Procedure-related complications

ORAL APPLIANCES

Alternatives to PAP therapy and tracheostomy must be considered for many patients. Whether it is due to intolerance, emotional or cultural barriers, or physical barriers, a patient with untreated sleep-disordered breathing should have treatment options to control sleep apnea and ideally prevent further exacerbation of potential comorbidities.[17]

Oral appliance therapy is a treatment of choice for many patients. Typically, these devices strive to advance the mandible and thus open the airway during sleep (Figures 13-18 and 13-19). There are also devices on the market that hold the tongue forward.

Research studies conducted to test the efficacy of these devices showed less effectiveness in patients with severe OSA.[17] Studies have varied widely regarding how effectiveness was determined. Some used a success factor defined as an apnea-hypopnea index (AHI) of less than 10, whereas others used a

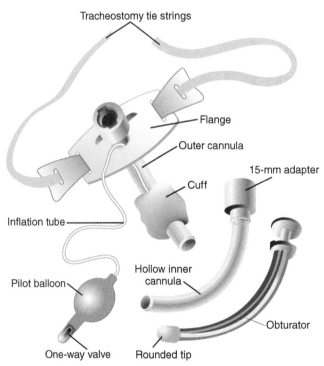

Tracheostomy tie strings

Flange

Outer cannula

15-mm adapter

Cuff

Inflation tube

Hollow inner cannula

Pilot balloon

Obturator

One-way valve   Rounded tip

FIGURE 13-17 Tracheostomy tube. *From Kacmarek RM, et al:* Egan's fundamentals of respiratory care, *ed 10, St Louis, 2013, Elsevier.*

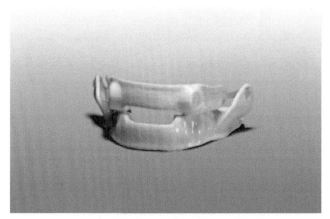

FIGURE 13-18 Narval oral appliance. *Used with permission from ResMed Corp., San Diego, California. www.resmedialibrary.com.*

reduction in AHI of at least 50%. Mandibular advancement devices vary widely on the degree of advancement titration. Consequently, it is somewhat difficult for an objective comparison of oral appliances currently on the market. Certainly, more studies are needed at this time.

Most importantly, current studies have demonstrated that the oral appliance is an option for patients with mild OSA. The patient, along with the family and support team, must work with a sleep physician or sleep dentist to make a decision regarding the use of an oral appliance as a treatment option. Many patients with mild OSA have enjoyed success with oral appliances, especially when PAP therapy was not a viable treatment option.

SURGICAL PROCEDURES

Surgical procedures for the treatment of OSA date back many years. Stanford physicians started performing multilayered surgeries in the mid-1980s to treat OSA. Uvulopalatopharyngoplasty concomitant with maxillomandibular advancement has been safely performed on many patients with good results, including a low risk of developing velopharyngeal insufficiency.[18]

The first line of treatment for pediatric OSA is adenotonsillectomy and has been shown to be quite beneficial in 75% to 100% of children, even those with increased BMI, based on the review of studies performed to evaluate the surgery.[19]

OUTCOME MANAGEMENT FOR POSITIVE AIRWAY PRESSURE THERAPY

The use of PAP in the home setting presents challenges for most patients. With breathing occurring naturally as an intrathoracic negative pressure gradient experience, the application of positive pressure to the airways is foreign to the human body. Many patients are motivated by the initial response that occurs with the use of positive pressure evidenced by the improvement in sleep continuity and waking hour alertness.

MANAGEMENT OF SIDE EFFECTS

Once in the home setting, many patients experience negative side effects related to PAP use. These side effects may include congestion, runny nose, ear pressure, facial soreness, pressure discomfort, skin

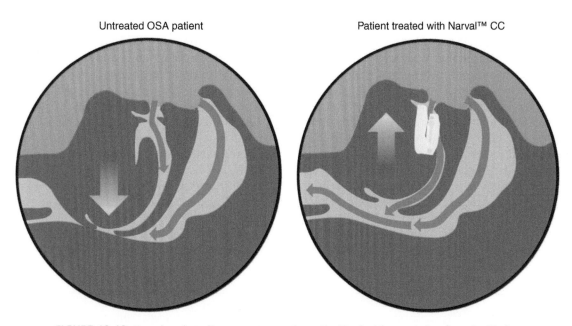

Untreated OSA patient   Patient treated with Narval™ CC

FIGURE 13-19 Narval oral appliance anatomy schematic. *Used with permission from ResMed Corp., San Diego, California. www.resmedialibrary.com.*

breakdown, claustrophobia, anxiety, and aerophagia, among others. Educating PAP users prior to initial home use is extremely important to prepare them for the risk of the side effects and to provide the patient with solutions and options prior to onset. The educated patient will not be surprised by the onset of potential side effects and should be prepared to deal with any that occur. The patient using PAP should be encouraged to contact a specified clinician for any related problems arising once home therapy is implemented.

EMERGING ROLE OF CLINICAL SLEEP EDUCATOR

The role of the **clinical sleep educator** is rapidly gaining recognition in sleep disorders programs. This skilled health care worker will spend significant time educating a new PAP user. This clinician must have the skills necessary to assess the learning methods most effective for each patient and apply techniques to ensure that learning and comprehension take place.

Allowing a patient and the family sufficient time for education contributes to their ability to understand the disease process, the required therapy, and the influence of therapy on sleep-disordered breathing, including associated areas of improved quality of life. Improvements may be experienced related to cognitive function, daytime alertness, oxygen levels, heart disease, metabolic syndrome, and weight control. A thorough understanding by the patient of the effect of noncompliance, or nonuse of treatment, must also be an integral part of the learning curriculum and reinforced by each member of the health care team.

EFFICACY MONITORING

Health care clinicians now have the ability to remotely monitor the usage of PAP therapy in the home setting (Figure 13-20). The major manufacturers of home PAP equipment have introduced technology that allows wireless and wired monitoring through secure websites and servers compliant with the privacy requirements of the Health Insurance Portability and Accountability Act (HIPAA) (Figures 13-21 and 13-22). Monitoring use allows the clinician real-time access to the patient's compliance data and immediately reveals issues such as nonuse, high leak, high AHI, central apnea activity, and snoring levels, depending on the mode of therapy.[20]

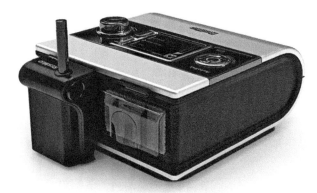

FIGURE 13-20 ResMed CPAP Model S9 with wireless modem monitoring. *Used with permission from ResMed Corp., San Diego, California. resmedialibrary.com.*

Based on the real-time review of information, the clinician may contact the patient with timely solutions to problems and issues. The clinician can also easily communicate with the attending physician if changes in therapy are warranted. Pressure changes can easily be made through this remote access, thereby addressing the issue in real time. The enormous benefit of this technology to the patient with sleep-disordered breathing cannot be overemphasized. The timely addressing of issues may be the key to maintaining a patient on therapy during the early and most challenging phase of PAP therapy.

Effect of Heated Humidification and Nasal Congestion

- Nasal resistance makes PAP difficult to tolerate.
- Heated humidification decreases nasal resistance.
- Consider a heated wire circuit for significant nasal issues.

Unintentional Leak

The unintentional mouth or mask leak must be addressed. The following are considerations when dealing with an unintentional leak.
- Mask refit or readjustment should be performed.
- The addition of a chinstrap may help mouth leak.
- Switch to an oronasal mask for mouth leak.
- Switching to a direct nasal mask may reduce leak.
- Increased heated humidification may resolve over time.
- Requires time and a patient health care provider.

See Figures 13-21 and 13-22 for sample efficacy monitoring reports.

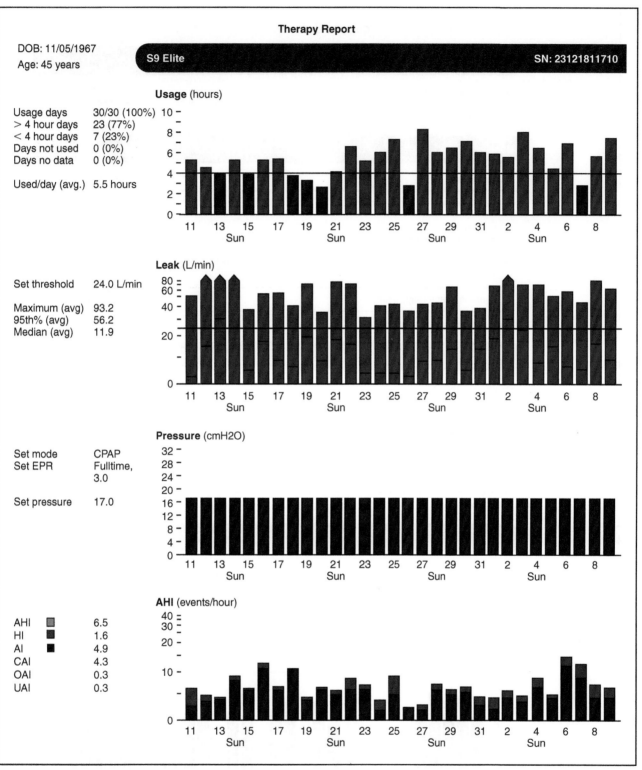

FIGURE 13-21 Detailed positive airway pressure (PAP) therapy report from a Philips Respironics
PAP device compliance report detailing:
Continuous PAP setting of 15 cm H_2O
Average obstructed airway apnea index of 1.5
Average hypopnea index of 1.5
Average apnea-hypopnea index of 3
Average vibratory snore index of 0.8
Average 90% mask leak of 82
This patient would benefit from an evaluation of his mask to address the leak issues.
Courtesy Philips Respironics, Inc., Andover, MA.

Compliance Report

Age: 43 years

30 day compliance	10/04/2012 - 11/02/2012
Compliance met	Yes
Compliance percentage	70%

Usage	10/04/2012 - 11/02/2012
Usage days	**22/30 days (73%)**
>= 4 hours	**21 days (70%)**
< 4 hours	**1 days (3%)**
Usage hours	164 hours 11 minutes
Average usage (total days)	5 hours 28 minutes
Average usage (days used)	7 hours 28 minutes
Median usage (days used)	7 hours 38 minutes

S9 AutoSet	
Serial number	23121535174
Mode	AutoSet
Minimum pressure	4 cmH2O
Maximum pressure	12 cmH2O
EPR	Fulltime
EPR level	2

Therapy					
Pressure - cmH2O	Median:	9.1	95th percentile:	11.3	Maximum: 11.8
Leaks - L/min	Median:	4.5	95th percentile:	13.5	Maximum: 25.0
Events per hour	A1:	0.7	HI:	0.0	AHI: 0.7
Apnea index	Central:	0.3	Obstructive:	0.3	Unknown: 0.0

Usage (hours)

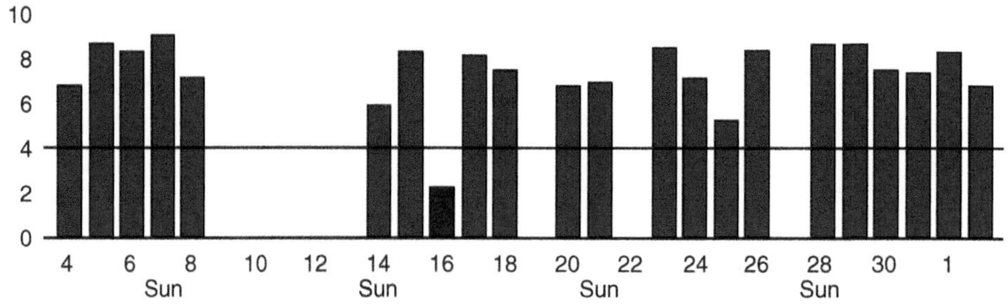

FIGURE 13-22 This summary 30-day compliance report is from a ResMed S9 Elite. The patient used the device 22 of 30 days with 21 days of more than 4 hours per day. The patient is using an autotitrating device with settings of 4-12 cwp. The patient's apnea-hypopnea index is under control with a value of 0.7 events per hour. The overall compliance percentage is 70%. The leak is in an acceptable range. *Data from ResMed Corp., San Diego, California. resmedialibrary.com.*

CHAPTER SUMMARY

- The technologist uses a variety of skills and knowledge to assist in the therapy of the patient with sleep-disordered breathing.
- Patient history must be reviewed and a face-to-face assessment must be done once the patient presents to the sleep laboratory for testing.
- The technologist must have respiratory event recognition skills and must grasp the titration algorithms used with the various PAP modalities for treatment of the patient's specific disease process.
- Protocols must be followed and evidence-based decisions made relating to titration steps.
- The sleep test provides valuable information for the physician, allowing a therapeutic decision that will optimally benefit the compliant patient in terms of improved health and well-being.
- The entire health care team will assist the patient in managing outcomes to the prescribed therapy and adjusting the treatment as required, based on the patient's physical and emotional needs.

References

1. Young, T, Peppard PE, Gottlieb DJ: Epidemiology of obstructive sleep apnea: a population health perspective, *Am J Respir Crit Care Med* 165:1217-1239, 2002.
2. Kushida, C, et al: Practice parameters for the use of continuous and bilevel positive airway pressure devices to treat adult patients with sleep-related breathing disorders, *Sleep* 29(3), 375-378, 2006.
3. American Sleep Disorders Association Task Force: The Chicago criteria for measurements, definitions, and severity of sleep related breathing disorders in adults. Presented at the Association of Professional Sleep Societies Conference, June 20, 1998, New Orleans, LA.
4. Javaheri S, Parker T, Wexler L, et al: Occult sleep-disordered breathing in stable congestive heart failure, *Ann Intern Med* 122(7), 487-492,1995.
5. Kaneko Y, Floras J, Usui K, et al: Cardiovascular effects of continuous positive airway pressure in patients with heart failure and obstructive sleep apnea, *N Engl J Med* 348: 1233-1241, 2003.
6. Berry RB, Brooks R, Gamaldo CE, et al., for the American Academy of Sleep Medicine: *The AASM manual for the scoring of sleep and associated events: rules, terminology and technical specifications,* Version 2.0, Darien, Ill., 2012, American Academy of Sleep Medicine. Accessed at www.aasmnet.org.
7. Morgenthaler TI, Kagramanov V, Hanak V, et al: Complex sleep apnea syndrome: is it a unique clinical syndrome? *Sleep* 29: 1203-1209, 2006.
8. NPPV Titration Task Force for the AASM: Best clinical practices for the sleep center adjustment of noninvasive positive pressure ventilation (NPPV) in stable chronic alveolar hypoventilation syndromes, *J Clin Sleep Med* 6(5), 491-508, 2010.
9. Silva RS, Truksinas V, de Mello-Fujita L, et al: An orientation session improves objective sleep quality and mask acceptance during positive airway pressure titration, *Sleep Breath* 12:85-89, 2009.
10. AASM PAP Titration Task Force: Clinical guidelines for the manual titration of positive airway pressure in patients with obstructive sleep apnea, *J Clin Sleep Med* 4(2), 157-168, 2008.
11. Teschler H, Stampa J, Ragette R, et al: Effect of mouth leak on effectiveness of nasal bilevel ventilatory assistance and sleep architecture [comment], *Eur Respir J* 14:1251-1257, 1999.
12. Gilmartin GS, Daly RW, Thomas RJ: Recognition and management of complex sleep-disordered breathing, *Curr Opin Pulm Med* 11:485-493, 2005.
13. Yoder EA, Klann K, Strohl KP: Inspired oxygen concentrations during positive pressure therapy, *Sleep Breath* 8:1-5, 2004.
14. Teschler H, Dohring J, Wang YM, et al: Adaptive pressure support servo-ventilation: a novel treatment for Cheyne-Stokes respiration in heart failure, *Am J Respir Crit Care Med* 164:614-619, 2001.
15. Morgenthaler TI, Gay PC, Gordon N, et al: Adaptive servoventilation versus noninvasive positive pressure ventilation for central, mixed, and complex sleep apnea syndromes, *Sleep* 30:468-475, 2007.
16. Scano G, Spinelli A, Duranti R, et al: Carbon dioxide responsiveness in COPD patients with and without chronic hypercapnia, *Eur Respir J* 8:78-85, 1995.
17. Ferguson KA, Cartwright R, Rogers R, et al: Oral appliances for snoring and obstructive sleep apnea: a review, *Sleep* 29(2), 244-262, 2006.
18. Li KK, Troell RJ, Riley RW, Powell NB, Koester U, Guilleminalut C: Uvulopalatopharyngoplasty, maxillomandibular advancement, and the velopharynx, *Laryngoscope* 111(6):1075-1078, 2001.
19. Schechter MS, Section on Pediatric Pulmonology, Subcommittee on Obstructive Sleep Apnea Syndrome: Technical report: diagnosis and management of childhood obstructive sleep apnea syndrome, *Pediatrics* 109(4):e69, 2002.
20. Taylor Y, Eliasson A, Andrada T, Kristo D, Howard R: The role of telemedicine in CPAP compliance for patients with obstructive sleep apnea syndrome, *Sleep Breath* 10:132-138, 2006.

REVIEW QUESTIONS

1. Proper application of respiratory airflow and effort monitoring equipment provides:
   a. Event identification specific to disease state
   b. Blood gas values
   c. Seizure detection
   d. On-going adherence monitoring for PAP use

2. An obstructive apnea is:
   a. A complete cessation of airflow in the presence of continued effort
   b. A partial reduction of airflow in the presence of continued effort
   c. A partial reduction of airflow in the absence of effort
   d. A complete cessation of airflow in the absence of effort

3. A central apnea is:
   a. A complete cessation of airflow in the absence of effort
   b. A complete cessation of airflow in the presence of continued effort
   c. A partial reduction of airflow in the absence of effort
   d. A partial reduction of airflow in the presence of continued effort

4. Supplemental oxygen is used to treat:
   a. REM sleep behavior disorder
   b. Insomnia
   c. Hypoventilation
   d. Obstructive sleep apnea

5. CPAP is the treatment of choice for:
   a. Neuromuscular disease
   b. CSA
   c. OSA
   d. Hypoventilation

6. The best choice of treatment for CSR is:
   a. Adaptive servo ventilation
   b. CPAP
   c. Phrenic nerve stimulator
   d. Wireless monitoring

7. The best choice of treatment for sleep-related hypoventilatory states is:
   a. CPAP at a high-pressure setting
   b. Hypoglossal nerve stimulator
   c. NPPV
   d. BPAP with narrow IPAP and EPAP delta

8. A critical factor for successful PAP adherence is:
   a. Patient education
   b. Length of tubing
   c. Varied work hours
   d. Varied sleeping hours

9. The monitoring of home PAP use provides:
   a. A detailed report of medication usage
   b. A method for addressing issues
   c. A detailed report of work hours
   d. A method to assess sleepiness

10. On-going support for patients with sleep-disordered breathing is necessary because:
    a. Annual reports must be sent to their employer
    b. Sleep-disordered breathing is a chronic health condition
    c. Patients always follow their doctors' recommendations
    d. PAP equipment will last a lifetime

Chapter 14

Infection Control and Emergent Response in the Sleep Center

Kimberly Trotter • Bonnie Robertson • Buddy Marshall

OUTLINE

LEARNING OBJECTIVES

After reading this chapter, you will be able to:
1. Describe the principles of infection control.
2. Understand the definition of standard precautions.
3. List the most common infections in humans that may be seen in the sleep laboratory.
4. Know the different circumstances in which to clean hands.
5. Describe the proper cleaning techniques for electrodes and sensors.
6. Identify soiled electrode artifacts.
7. Explain positive airway pressure equipment cleaning techniques.
8. Understand how to interpret the material safety data sheet.
9. Respond to patient life-threatening emergencies.
10. List fire safety measures.
11. Identify ways to maintain a safe environment through electrical safety.

KEY TERMS

barrier measures
common vehicle transmission
disinfection
fomites
gluteraldehyde
host
idioventricular

material safety data sheet
  (MSDS)
nosocomial infections
parenteral infections
PASS
pasteurization
pathogen

personal protective equipment
  (PPE)
prion
RACE
standard precautions
sterilization
uninterruptible power supply (UPS)

INFECTION CONTROL OVERVIEW

Infection occurs when a microorganism capable of producing a disease, known as a **pathogen**, is transmitted to and overcomes the barriers of a **host** organism that is invaded by the pathogen (Figure 14-1). The principles of infection control can be described as a chain: (1) pathogenic source; (2) transmission of pathogen to host; and (3) host susceptibility. The primary goal of infection control is to cause a break in this chain of events by eliminating the source, obstructing the transmission route, or reducing the susceptibility of the host. More specifically, infection control procedures aim to decrease the host's susceptibility by eliminating or minimizing the source of infectious agents, creating barriers and processes to interrupt the transmission of pathogens, and providing health and infection control knowledge to the individuals involved in the provision of health care, thus protecting those at elevated risk.[1]

TRANSMISSION OF INFECTION

The source of an infection can be either an animate source, such as a patient, staff member, or visitor, or inanimate objects such as medical equipment, sensors, preparation material, linens, clothing, surfaces, and even barriers meant to protect from infection like a box of contaminated gloves. Microorganisms are often directly transmitted through body surface–to–body surface contact (person-to-person), or transmission may be through indirect means in which contact is made with a contaminated object, most often the hands. This can result in hands-to-nose, hands-to-eyes, or hands-to-mouth self-infection, or contamination of surfaces or other persons.[1]

Droplet transmission of pathogens, also known as **fomites**, occurs when contaminated respiratory droplets are discharged into the air during coughing, sneezing, and even talking. Released droplets from the infected person can then be deposited onto a nearby host's mucosal surfaces, such as those in or around the mouth, nose, and eyes. Small droplets can be inhaled directly into the lungs where they are deposited. Droplet transmission is responsible for the spread of *Haemophilus influenza,* which is often responsible for pneumonia and epiglottitis; the common influenza (flu) virus; and rubella, which results in infection with the German measles. Other common diseases spread by airborne transmission include mycobacterium tuberculosis (TB) and varicella-zoster (chickenpox).

Although less common in the sleep testing facility, pathogens may also be ingested within food and water or on the surface of medications. Known as **common vehicle transmission**, this pathway is responsible for the spread of diseases such as salmonellosis, hepatitis A, and cholera. The least likely method of transmission of nosocomial, or hospital-acquired, infections is vector-borne transmission of pathogens, which includes transfer by animals or insects of pathogens such as West Nile virus, rabies, and malaria.

For the infectious agent to fully develop, a susceptible host must be present. Infection of the host depends on both the virulence of the organism and the resistance of the host. For this reason, persons with a medical condition that suppresses the immune system, such as cancer, human immunodeficiency virus (HIV) or acquired immune deficiency syndrome (AIDS), any organ transplant patient, or patients with other autoimmune disorders, are at increased risk of becoming infected when exposed to a pathogen.[2] The very young and older adults, individuals with diabetes mellitus, leukemia, or any other debilitating or chronic disease are also more susceptible to infection.[2] Likewise, when being treated with corticosteroids, radiation, certain antimicrobials, and immunosuppressive agents, individuals have diminished immune defenses against infection. When exposed to a virulent organism, even those with healthy

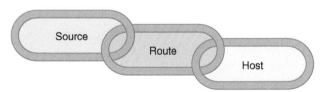

FIGURE 14-1 Spread of infection. *From Kacmarek RM, et al: Egan's fundamentals of respiratory care, ed 10, St Louis, 2013, Elsevier.*

immune function will become infected if adequate precautions are not employed. Sleep technologists and other health care workers must vigilantly protect patients and themselves against the risk of infection by consistently following established infection control procedures.

Some common infections that may be encountered in the sleep laboratory, with or without the technologist's knowledge include:

- AIDS
- HIV
- *Pediculus capitis* (head lice)
- Hepatitis B and hepatitis C
- *Herpes simplex*; *Herpes zoster* (shingles)
- Methicillin-resistant *staphylococcus aureus* (MRSA; antibiotic resistant staphylococcus)
- Conjunctivitis (pink eye)

STANDARD PRECAUTIONS

Standard precautions are designed to reduce the risk of transmission of microorganisms from all sources of infection in health care settings. Standard precautions, also commonly called universal precautions, are applied to all patients and in all situations, regardless of diagnosis or presumed infection status. Because any patient can serve as a reservoir for infectious agents, following standard precautions during the care of all patients is essential to interrupting the transmission of microorganisms. In essence, all patients should be treated as if they are potentially infectious.[3]

Standard precautions are practices to reduce health care–associated infections. They are intended to be used during interaction with every patient, regardless of diagnosis or isolation status, and apply to any potential contact with blood, body fluids, secretions, and excretions, except sweat. This set of procedures should be followed regardless of whether fluids contain visible blood, nonintact skin is present, or procedures require direct contact with mucous membranes.

HAND HYGIENE

Hand hygiene includes hand washing any time there exists visible soiling of the hands or gloves, or using an approved antimicrobial between each patient prior to donning gloves and after removal of gloves when hands are not soiled. Hand hygiene should also be performed following equipment processing and exposure to potentially infectious linens, surfaces, and equipment. For the benefit of both the health care professional and the patient, hand washing is always indicated after using the restroom and before eating. Proper hand hygiene is the most effective preventative measure toward reducing the occurrence of nosocomial infections.[4]

Hands must be cleaned:
- At the beginning of work
- When entering and exiting the patient room or environment even if there is no contact with the patient
- Before and after patient contact, including contact with intact skin
- Before donning gloves to provide direct patient care
- To prevent infection of the box of clean gloves
- After removal of gloves
- Before and after performing procedures
- Before and after contact with wounds
- Before handling sterile or clean supplies
- Before handling food
- Before handling medication
- When moving from a contaminated body site to a clean body site during patient care
- During care between completing a "dirty" task and starting a clean task (e.g., assisting with a urinal, and doing a blood glucose check, or transferring the patient and getting him or her water)
- After contact with the patient's environment even if there is no direct contact with the patient
- After contact with any bodily substances
- After handling equipment, supplies, or linen that are soiled or even potentially contaminated
- After using the restroom or performing any type of personal hygiene
- After touching one's face, nose, hair, or personal device (i.e., pager, mobile phone)
- Before leaving the work area

Use soap and water when hands are visibly soiled, upon removal of gloves, before preparing or eating food, or after using the restroom. Alcohol gel may be used in all other situations. There is no maximum number of gel uses before soap and water wash is required.[9]

Recommendations for Hand Hygiene in Ambulatory Care Settings[5]

Key situations in which hand hygiene should be performed include:
- Before touching a patient, even if gloves will be worn
- Before exiting the patient's care area after touching the patient or the patient's immediate environment
- After contact with blood, body fluids or excretions, or wound dressings
- Prior to performing an aseptic task (e.g., placing an intravenous line, preparing an injection)
- If hands will be moving from a contaminated body site to a clean body site during patient care
- After glove removal

Use soap and water when hands are visibly soiled (e.g., blood, body fluids), or after caring for patients with known or suspected infectious diarrhea (e.g., *Clostridium difficile,* norovirus); otherwise, the preferred method of hand decontamination is with an alcohol-based hand rub.

DISINFECTION

Disinfection of all surfaces, equipment, and sensors between patients is imperative. Disinfection is the elimination of most disease-producing microorganisms, including bacteria, viruses and fungi. Surfaces including countertops, equipment housing, railing, chairs, and all other surfaces should be wiped down using a hospital-approved disinfectant. At minimum, sensors that do not come into contact with mucous membranes should be cleaned and wiped down with 70% isopropyl alcohol or another low-level disinfectant. Equipment, particularly where there is a potential for contact with mucous membranes, requires high-level disinfection, which is covered later in this chapter.

PERSONAL PROTECTIVE EQUIPMENT (PPE)

The appropriate use of **personal protective equipment (PPE)** (e.g., gowns, gloves, mask, and eye protection) should be employed for reasonably anticipated contact with body substances or contaminated equipment. **Barrier measures** place protection between the health care professional and the source of infection. Gloves should be worn anytime the potential for contamination exists, including during measurement for electrode placement, affixing electrodes, electrode removal, and equipment processing. In addition, gloves and additional barrier measures should be applied any other time the situation necessitates contact with body substances or fluids, including those present on used linens.

In many sleep laboratories and neurodiagnostic testing departments, latex gloves continue to be used because of the effect chemicals used in these professions have on gloves made of alternative materials. In the event of latex glove use in a facility, be cognizant of the wearer's response to latex and, most importantly, patients with a known latex allergy. In the event a patient is sensitive to latex, consider applying multiple layers of nonlatex gloves to protect the technologist's skin when applying electrodes with collodion, and removing electrodes using acetone. The technologist should routinely wear gloves during preparation for patient testing for both infection control and personal health-related concerns. It is possible for even light preparation of the skin with abrasive material to result in broken skin and exposure to small, but potentially infectious, amounts of blood. Furthermore, prolonged skin exposure or inhalation of collodion may result in both kidney and nervous system damage.[6] Even short-term exposure can cause irritation to the eyes, nose, and throat.

RESPIRATORY HYGIENE AND COUGH ETIQUETTE

Patients should be instructed, and technologists should practice, all methods to reduce the spread of respiratory droplets when coughing, talking, and sneezing. Tissues and a disposal container should be supplied to patients with a chronic cough and those with an acute respiratory infection, runny nose, or cough. At minimum, the mouth and nose should be covered anytime one coughs or sneezes. When possible, patients with a chronic cough should be given a mask to wear while in common patient areas. According to the Centers for Disease Control, a mask should be worn any time the technologist is 3 feet or less from an individual with a productive cough. Current recommendations suggest it may be prudent to don a mask when within 6 to 10 feet of the patient or upon entry to the room to reduce the spread of infection through respiratory droplets.[7]

TRANSMISSION-BASED PRECAUTIONS

Used in addition to standard precautions, transmission-based precautions are implemented in regard to the specific route by which a particular pathogen is spread. These are always employed alongside standard precautions as an additional measure in the battle against the spread of infection. In the health care setting, the most common of these precautions are (1) airborne precautions, (2) droplet precautions, and (3) contact precautions.

AIRBORNE PRECAUTIONS (<5 MICRONS)

Because infections requiring airborne precautions are caused by pathogens small enough to remain suspended in air, these patients require physical isolation in a room with negative airflow with at least six air exchanges per hour and direct exhaust to the outside (or high-efficiency particle air filtration if air recirculation is unavoidable). When entering the room, respiratory protection using a certified N95 or higher level respirator is recommended when there is known or suspected pulmonary TB, rubeola (measles), or varicella (chickenpox) present.[7]

DROPLET PRECAUTIONS (>5 MICRONS)

Because some droplets are too large to enter the lower airways, they are typically deposited on the mouth or nose. Transmission can occur during talking, coughing, sneezing, suctioning, and intubation. Physical isolation is recommended. Because droplets do not remain suspended in the air, maintaining a distance of 3 feet or greater from the patient reduces the chance of transmission. When it is necessary to be within 3 feet of the patient, a mask is recommended, although the option remains to don a mask when within 6 to 10 feet of the patient or upon entry to the room. A mask should also be placed on the patient at all times during transit outside the patient room, according to the criteria previously discussed.[7]

CONTACT PRECAUTIONS

Wear clean gloves when entering the patient's room and remove gloves before exiting, taking care not to touch any potentially contaminated surfaces inside the room. Immediately wash hands with facility-approved antimicrobial soap. Inside the room, gloves should be changed each time they are contaminated.

Wear a clean, nonsterile gown when entering the patient's room any time it is anticipated that personal clothing may contact the patient or soiling is likely. Remove the gown before leaving the room, thus ensuring personal clothing does not contact potentially contaminated surfaces or supplies.

Equipment should not be shared between patients with contact precautions and others whenever possible. After discontinuation of use of reusable items, equipment should be cleaned and adequately disinfected to ensure the safety of others.[7]

NOSOCOMIAL AND PARENTERAL INFECTIONS

Nosocomial infections are infections that are acquired in the hospital. **Parenteral infections** are acquired intravenously. By definition, these hospital and procedure-acquired infections are usually seen in the inpatient population. However, when a patient who was recently discharged from the hospital is being studied in the sleep center, one must keep in mind that the patient may have become infected during the in-patient admission. Likewise, serious infectious diseases have become more prevalent within the community in recent years.[3,7] Most importantly, sleep technologists must remember that infection can easily be spread from one sleep disorders–testing patient to another, or from the technologist to the patient, if standard precautions are not meticulously followed. This includes hand hygiene between each patient and removal of PPE before stepping outside the patient room.

More often than not, sleep technologists are uninformed regarding the active infection status of a sleep center patient regarding nondisclosure (privacy) laws or because the patient is otherwise unaware of the issue.

As an example of a new community-acquired pathogen, during the past few years methicillin-resistant *Staphylococcus aureus* (MRSA), a historically hospital-acquired infection with limited evidence of spread outside of the health care setting, has become a major health concern within the general population. MRSA remains a significant problem both within the hospital and the community. Because of the prevalence of MRSA in the community, it is likely that these cases will be seen in the sleep-testing facility.[8]

Because the procedures performed by sleep technologists are noninvasive, a procedure-acquired infection is unlikely to occur. Failure of the sleep technologist to follow standard precautions with every patient and to implement additional precautions on an as-needed basis is no less than negligence. A patient should never leave the sleep center with an infection that could have been prevented through the practice of reasonable precautions.

PRIONS

A **prion** is an infectious particle of protein that, unlike a virus, contains no nucleic acid, does not trigger an immune response, and is not destroyed by extreme heat or cold. These particles are considered responsible for such diseases as scrapie, bovine spongiform encephalopathy (mad cow disease), and Creutzfeldt-Jakob disease.[7] These particles are very rare, but still a concern, and are an example of why infection control precautions are so important.

CLEANING, DISINFECTION, AND STERILIZATION

The continuum of equipment processing includes cleaning, disinfection, and **sterilization**.[9]

- Cleaning is the physical removal of soil and organic material. Cleaning is the first step in the continuum to disinfection and sterilization of objects. Cleaning *must* be done before disinfection and sterilization for those processes to be effective.
- Disinfection is the level of processing between cleaning and sterilization that includes the elimination of disease-producing microorganisms, but not spores, from inanimate objects via **pasteurization** or use of liquid chemicals. Pasteurization is a high-level disinfection process using water heated above 166 degrees Fahrenheit.
- Sterilization is a process by which all forms of microbial life, including bacteria, viruses, spores, and fungi, are destroyed. An autoclave is a device that can be used to accomplish equipment sterilization.

BARRIER MEASURES

Barrier measures rely on the use of PPE, including gloves, an eye shield, mask, and gown, to prevent exposure of the health care worker and patient to pathogens. These should all be removed before entering common areas, such as the control room, hallways, and elevators. In fact, gloves should be donned at entry to the patient's room and removed at exit.

ELECTRODES AND SENSORS

Reusable electrodes and other sensors are used on multiple patients. It is important to properly clean and disinfect them to avoid infecting others with pathogens left behind from previous use.[10] Box 14-1

BOX 14-1
Cleaning of Electrodes and Sensors

CUP ELECTRODES AND ELECTROCARDIOGRAPHY LEAD WIRES

1. Inspect electrode lead wires for adhesive residue and clean with adhesive remover or alcohol.
2. Wash electrode cups and lead wires using warm water and a mild detergent using a small, soft-bristled brush to remove electrode cream or gel, organic material, and fixative from the electrode surface.
3. Soak the electrode cup only in 1:10 bleach and water solution for 10 minutes, then thoroughly rinse the electrodes and lead wires and allow to air dry.
4. For reusable electrocardiography lead wires used with disposable electrodes, inspect for tape residue and clean with adhesive remover or alcohol.
5. Disinfect the length of the wire and electrode connector with alcohol or an antimicrobial wipe, according to lead wire composition and facility policy.
6. Ensure recessed female connectors are dry prior to inserting into the electrode input board.

THERMAL SENSORS, PRESSURE SENSORS, EFFORT SENSORS, AND SNORE MICROPHONES

1. Following each use, and prior to application to the patient, sensors and wires should be inspected for tape residue, which should be removed using adhesive remover or alcohol.
2. Sensors and wires should be gently cleansed and disinfected using alcohol or a facility approved antimicrobial cleanser that is safe for patient contact once dry.
3. Allow sensors to air dry in a designated "clean" area prior to next use.
4. Sensors and interface boxes should never be immersed in liquid or saturated with cleanser, water, or disinfectant. Exceptions exist, but as a general rule this practice should be followed.

provides an example policy for processing electrodes. Each facility should develop a policy to be habitually followed that is specific to the types of equipment and sensors used and to the local infection control policy. The technologist must know and follow all facility policies regarding electrode and sensor cleaning and disinfection. To ensure separation between articles being processed and those for which disinfection has already been accomplished, a dedicated place to clean equipment, electrodes, and sensors (decontamination area), and signage denoting a "dirty area" or "soiled utility" is recommended. Likewise, a "clean area" or "clean utility" should be available and clearly labeled for decontaminated articles prior to them being put away in the storage area.

Artifacts Caused by Soiled Electrodes

Using soiled or dirty electrodes can cause a number of artifacts on the polysomnogram (PSG), including electrode popping, baseline sway, and 60 Hz artifact.[11] By visually inspecting the electrodes before placement, and ensuring an appropriate impedance level once in place, many of these artifacts will be avoided. Dried electrode cream in the electrode cups is a main cause of these artifacts as it causes an unstable battery effect.

POSITIVE AIRWAY PRESSURE EQUIPMENT CLEANING AND DISINFECTION

In the laboratory, positive airway pressure (PAP) therapy devices require many components, including headgear, an interface, tubing, and a humidifier chamber. To avoid mineral build up, it is recommended that distilled water be used in the humidifier chamber. Many sleep laboratories are using disposable humidifier chambers and discard them after one use, although other facilities find this cost prohibitive. Reusable chambers can be disinfected either by chemical means using an agent such as **gluteraldehyde**, or by pasteurization. When using a chemical disinfectant, it is critical that the chamber be thoroughly rinsed or the patient will inhale residual chemical fumes. In a field in which success relies on initial acceptance and long-term compliance to therapy, it is imperative that the patient does not have an initial negative reaction to therapy because of fumes. For this reason, the mask and tubing must be completely rinsed of chemical residue. Headgear should be washed with warm water and soap between patients. The interface, mask, and tubing should be soaked in a moderate-to-high level disinfectant, according to the manufacturer's guidelines.

PAP Interface

After each use, the PAP interface must be thoroughly washed to ensure organic material has been removed and completely rinsed using clean water. Failure to remove all organic material will yield subsequent disinfection or sterilization procedures ineffective.

Acceptable methods of disinfecting PAP interfaces in the sleep laboratory setting include various chemical disinfectants made specifically for health care use, and pasteurization. Most chemical disinfectants are a formulation of activated alkaline gluteraldehyde. Pasteurization consists of placing equipment in a hot water bath (typically 167° F) for a minimum of 30 minutes. In either case, the equipment must be fully submerged and free of air bubbles to ensure all surfaces are in contact with the liquid.

In many laboratories, only PAP interfaces are disinfected using one of these methods because other components of the PAP circuit do not typically come in contact with the mucous membranes or patient secretions; however, because an amount of exhaled gas does flow into the circuit, some facilities require that a bacterial filter be placed at the machine outlet to prevent exhaled gas from entering the PAP machine.

PAP Devices Used in the Home

PAP devices used in the home can be cleaned using less stringent methods than those used in a health care facility because the device is used by the same patient every night. Most PAP device manufacturers recommend washing the single-patient, multiple-use mask daily in soap and warm water followed by air drying. Tubing can be cleaned weekly, using the same cleaning instructions. The humidifier chamber can be cleaned using warm water and soap, although many manufacturers now recommend washing in the top rack of a dishwasher.

To prevent the humidifier, tubing, and interface from harboring bacteria or providing a medium for mold growth, all components of the PAP circuit should be disinfected at least weekly in the home. Homecare providers recommend that this be accomplished by physical cleaning using soap and water, followed by a 30-minute soak in a 1:3 vinegar-to-water solution. Distilled white vinegar is acetic acid and provides adequate disinfection of single-patient multiuse equipment. Headgear should be cleaned when soiled, using soap and warm water followed by air drying.

Because patients may not clean their equipment as often as they should, regular cleaning should be encouraged by the sleep technologist. Daily cleaning is necessary to avoid facial skin irritation or infection, mask breakdown, discoloration of mask, and hardening of mask, which is caused by exposure to skin oils. When the mask material becomes less pliable, mask leaks become a chronic problem and the interface should be replaced.

MATERIAL SAFETY DATA SHEET

A **material safety data sheet (MSDS)** is a technical bulletin prepared by the manufacturer of a chemical product and is the primary source of information on the hazardous properties of the material, including information on its safe handling, storage, and disposal (Figure 14-2). It provides information needed to work safely with the material, and instructions for what to do when exposure exceeds normal limits. Any time a potentially hazardous material is purchased, the manufacturer is required to send the MSDS along with the product.

The MSDS for a given product can usually be located online and it is recommended that a hard copy be available to staff at all times. Most sleep center accrediting agencies require this information be made available to employees. Figure 14-2 is a sample MSDS for EC2 electrode cream.

EMERGENCIES IN THE SLEEP CENTER

RESPONSE TO LIFE-THREATENING EMERGENCIES

Every sleep testing facility should have a comprehensive emergency-preparedness policy. The plan should be facility specific, taking patient demographics, facility location, access to other health care professionals, and other related issues into consideration. When a patient emergency occurs within a hospital-based testing facility, the technologist is typically the first responder and relies on other hospital-employee responders to arrive very quickly. When the laboratory is offsite, the scenario is very different. Here the technologist would be the first responder, but this role may be extended as compared with the hospital setting.

In the United States, emergency services are usually contacted by calling 9-1-1. After contacting emergency services, the technologist may be responsible for providing basic life support for an extended period. Patient care policies should provide clear direction on what the technologist is expected to do in response to cardiac dysrhythmias, cardiorespiratory arrest, severe oxyhemoglobin desaturation, epileptiform activity, seizures, parasomnia-related manifestations, and suicidal ideation. See Figures 14-3 to 14-6 for emergency scenario responses.

FACILITY EMERGENCY POLICIES

The facility policy manual should also list the names and phone numbers of staff members and providers to call during an emergency, along with staff responsibilities. The American Academy of Sleep Medicine has specific guidelines for emergencies in the sleep laboratory.[12] Policies should be reviewed annually, and an annual drill should be completed and documented.

In addition to patient care policies, facilities' policies should minimally include protocols on violence in the center regardless of whether the violence is caused by a patient acting out, a family member, or an external party who has entered the building. Both patient and staff member safety should be addressed.

Material Safety Data Sheet
May be used to comply with
OSHA's Hazard Communication Standard,
29 CFR 1910.1200. Standard must be
consulted for specific requirements.

U.S. Department of Labor
Occupational Safety and Health Administration
(Non-Mandatory Form)
Form Approved
OMB No. 1218-0072

IDENTITY (As Used on Label and List) EC2 ELECTRODE CREAM	*Note: Blank spaces are not permitted. If any item is not applicable, or no information is available, the space must be marked to indicate that.*

Section I

Manufacturer's Name GRASS TELEPACTOR PRODUC GROUP/ASTRO-MED,INC.	Emergency Telephone Number (781) 848-2970
Address (Number, Street, City, State, and ZIP Code) 600 E. GREENWICH AVENUE	Telephone Number for Information (401) 828-4000
	Date Prepared 9-29-05
W. WARWICK, RHODE ISLAND 02893	Signature of Preparer (optional)

Section II - Hazardous Ingredients/Identity Information

Hazardous Components (Specific Chemical Identity; Common Name(s))	OSHA PEL	ACGIH TLV	Other Limits Recommended	%(optional)
NO HAZARDOUS COMPONENTS.				
THIS PRODUCT DOES NOT CONTAIN ANY NICKEL, LATEX, OR SILICONE.				

Section III - Physical/Chemical Characteristics

Boiling Point N/A		Specific Gravity (H2O = 1) 1.41	
Vapor Pressure (mm Hg) UNKNOWN		Melting Point N/A	
Vapor Density (AIR = 1) N/A		Evaporation Rate (Butyl Acetate = 1) N/A	
Solubility in Water DISPERSES IN WATER			
Appearance and Odor WHITE CREAM - ODORLESS			

Section IV - Fire and Explosion Hazard Data

Flash Point (Method Used) N/A	Flammable Limits	LEL N/A	UEL N/A
Extinguishing Media N/A			
Special Fire Fighting Procedures NOT A FIRE HAZARD			
Unusual Fire and Explosion Hazards N/A			

(Reproduce locally)	OSHA 174, Sept. 1985

FIGURE 14-2 Sample material safety data sheet. *From U.S. Department of Labor, Occupational Safety and Health Administration.*

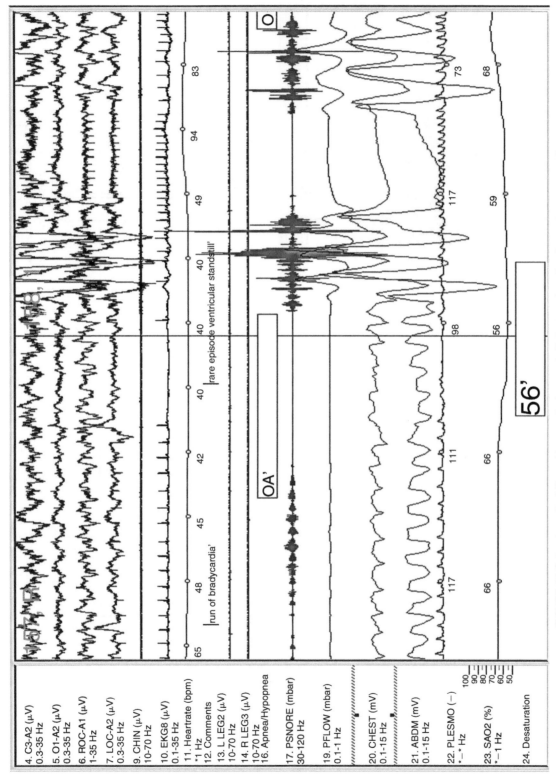

FIGURE 14-3 Bradycardia followed by ventricular standstill during a lengthy obstructive apnea with severe oxygen desaturation to 56%. The technologist should assess the patient. Intervention with continuous positive airway pressure is indicated because of the severity of the apnea combined with the cardiac response. The technologist should document and inform the attending physician as indicated by sleep center policy.

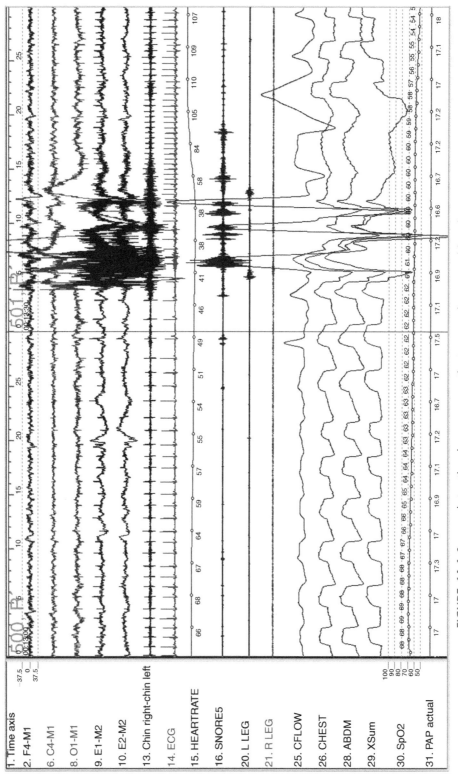

FIGURE 14-4 Severe obstructive sleep apnea patient on continuous positive airway pressure therapy level of 17 cm H_2O. This is most likely a hypoventilation response as indicated by severe prolonged desaturation into the 50 percent range. The technologist must assess the patient. Most likely supplemental oxygen, bilevel therapy, or both in tandem will be considered to effectively treat this severe condition. The technologist should document and inform the attending physician as indicated by sleep center policy.

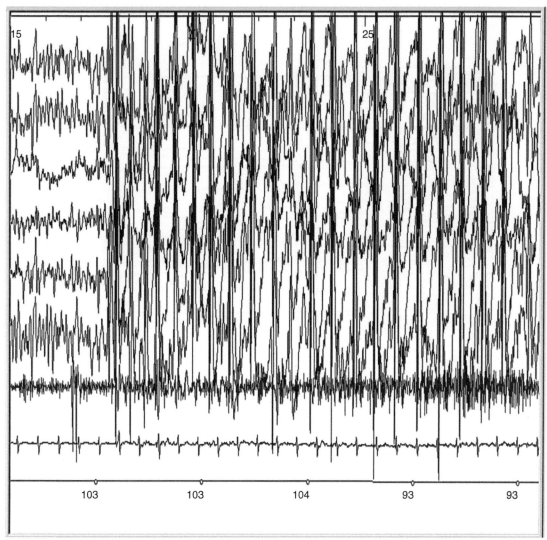

FIGURE 14-5 Seizure manifesting as evidenced by this electroencephalogram sample. The technologist should assess the patient, ensure his or her safety, and initiate emergency response if seizure continues longer than 5 minutes, or according to departmental policy. The technologist should document and inform the attending physician as indicated by sleep center policy.

Potential issues with the facility itself should also be considered and policies for dealing with them drafted before they are needed. Some examples include a power failure; inclement weather and weather-related emergencies; internal disasters; external disasters; security system and lock failure; and lack of water, sewer systems, heat, or air conditioning.

PROTOCOL: CARDIAC DYSRHYTHMIA INTERVENTION FOR THE SLEEP TECHNOLOGIST

This section represents an example protocol for technologist response to various cardiac dysrhythmias developed by Baptist Health Schools Little Rock–School of Sleep Technology and is used by permission. This is a guideline for training entry-level sleep technologists.

This guideline is not intended to replace any existing policy; rather it is to be considered in the absence of a comprehensive facility policy. This example protocol was drafted by the school's program director, medical director, and medical consultant for cardiology with the sleep-testing patient's safety in mind.

Each sleep testing facility should establish guidelines for technologist response regarding abnormal cardiac rhythms; however, such guidelines are not always available. The following protocols outline possible interventions for students and technologists when other guidance is not provided. The technologist should follow the policies of his or her employer, if available.

The protocol for cardiac dysrhythmias is divided into three separate groups (I, II, III) and the guidelines are determined by the type of condition.

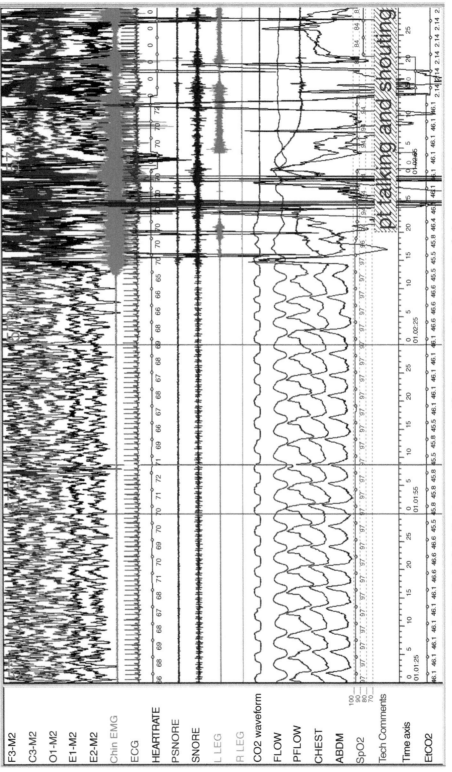

FIGURE 14-6 Pediatric parasomnia manifesting as vocalizations out of slow-wave sleep. The technologist should assess the patient, ensure safety, and document the event.

BOX 14-2
Group I: Document and Continue to Monitor

Normal sinus rhythm	Atrial fibrillation (*MD if new onset*)
Sinus arrhythmia	First degree AV block
Sinus tachycardia	Second degree AV block, type I
Sinus bradycardia	Premature atrial complexes
Bundle branch block	Premature junctional complexes
Atrial flutter (MD if new onset)	Unifocal premature ventricular complexes

AV =Atrioventricular

Group I

When the patient exhibits a pattern or complex listed in group I and no additional electrocardiographic (ECG) abnormalities are present, it is the technologist's responsibility to simply recognize and document the occurrence (Box 14-2). Because these patterns are considered benign, there is no indication to contact the physician or emergency services. The recording technologist should continue to monitor the patient and PSG data for abnormalities as the study progresses. Note, however, that if atrial flutter or atrial fibrillation emerge as a new variant during testing, the attending physician should be contacted. This is because new onset of these rhythms can cause blood clots to break loose and lodge in the lung, resulting in pulmonary emboli. The physician or other attending practitioner should determine how to proceed and may ask the technologist to describe the patient's appearance when contacted.

Figures 14-7 and 14-8 demonstrate cardiac dysrhythmias in group I of the protocol. The heart rate and rhythm represent a phenomenon known as the *mammalian diving reflex.* When a whale, or any other mammal for that matter, dives, metabolic function decreases in an attempt to conserve energy and much-needed oxygen. When these mammals resurface, the heart rate speeds up along with breathing to deliver oxygen to the tissue throughout their bodies. When humans have hypopneas and apneas, particularly those caused by airway narrowing or obstruction, these patterns often appear on the PSG. As airflow becomes diminished or absent, the heart rate slows down to conserve resources. As breathing normalizes, the heart rate speeds up in an attempt to deliver oxygen to the vital organs and other tissues of the body.

Because this pattern, commonly referred to as a *bradytachy rhythm,* is normal in the patient with sleep disordered breathing and does not pose an immediate threat, it falls into group I (sinus bradycardia and sinus tachycardia). The technologist must document the occurrence. In the presence of underlying disease, or when these periods of diminished airflow and oxygenation are extended, dangerous dysrhythmias may quickly emerge. The recording technologist must be vigilant even when only benign patterns are being monitored.

Group II

When patterns or beats listed in group II are identified, the responsibility of determining the course of action belongs to the physician (Box 14-3). Depending on the frequency of abnormal beats and the patient's history and underlying pathologic conditions, appropriate actions can vary greatly. The technologist's primary role is to accurately identify the abnormal beats or rhythm and contact the physician for guidance. As noted previously, the technologist should do a basic assessment of the patient prior to seeking physician support. The physician may ask for an assessment of the patient prior to determining what should be done. The technologist should document what was observed on the recording, who was contacted, the time, and a concise narrative describing the conversation with the physician. The patient should be continuously monitored to ensure the abnormality does not progress to something worse that may require additional support. Figure 14-9 represents a dysrhythmia from group II.

Group III

The technologist must assess the patient prior to responding to the rhythms, or lack thereof, listed in group III (Box 14-4). These are considered the life-threatening, or at least potentially life-threatening, dysrhythmias. A common pitfall in emergencies is responding to the monitor instead of the patient. It is

---

BOX 14-3
Group II: Contact the Physician, Document, and Continue to Monitor

Sinus arrest	Multifocal atrial tachycardia
Sinoatrial block	Paroxysmal supraventricular tachycardia (new onset)
Junctional escape beats	Sustained supraventricular tachycardia
Junctional escape rhythm	Second degree AV block, type II
Junctional bradycardia	Second degree AV block, 2:1 conduction
Junctional tachycardia	Third degree AV block
Accelerated junctional rhythm	Multifocal premature ventricular contractions
Ventricular escape beats	R-on-T premature ventricular contractions
Ventricular tachycardia (< 30 sec)	

AV = Atrioventricular

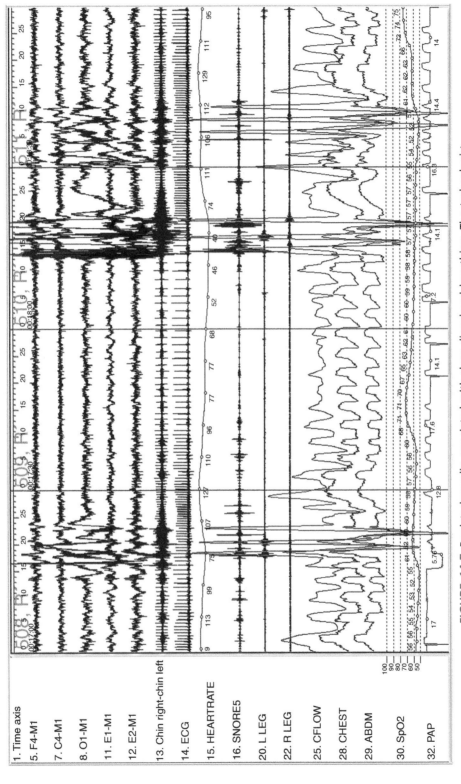

FIGURE 14-7 Bradytachycardia associated with sleep-disordered breathing. The technologist should assess the patient, ensure his or her response, and adjust positive airway pressure settings as indicated by the sleep centers policy. The technologist should document and report to the attending physician as indicated by protocol.

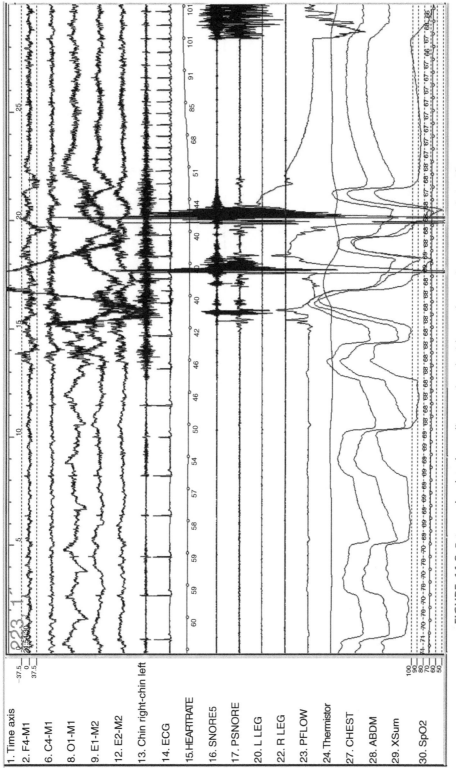

FIGURE 14-8 Extreme bradytachycardia associated with an obstructive apnea and significant oxygen desaturation. Technologist should assess patient, ensure patient's response, and place patient on continuous positive airway pressure per sleep center's protocol. The technologist should document and report to the attending physician as indicated by the sleep center's policy.

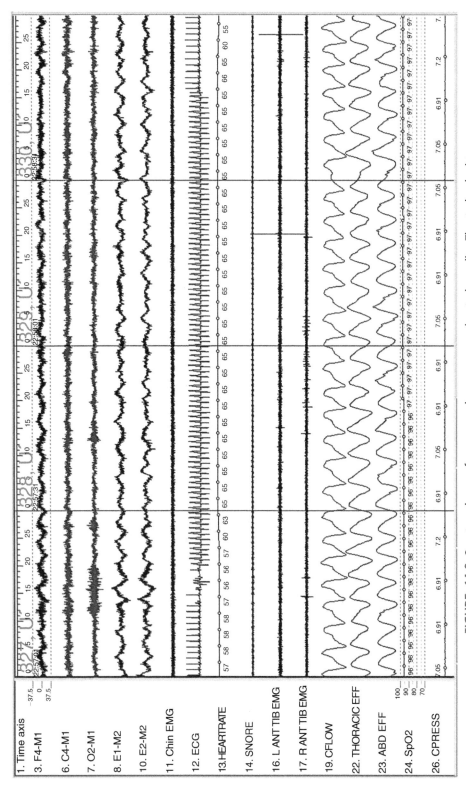

FIGURE 14-9 Onset and run of paroxysmal narrow complex tachycardia. The technologist should assess the patient, ensure his or her response, and document the event. The technologist should notify the attending physician per protocol.

BOX 14-4

Group III: Contact EMS and Attending Physician, Document, and Continue to Monitor

Ventricular tachycardia (sustained > 30 sec)	Asystole
Ventricular fibrillation—use AED if available	Ventricular flutter
Third-degree AV block with wide QRS	Idioventricular rhythm
Accelerated idioventricular rhythm	

AED = Automatic external defibrillator

---

possible for recording faults to resemble life-threatening ECG patterns; therefore, the patient must be assessed for pulse, breathing, and responsiveness prior to intervention. During the excitement of an emergency it can be difficult to palpate a pulse or even sense breathing airflow. Remember that if the patient responds, he or she has a pulse and is breathing. In the sleep center, it should be possible to awaken even the sleepiest patient to get a response.

In the event of a true group III emergency, sleep center staff should begin cardiopulmonary resuscitation until more advanced responders arrive. If more than one technologist is working, someone should contact emergency medical services and the attending physician, and continue monitoring the other patients while two or more technologists begin resuscitation efforts. Once advanced-level responders arrive, the recording technologist must document what occurred with help from other staff members.

Idioventricular Rhythms

Idioventricular rhythms are abnormal ventricular heart rhythms of unknown origin. The idioventricular rhythms (IVRs) and accelerated IVRs may not be life threatening. However, given the limited nature of the single, modified lead II ECG derivation used for sleep testing, it may be difficult to differentiate IVRs from other immediately life-threatening ventricular rhythms. Definitive ventricular flutter probably warrants the same response as ventricular tachycardia in the sleep laboratory and true IVR may imply more serious conduction disease requiring an aggressive medical approach. Given these limitations and considerations, emergency services should be contacted, and the patient should be assessed for responsiveness, pulse, and breathing, as consistent with other potentially life-threatening rhythms.

FIRE SAFETY

Sleep-testing facilities within a hospital setting will likely follow the hospital's fire safety procedure.

Sleep centers not associated with a hospital or in an offsite location should create their own policies or adapt existing policies specific to the needs of the facility. All fire safety policies should minimally include fire prevention guidelines, fire preparedness, fire response and evacuation, fire drills, use of extinguishers, and use of fire hoses if available.[13,14] It is important that these procedures be reviewed annually and that training is documented for all staff members.

Fire Prevention

The goal of a fire prevention policy is to create and maintain a fire-safe environment by following guidelines such as:

- Enforcement of no smoking policy
- Staff education (new employee and annually)
- Proper maintenance of medical equipment and facility systems
- Building features
  - Containment of smoke and fire
  - Safe passage in hallways and stairs
  - Automatic fire detection and suppression systems
- Annual safety inspection
- Fire prevention guidelines for staff
  - Maintain a smoke-free facility.
  - Ensure fire doors and alarm pull stations are free of obstruction.
  - Perform scheduled fire extinguisher maintenance checks.
  - Assess safety of power cords and remove equipment as warranted.
  - Use equipment in accordance with manufacturers' guidelines.
  - Remove faulty equipment from service and report to the supervisor.
  - Using a wedge or block to hold open doors that have automatic closers or open to an exit corridor negates fire safety controls.
  - Store flammable items such as collodion and acetone in an approved flammables cabinet that meets local code.
  - Follow MSDS recommendations for hazardous materials.
  - Secure compressed gas cylinders upright in designated storage areas.
  - Purchase only flame-resistance furniture, fabrics, and equipment.
  - Use only flame-retardant decorations.
  - Do not store anything within 18 inches of sprinkler heads because this may prevent full coverage of the room with water during a fire.

Fire Preparedness

The goal of this policy is to ensure building systems and employees are adequately prepared to respond quickly in the event of a fire. Aspects of fire preparedness include:

- Clearly marked evacuation routes
- Locations of fire alarm pull stations and fire extinguishers
- Staff education on specific evacuation steps at the fire's point of origin
- Procedures to follow once away from the fire's point of origin
- Knowledge about smoke compartment locations and emergency assembly points
- Yearly drills for both day and night shift staff members
- Regular inspection of exits and corridors
- Monthly fire extinguisher checks and annual maintenance
- Testing and inspection in accordance with codes and regulations
  - Fire alarms
  - Communication systems
  - Automatic fire extinguishing systems
  - Automatic fire detection systems

Fire Response and Evacuation

At fire's point of origin: Most hospital-based and offsite sleep centers use the acronym **RACE** for the steps taken at the fire's point of origin.

- REMOVE patients in immediate danger if it is safe to do so.
- ANNOUNCE or activate the fire alarm system.
- CONTAIN the smoke and fire by closing all doors.
- EXTINGUISH if safe to do so, or evacuate.

Away from the fire's point of origin: When the fire alarm is activated, but no evidence of fire or smoke is present, different steps are to be taken depending on the facility setting.

- During testing, close all doors (defend in place) and prepare to evacuate.
- When no patients are in the facility and only clinical and administrative staff are present, evacuate and wait for "all clear" from the fire department.
- When no testing is being performed, but patients incapable of self-evacuation are present, close all doors (defend in place) and prepare to evacuate.

Fire Drills

The sleep center should conduct at minimum, yearly fire drills for day shift, night shift, and administrative staff. These should be evaluated and documented. If any steps of the procedure are failed, further education should be performed and documented along with more frequent drills.

Fire Extinguishers and Fire Hoses

Fire extinguishers must be available in a health care facility. Hospital-based centers have fire extinguishers that are tested on a regular schedule. If the facility is offsite, it is the responsibility of the manager to ensure

extinguishers are being properly tested and maintained. Staff must be trained on using fire extinguishers, and a common acronym for the steps to using a fire extinguisher is **PASS**.

Pull the pin.
Aim the extinguisher at the base of the fire.
Squeeze the trigger slowly.
Sweep from side to side.

When fire hoses are available, it is important that only trained personnel use them.

ELECTRICAL SAFETY

It is important for the sleep technologist to have a cursory understanding of electricity and how it can be dangerous if the patient environment is not safe or equipment is not maintained or used properly.[15] Chapter 3 provides a thorough review of concepts related to electricity. Other chapters presented earlier in this book discuss electricity and electronics specific to the practice of polysomnography.

Creating a Safe Environment

All power outlets should be regularly tested for leaks or damage by a qualified technician such as a hospital clinical (biomedical) engineer or electrician. Confirming outlet-ground patency is another essential component of electrical safety testing. If the ground wire connecting the outlet to the building ground, and eventually the earth, is faulty, it cannot prevent one from being electrocuted or "shocked" when exposed to electrical current. If excessive electrical leakage current develops within the recorder, regardless of the cause, it will have no path to ground, and will present a risk of electrocution to the patient and technologist.

Many facilities insist that testing be performed every 6 months, but it should be performed at least annually.[15] Outlets that are not used should be blocked with a plastic child-safety plug. This should especially be the case for any rooms used by pediatric patients. Power cords should be checked for any fraying or damage to the cord or the plug. Only three-prong plugs should be used, and only three-prong power outlets should be installed. As described previously, outlets without a patent ground lack the ability to protect the patient or technologist from electrical leakage current.

Most hospitals use red power outlets for medical equipment; if these are available, the equipment should be plugged into them. Red power outlets are attached to an emergency power generator. In the event of power failure, the equipment plugged into these outlets will continue to work. If red outlets are not available, using an **uninterruptible power supply (UPS)** will provide temporary power. A UPS contains a battery that enables the equipment plugged into the unit to continue to work for a specified period. This allows the technologist to at least close the monitoring system down properly, saving the collected data, before complete loss of power. The laboratory will want to purchase a UPS for each recording system that provides the maximum run time on battery.

Equipment Safety Checks

Safety checks on all electrical equipment should be performed at least annually.[15] If the laboratory is hospital-based, the clinical engineering (biomedical engineering) department should conduct these checks and keep track of when they are due and the amount of leakage current generated by each piece of equipment. If the laboratory is not affiliated with a hospital, these checks will need to be performed by a qualified technician, electrician, or contracted biomedical engineer. The date testing is performed and the results of these checks must be kept on record by the sleep facility.

Electricity and the Patient

Patients are discouraged from bringing electrical devices from home such as a heating pad, fan, or even a hair dryer to the testing facility. Many facilities have policies governing both inpatient and outpatient admissions that forbid the use of a home electronic device by the patient until the biomedical engineering department has performed electrical safety testing and approved it for use. In the event a policy is not in place, or the item has not been approved, and the patient brings a personal electronic device into the testing area, it may present problems during testing.

If the technologist notices electrical noise artifact on the recording, it may be due to the patient's item. Electrical noise in the form of 50 Hz in many European countries and 60 Hz in the United States can also invade the recording if the patient ground electrode is not adequately attached, has loosened from the skin, contains dried out conductive material, or the lead wire has been broken inside the casing. Chapter 10 in this text addresses strategies for avoiding and minimizing recording artifacts.

It is essential that the sleep technologist keep all electrode wires and sensor cables away from other electrical equipment and, especially, wet conductive surfaces. These small conductive wires pose a potential danger to the patient if not treated with respect by the technologist. No appreciable risk exists to the patient as long as electrodes are applied correctly, equipment and sensors are knowledgeably used, and other sources of electricity are isolated from the patient and testing circuit.

CHAPTER SUMMARY

- Infection begins with a pathogen and will spread unless a break in the transmission cycle is implemented.

- Standard precautions and transmission-based precautions protect health care providers and patients.
- Hand hygiene is the single most important step in controlling the spread of infection.
- Electrodes and sensors must be cleaned and disinfected properly to avoid cross-contamination between patients and to reduce the likelihood of sleep testing artifact.
- Electrical equipment used on patients must be routinely inspected and maintained.
- Sleep testing facilities need detailed emergency response protocols.

References

1. Goodman RA, Solomon SL: Transmission of infectious diseases in outpatient health care settings, *JAMA* 265:2377-2381, 1991.
2. Wilkins RL, Stoller JK, Kacmarek RM: *Egans's fundamentals of respiratory care*, ed 9, St. Louis, 2009, Elsevier/Mosby.
3. Jarvis WR: Infection control and changing health-care delivery systems, *Emerg Infect Dis* 7:17-173, 2001.
4. Maki DG, Crnich CJ: History forgotten is history relived: nosocomial infection control is also essential in the outpatient setting, *Arch Int Med* 165:2565-2567, 2005.
5. http://www.cdc.gov/HAI/prevent/prevent_pubs.html
6. http://www.sciencelab.com/msdsList.php
7. Siegel JD, Rhinehart E, Jackson M, Chiarello L, and the Healthcare Infection Control Practices Advisory Committee: 2007 guideline for isolation precautions: preventing transmission of infectious agents in healthcare settings (website). http://www.cdc.gov/ncidod/dhqp/pdf/isolation2007.pdf.
8. Centers for Disease Control and Prevention: Methicillin-resistant *staphylococcus aureus* (MRSA) infections (website). http://www.cdc.gov/mrsa/statistics/index.html.
9. Rutala WA, Weber DJ: Disinfection and sterilization in health care facilities: what clinicians need to know, *Clin Infect Dis* 39(5):702-709.
10. Sullivan LR, Altman CL: Infection control: 2008 review and update for electroneurodiagnostic technologists, *Am J Electroneurodiagnostic Technol* 48:148, 2008.
11. Butkov N: *Atlas of clinical polysomnography*, 1996, Synapse Media 330-331.
12. American Academy of Sleep Medicine Center accreditation fact sheet: emergency procedures (website). www.aasmnet.org/resources/pdf/accred/emergency.pdf.
13. Occupational Safety and Health Association fact sheet: Fire safety in the workplace. *Title 29 of the Code of Federal Regulations*, 2002.
14. Occupational Safety and Health Association: Exit routes, emergency action plans, and fire prevention plans, Title 29, Subpart E, Part 1910.
15. Hobby MK: Safety considerations in the sleep center. In Butkov N, Lee-Chiong T, editors: *Fundamentals of sleep technology*, Philadelphia, 2007, Lippincott Williams and Wilkins.

REVIEW QUESTIONS

1. Minimum droplet size that is considered for droplet precautions is:
   a. >10 microns
   b. <5 microns
   c. >5 milliliters
   d. >5 microns

2. Which of the following is not a common human infection?
   a. Prion disease
   b. AIDS
   c. HIV
   d. Herpes zoster

3. Electrode artifact that results from dried-on conductive material functions like which of the following?
   a. An unstable battery
   b. An electrode with a broken wire
   c. A salt bridge
   d. A wet electrode

4. PAP equipment for multiple-patient use in sleep testing can be processed by washing with soap, rinsing, and:
   a. Soaking in bleach and rinsing with water
   b. Soaking in vinegar and rinsing with water
   c. Soaking in disinfectant and rinsing with water
   d. Soaking in water and then an autoclaving

5. MSDS stands for:
   a. Medical standard data source
   b. Material safety data sheet
   c. Material safety document source
   d. Medical standard data sheet

6. By nationally accepted guidelines, patient emergency protocols should *minimally* contain which of the following elements?
   a. Disaster preparedness, cardiac dysrhythmias, low oxygen saturation, and suicidal ideation
   b. Seizure response, fire safety, disaster preparedness, and low oxygen saturation
   c. Suicidal ideation, cardiac dysrhythmias, seizures, and low oxygen saturation
   d. Cardiac dysrhythmias, seizure, suicidal ideation, apneas, and equipment failure

7. Which fire safety measure is *most* effective when reinforced through staff education?
   a. Fire preparedness
   b. Fire recovery
   c. Fire prevention
   d. Fire response

8. Which of the following technologist's responsibilities would be *most* beneficial toward protecting the patient from an electrical hazard?
   a. Performing the biannual electrical ground safety checks
   b. Keeping electrodes away from other power sources
   c. Measuring the patient's home PAP setting
   d. Maintaining documentation on biannual safety checks

FUNDAMENTAL MATH CONCEPTS

VOCABULARY

Constant: A number that is assumed not to change value in a given mathematical discussion.

Expression: A mathematical sentence containing constants, variables, and a finite number of algebraic operations (addition, subtraction, multiplication, division and exponentiation by an exponent that is a rational number). For example, $3x^2 - 2xy + c$ is an algebraic expression.

Exponent: A symbol written above and to the right of a mathematical expression to indicate the operation of raising it to a power.

Fraction: A part of a whole or, more generally, any number of equal parts.

Integer: A member of the set of whole positive numbers, whole negative numbers, and zero.

Mean: The arithmetic average, or simply the average of a set of numbers.

Median: The numerical value separating the higher half and lower half of a set of numbers.

Mode: The value that appears most often in a set.

Proportion: A part considered in relation to the whole.

Ratio: the relationship in quantity, amount, or size between two or more things.

Variable: A letter representing an unknown quantity; a value that may change within the scope of a given problem or set of operations (e.g., x).

FRACTIONS, RATIOS, AND PROPORTIONS

By definition a fraction is a portion of the whole. Fractions are most commonly expressed by placing the numerator over the denominator as exemplified below:

$$\frac{3}{5}$$

In the sciences, including the health care sciences, these are most often documented in the decimal form. A decimal form of a fraction can simply be thought of as a division problem in which the numerator is divided by the denominator. The decimal form of a fraction is much more user friendly when used to perform calculations.

$$\frac{3}{5} = 3 \div 5 = 0.6$$

Fractions, ratios, and percentages can be thought of as one in the same. A ratio is simply the comparison of two variables. In the previous fraction, ⅗ is actually three parts of the total five parts, or a ratio of 3:5. A fraction in decimal form multiplied by 100 provides the corresponding percentage. Review the following examples of fractions, ratios, and percentages.

$$\frac{1}{5} = 0.20 = 20:100 = 20\%$$
$$\frac{1}{4} = 0.25 = 25:100 = 25\%$$
$$\frac{1}{20} = 0.05 = 5:100 = 5\%$$

Any time a number is written with a value less than 1, add a leading zero as in the following example:

$$\frac{1}{4} = 0.25$$

When using scientific notation, round the number off two places to the right of the decimal. When dealing with whole numbers or others that do not extend to the hundredths place, add zeros two places to the right of the decimal, as place holders. When the number in the thousandths place is 5 or greater, round the number in the hundredths place up, as shown:
1.235 becomes 1.24
1.239 becomes 1.24
When the number in the thousandths place is less than 5, round the number in the hundredths place down:
0.231 = 0.23
0.234 = 0.23

ADDITION AND SUBTRACTION OF INTEGERS

Adding two positive numbers is basic addition and will always yield a positive sum. Adding a positive number and a negative number is basic subtraction with a positive sum when the positive number is larger than the negative number or a negative sum when the negative number is larger than the positive number. Any time two negative numbers are added together, the sum will be negative. This simply requires adding the two numbers together and placing the negative sign before the sum.

MULTIPLICATION OF POSITIVE AND NEGATIVE NUMBERS

The product of two positive numbers is always positive. This is multiplication in its simplest terms. When both numbers are negative, the product will be positive as well. However, multiplication of one positive number and one negative number will always result in a negative product.

ALGEBRA BASICS

Algebra is the mathematics of logic that relies on a step-by-step approach to problem solving using variables and constants. A variable is a letter that represents an unknown quantity. A constant is a number that cannot change. Using the operations of addition, subtraction, multiplication, and division, algebra can be used to determine the value of unknown quantities. Two algebra concepts covered in this section are evaluating expressions and solving equations for a specific variable.

Algebraic expressions must be evaluated using the "order of operations:"
1. Evaluate numbers within parentheses.
2. Multiply numbers with exponents.
3. Multiply and divide numbers from left to right.
4. Add and subtract numbers from left to right.
The acronym *PEMDA* may be helpful for remembering the order in which values are calculated. *PEMDA* stands for *Parentheses*, *Exponents*, *Multiplication*, *Division*, and *Addition and subtraction*.

EVALUATING THE EXPRESSION

When a specific value is substituted for each variable in the expression, followed by performing the operations, it's called "evaluating the expression."
Evaluate the expression $ab + c$, if $a = 4$, $b = -2$, and $c = 7$
Substitute the numbers into the given expression (use parentheses when inserting numbers).
Multiply $4 \times -2 = -8$
Add $-8 + 7 = -1$

SOLVING EQUATIONS FOR A SPECIFIC VARIABLE

To solve equations for a specific variable, perform the operations in the reverse order in which you evaluate expressions.

$$2x + 5 = 15$$

To solve, the "x" must be isolated on one side of the equal sign.
First, subtract 5 from the left side of the equation. To keep the equation balanced, 5 must be subtracted from the right side as well.

$$2x + 5 - (5) = 15 - (5)$$

This leaves:

$$2x = 10$$

Now, divide both sides by 2:

$$\frac{2x}{2} = \frac{10}{2}$$
$$x = 5$$

Finally, to ensure the answer is correct, replace "x" with "5" to ensure it balances the original equation:

$$2x + 5 = 15$$
$$2(5) + 5 = 15$$
$$10 + 5 = 15$$
$$15 = 15$$

To solve more complex problems, the order of operations represented by PEMDA is essential. Consider the following equation:

$$(3 + 4)^2 - (4 - 2) = x \div 2$$

Parenthesis

$$(7)^2 - (2) = x \div 2$$
$$(7)^2 - 2 = x \div 2$$

Exponents

$$49 - 2 = x \div 2$$

Multiplication/Division

$$2(49 - 2) = (x \div 2)2$$
$$2(49 - 2) = x$$

Addition/Subtraction

$$2(47) = x$$
$$94 = x$$

MEAN, MEDIAN, AND MODE

The **mean** is the arithmetic average. To calculate the mean, simply add all items together and divide by the number of items. Of these three concepts, the mean is most important to sleep technologists. The mean sleep latency is a common parameter calculated following the multiple sleep latency test. The median and mode are mentioned here only to avoid confusion. The **median** is the middle number in a series of numbers, and the **mode** is the number that occurs most frequently within a series.

Consider the group of numbers: 1, 2, 2, 6, 8, 9, 9, 9, 12, and 45

$$1 + 2 + 2 + 6 + 8 + 9 + 9$$
$$+ 9 + 12 + 45 = 103$$
$$103 \div 10 = 10.3$$

The arithmetic average, or mean is 10.3

Using the same example, the fifth and sixth numbers represent the middle of the series. Add 8 and 9 together and divide by 2 for a median of 8.5. When an uneven number of values are in a series, the median is simply the middle number.

Because 9 occurs three times, 2 twice, and all other numbers only once in this example, 9 is the mode.

APPENDIX II
COMMON REPORT PARAMETERS AND RECOMMENDED SETTINGS

MULTIPLE SLEEP LATENCY TESTING

INITIAL SLEEP LATENCY

The initial sleep latency (ISL) for both the multiple sleep latency test (MSLT) and polysomnogram report is defined as the time from lights out (LT) to the first epoch that can be scored as sleep. An epoch is scored as sleep when it contains greater than 15 cumulative seconds of sleep.

$$ISL = (\text{sleep onset}_{epoch} - LT_{epoch}) \div 2$$

or

$$ISL = \text{sleep onset}_{epoch} - LT_{time}$$

THE MEAN SLEEP LATENCY

The MSLT is a daytime procedure used along with other data and clinical judgment in the evaluation of patients suspected of having narcolepsy or idiopathic hypersomnia. The mean sleep latency from the MSLT must be less than 8 minutes to support one of these diagnoses. At the conclusion of testing, the sleep technologist calculates the mean sleep latency in minutes. The mean is the arithmetic average. When data are provided according to the number of epochs, first divide by 2 because the standard epoch size for sleep testing is 30 seconds. Consider the following data from the five MSLT nap trials:

Individual sleep latencies: 5, 9, 20, 4, and 6 minutes

$$5 + 9 + 20 + 4 + 6 = 44 \text{ minutes}$$
$$44 \div 5 = 8.80$$
$$\text{mean sleep latency} = 8.80 \text{ minutes}$$

POLYSOMNOGRAPHY

TOTAL RECORDING TIME

Total recording time (TRT) is the amount of time that elapses between the start of a sleep study, LT, and the end of testing, lights on (LN). The easiest way to do this without errors is to multiply the full hours of testing by 60, add this to the minutes between LT and the beginning of the full hour of recording, and finally add the minutes of testing following the final full hour of testing for total recording time in minutes. If the TRT needs to be documented as whole hours and the decimal form of the fraction of hours, simply divide the value in minutes by 60. For a sleep study with LT at 10:35 p.m. and LN at 7:07 a.m., TRT can be determined as:

Time from 11:00 p.m. and 7:00 a.m. is 8 hours. 8 hours = 480 minutes.

From LT to 11:00 p.m., 25 minutes elapses.

Finally, there are seven minutes between 7:00 a.m. and LN.

$$480 + 25 + 7 = 512 \text{ minutes}$$
$$512 \text{ minutes divided by } 60 = 8.53 \text{ hours}$$

WAKE AFTER SLEEP ONSET

Wake after sleep onset (WASO) includes all wake time, including time out of bed, between ISL and LN.

$$WASO_{min} = SP_{min} - TST_{min}$$

or

$$WASO_{min} = TRT_{min} - ISL_{min} - TST_{min}$$

TOTAL SLEEP TIME

Total sleep time (TST) is the amount of time the subject sleeps during TRT. According to sleep-stage scoring rules, an epoch must contain greater than 15 seconds of cumulative sleep to qualify as stage N1, N2, N3, or rapid eye movement (REM) sleep. Therefore TST in minutes can be derived by adding up all 30-second epochs scored as any sleep stage, and dividing the total by 2. If already tallied, adding up the time in minutes that represents all substages of sleep will provide the same information. TST can also be determined by subtracting all wake time between LT and LN, from TRT. This includes all WASO and the ISL. Total sleep time in minutes divided by 60 yields TST in hours.

$$TST_{min} = TRT_{min} - ISL_{min} - WASO_{min}$$
$$TST_{min} = N1_{min} + N2_{min} + N3_{min} + REM_{min}$$

or

$$TST_{min} = (TRT_{epoch} - ISL_{epoch} - WASO_{epoch}) \div 2$$
$$TST_{min} = (N1_{epoch} + N2_{epoch} + N3_{epoch} + REM_{epoch}) \div 2$$

THE SLEEP PERIOD

The sleep period (SP) is the time from the first epoch scored as sleep through the end of testing at LN. Total SP time can be determined by subtracting the ISL from TRT. It can also be identified by adding the TST to the WASO time.

$$SP_{min} = TRT_{min} - ISL_{min}$$
$$SP_{min} = TST_{min} + WASO_{min}$$

or

$$SP_{min} = (TRT_{epoch} - ISL_{epoch}) \div 2$$
$$SP_{min} = (TST_{epoch} + WASO_{epoch}) \div 2$$

SLEEP EFFICIENCY

Sleep efficiency (SE) represents the percentage of sleep relative to the amount of time in bed available for sleep. A percentage can be calculated as TST divided by TRT and multiplied by 100.

$$\%SE = TST \div TRT \times 100$$

TOTAL WAKE TIME

Total wake time includes all wake time that occurs throughout TRT. Both the ISL and WASO are included in this calculation. Total wake time may be reported in minutes or as a percentage of the total recording time.

$$Wake_{min} = ISL_{min} + WASO_{min}$$
$$\%Wake = (ISL_{min} + WASO_{min} \div TRT_{min}) \times 100$$

or

$$Wake_{min} = TRT_{min} - TST_{min}$$
$$\%Wake = 100\% - SE$$

VARIOUS INDICES

In sleep medicine and technology, the index is the average number of times something occurs per hour. Most indices are based on total sleep time, although some indices, like those derived from home sleep testing data, may be calculated using total recording time. An index is calculated as follows:

$$\text{Total number of events} \div \text{time in minutes} \times 60$$

or

$$\text{Total number of events} \div \text{time in hours}$$

Example: On a sleep study with 4 hours and 51 minutes (291 min) of total sleep time, the patient exhibits a total of 204 apneas plus hypopneas. The apnea-hypopnea index (AHI) is calculated based on total sleep time.

$$AHI = 204 \div 291 \times 60 = 42.06$$

or

$$AHI = 204 \div 4.85 = 42.06$$

Settings for Sleep Study Recordings

Parameter	Derivation	LFF (Hz)	HFF (Hz)	Gain	Samples/s
EEG	F4-M1	0.3	*35	20,000	200/500
EEG	C4-M1	0.3	*35	20,000	200/500
EEG	O2-M1	0.3	*35	20,000	200/500
EOG	LIO-M2 (LOC)	0.3	35	20,000	200/500
EOG	RSO-M2 (ROC)	0.3	35	20,000	200/500
EMG	Chin (midline-inferior)	10	100	20,000	200/500
EMG	LAT	10	100	10,000	200/500
EMG	RAT	10	100	10,000	200/500
Snoring	Snore sensor or microphone	10	100	20,000	200/500
ECG	Modified lead II	0.3	70	10,000	200/500
Airflow	NC pressure transducer	0.1	15	10,000	25/100
Airflow	Thermal sensor	0.1	15	10,000	25/100
Effort	Thoracic RIP	0.1	15	10,000	25/100
Effort	Abdominal RIP	0.1	15	10,000	25/100
SpO$_2$	Pulse oximetry	DC		0-1 V input	10/25
Position	Sensor or manual input	DC		0-1 V input	1/1

DC, Direct current, direct coupled; ECG, electrocardiogram; EEG, electroencephalogram; EMG, electromyogram; EOG, electrooculogram; HFF, high-frequency filter, low-pass filter; Hz, Hertz, cycles per second; LFF, low-frequency filter; high-pass filter; NC, nasal cannula; RIP, respiratory inductance plethysmography; Samples, samples per second, American Academy of Sleep Medicine states Hz; SpO$_2$, oxygen saturation as measured using pulsatile data; V, volt.
*Attenuation of epileptiform spikes with a frequency of 14 to 50 Hz, and distortion of fast muscle spikes is possible at this setting.
Data from American Academy of Sleep Medicine.

APPENDIX III
MEASUREMENTS AND CONVERSIONS

THE METRIC SYSTEM

Many systems of measures have developed around the world throughout history. Common examples include the U.S. system of measurement and the imperial system of measurements, which were derived from the older English units of measure, and the metric system with its standardized structure and decimal features. In the sciences, including the health sciences, we routinely refer to use of the metric system. In fact, the system currently in use did evolve from the metric system, and was adopted in 1960 as the international system of units, with the international abbreviation SI. Upon adoption of the SI, the metric system was simplified with the establishment of seven base units. These include the meter for length, the kilogram for mass, the second for time, the ampere for electric current, the Kelvin for thermodynamic temperature, the mole for the amount of a substance, and the candela for luminous intensity. The first four of these base units will be used extensively in the study of sleep technology.

UNITS OF SCIENTIFIC MEASUREMENT

Dimension	Metric Unit	Symbol
length	meter	m
volume	liter	L
mass	gram (kilogram)	g (kg)
temperature	Kelvin (Celsius)	K (°C)
time	second	sec or s
EMF	volt	V

EMF, Electromagnetic frequency.

Macro prefix	Factor	Symbol
giga	billion (1,000,000,000)	G
mega	million (1,000,000)	M
kilo	thousand (1,000)	k
hecto	hundred (100)	h
deka	ten (10)	da

$$1,000 \text{ g} = 1 \text{ kg} = 10 \text{ hg} = 100 \text{ dag}$$

$$5,400 \text{ g} = 5.40 \text{ kg} = 54 \text{ hg} = 540 \text{ dag}$$

Micro prefix	Factor	Symbol
deci	tenth (1/10)	d
centi	hundredth (1/100)	c
milli	thousandth (1/1,000)	m
micro	millionth (1/1,000,000)	μ
Nano	billionth (1/1,000,000,000)	n

$$1 \text{ g} = 1,000 \text{ mg} = 1,000,000 \text{ μg}$$

$$2.30 \text{ g} = 2,300 \text{ mg} = 2,300,000 \text{ μg}$$

Factor	Symbol	Decimal	Exponent
tenth (1/10)	d	0.1	10^{-1}
hundredth (1/100)	c	0.01	10^{-2}
thousandth (1/1,000)	m	0.001	10^{-3}
millionth (1/1,000,000)	μ	0.000001	10^{-6}

PRACTICAL APPLICATION OF MEASUREMENTS

Both the distance and the height of data are important variables being assessed during acquisition and subsequent review of a sleep study. If given the recorder settings with which data are acquired, it is possible to determine how much voltage is being generated at the anatomic location being evaluated. This is a function of the measured height (aka *amplitude* or *deflection*) of the data and the recorder settings. Likewise, by measuring a distance and counting how many complete cycles occur in the space, the frequency and duration of the data can be extrapolated. Much of the material that follows is related to amplitude, voltage, frequency, and duration.

LENGTH (DISTANCE AND HEIGHT)

Horizontal length (distance) and vertical length (height) may be represented in both micro and macro units of meters. The meter, equivalent to 39.4 inches, is 1/1000 of the kilometer, which has been adopted by the SI as the measure of distance. As further comparison to the U.S. system of measurement, 1 kilometer is equal to 0.62 miles. In the study of human physiology, the meter and micro units of the meter are most commonly used for practical reasons.

DISTANCE CONVERSIONS

1 m = 39.37 (39.4) inches	#cm $\times$ 0.39 = #inches
1 inch = 2.54 cm	#inches $\times$ 2.54 = #cm
1 cm = 0.39 inches	#cm $\div$ 2.54 = #inches
1 km = 0.62 miles	1 mile = 1.61 km

1 cm	1 mm	1 μm
10 mm	0.10 cm	0.001 mm
10,000 μm	1000 μm	0.01 cm
		0.000001 m

Human height may be assessed in millimeters (thousandths of meters), whereas small blood vessels and airways of the lungs are measured in millionths of a meter, known as micrometers (μm). The metric units of distance commonly used in polysomnography are the millimeter (mm) and the centimeter (cm). One meter is equivalent to 1000 millimeters and 100 centimeters. The vertical height of sleep study parameters, also known as *signal amplitude* or *deflection*, is a representation of the voltage arising from the patient's body or the voltage generated by sensors in response to physiologic change. To determine how much voltage is represented by a given amount of amplitude, scale must be known. Amplitude scale is the product of amplifier settings used during data acquisition. When known, it is possible to determine the amount of voltage that was responsible for any deflection on the recording.

WEIGHT (MASS)

The SI unit for mass is the kilogram (kg), which is 1000 grams. In the practice of sleep technology, human body weight is typically expressed in kilograms, either directly measured or converted from a measurement obtained in pounds. Because the SI is preferred to the U.S. system of measurement, weights measured in pounds (lbs) must be converted to kilograms. This is a simple conversion that is routinely performed during practice in the health sciences. To convert weight measured in pounds to kilograms, simply divide the value in pounds by 2.205. To convert kilograms to pounds, multiply the weight in kilograms by 2.205.

1 g = 1 cc of water @ 4° C	# kg $\times$ 2.205 = # pounds
1 kg = 2.205 lbs	# lbs $\div$ 2.205 = # kg
# kg $\div$ 0.454 = # pounds	1 lb = 0.454 kg

TIME

The SI unit for time is the second. In the course of both collecting and evaluating sleep study data, the second and its micro units are of great importance. The most commonly used micro unit of time is the millisecond, which represents one one-thousandth (1/1000) of a second. The interpretation of data requires an assessment of how many waveforms or cycles occur within a specified amount of time. This is known as *frequency*. Another way to express time, *duration*, represents how long something lasts. The basic unit of time used to express both frequency and duration is the second. In the world of physiologic monitoring, a given vertical distance represents 1 second from which a frequency in cycles per second, or hertz (Hz) can be determined by counting the number of complete cycles that occur within the given distance. Likewise, the number of vertical distance measures can be counted between the start of something and its end to identify duration in seconds.

1 second	1 millisecond (msec)	1 microsecond (μsec)
1000 msec	1/1,000 sec	1/1,000,000 sec
1,000,000 μsec	0.001 sec 1000 μsec	0.000001 sec 1/1,000 msec

Frequency and duration possess a reciprocal relationship. When it is impractical to directly measure one of these values because of data that is either very slow or very fast, the reciprocal of the measurable unit of time can be used to calculate an average value of the other.

$$1 \div \text{frequency} = \text{average duration}$$

$$1 \div \text{duration} = \text{average frequency}$$

The need to extrapolate these values, particularly frequency, will become more apparent with experience recording data. During continued studies of amplifier filters, consider this: epileptiform spikes have a duration of 20-70 milliseconds or 0.02-0.07 seconds. This corresponds to an average frequency of 14-50 Hz.

VOLTAGE

The difference in electrical potential measured at two points within a circuit describes voltage. The volt is the unit used to measure the work required to move a charge between the two points. Differences in electrical potential measured from the surface of the skin known as *biopotentials* represent the cumulative effect of the rising and falling potentials of large groups of neurons. Physiologic data are obtained directly from the body in the range of millionths of volts known as *microvolts (μV)* and thousandths of volts known as *millivolts (mV)*. Likewise, most sensors attached to the body to measure airflow, breathing effort, snoring, body position, and other parameters generate data in this range.

1 Volt	1 millivolt (mV)	1 microvolt (μV)
1,000 mV	1/1,000 V	1/1,000,000 V
1,000,000 μV	0.001 V 1,000 μV	0.000001 V 1/1000 mV 0.001 mV

PRACTICAL APPLICATION OF S = V/D

The amplifier sensitivity control is used to increase or decrease the amplifier output of a recorded signal.

The units of sensitivity are μV/mm and range from 1 to 70. When any two of the three variables related to amplifier sensitivity are known, the third can be calculated using S = V/D or one of its three variations. Examples of why S = V/D is important follow:

The technologist must determine if the 0.5-2 Hz activity being recorded meets the voltage criteria for delta activity. If the scale or recording sensitivity setting is known, she or he can measure the deflection and determine how much voltage was generated by the patient to produce it.

$$\text{Voltage} = \text{Deflection} \times \text{Sensitivity}$$

When inputting a known voltage to calibrate the recorder, the technologist must know the expected deflection at a given sensitivity setting to evaluate instrument accuracy. This is one step he or she uses to determine if the equipment is operating properly and to make adjustments to the settings.

$$\text{Deflection} = \text{Voltage/Sensitivity}$$

Scale must be known to determine how much voltage the patient was generating. When evaluating a recording for which the scale is unknown, the technologist can measure the amplitude of a pretesting calibration signal of known voltage and determine the sensitivity setting that was employed during data acquisition

$$\text{Sensitivity} = \text{Voltage/Deflection}$$

DETERMINING MILITARY TIME

Because there are no colons in military time, the first step toward converting clock time to military time is to drop the colon. If before noon, add zeros on the left, as needed, to form a four-digit time. If after noon, add twelve to the clock hour time. Midnight is zero-hundred hours. Noon is twelve-hundred hours. Twenty-four-hundred hours does not traditionally exist.

8:31 a.m. becomes 0831 hours
Noon is 1200 hours
12:09 p.m. becomes 1209 hours
1:00 p.m. becomes 1300 hours
8:33 p.m. becomes 2033 hours
11:59 p.m. becomes 2359 hours
1:22 a.m. becomes 0122 hours

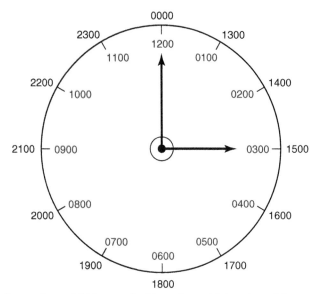

Comparison of 24 hours of military time with hourly positions on the clock face for civilian time. *From Potter PA, et al: Basic nursing, ed 7, St. Louis, 2011, Mosby.*

Many healthcare systems require documentation of 0000 in place of 2400 to denote midnight

VOLUME

1 cubic centimeter = 1 milliliter

30 mL = 1 ounce $\cong$ 2 T $\cong$ 6 tsp

1 liter = 1000 cc = 1000 mL $\cong$ one quart

CONVERTING TEMPERATURE SCALE

$$^\circ F = \frac{9}{5}\,(^\circ C) + 32$$

$$^\circ C = (^\circ F - 32)\,\frac{5}{9}$$

GLOSSARY

10-20 System: Formally the *International 10-20 System of Electrode Placement,* this manual provides a standardized means of cephalic measurement for electroencephalographic electrode application based on 10% and 20% of distances between anatomic landmarks. (Chapter 9)

acid-base balance: The balance between production and excretion of acid or alkali by the body, resulting in a stable concentration of hydrogen in body fluids, as determined from the pH value reported on an arterial blood gas analysis report. (Chapter 12)

actigraphy: The process of recording gross body movements over time using a small device similar to a watch that is worn on the wrist, known as an *actigraph.* Estimated sleep-wake time can be extrapolated from actigraphy data. (Chapter 2)

action potential: A rapid alteration in membrane potential, lasting 1 msec, during which the membrane changes from -70 μV to $+30$ μV and then returns to its original value. (Chapter 4)

adaptive servo ventilation: A mode of ventilation used to treat Cheyne-Stokes breathing, complex sleep apnea, and other central forms of sleep-disordered breathing by dynamically augmenting pressure support, as needed on a breath-by-breath basis, to ensure target minute ventilation is achieved. (Chapter 13)

adherence: The extent to which the patient continues the agreed-upon mode of positive airway pressure under limited supervision when faced with conflicting demands, as distinguished from compliance or maintenance. (Chapter 13)

adjustment insomnia: Acute insomnia characterized by a distinct change from the patient's normal sleep pattern caused by a stressor in the person's life. (Chapter 2)

airflow signal artifacts: When a thermal sensor falls out of the direct path of airflow or touches the skin for any reason, the relative change in temperature from which the signal is derived will be dampened, causing signal degradation, or complete loss. Pressure transducer data will also be distorted or lost when the sampling cannula is not in the direct path of flow, becomes partially occluded by organic material or moisture, or if moisture saturates the filter. During positive airflow pressure titration, a multiphasic airflow signal is likely the result of accumulation of large amounts of water in the tubing, and the flow and pressure fluctuations this will cause. (Chapter 10)

aliasing: Signal distortion resulting from the use of a lower than adequate sampling rate during data acquisition. (Chapter, 7)

alpha activity: Electroencephalographic data in the range of 8-13 Hz, most prominently recorded from the occipital region. Waveform morphologic characteristics are typically sinusoidal, often appearing in a crescendo-decrescendo pattern. (Chapter 5)

alternating current (AC) amplifier: A type of physiological amplifier designed for the recording of quickly changing variables such as electroencephalogram, electrooculogram, electromyogram, and others, with characteristics similar to those of alternating current electricity. (Chapter 4)

alternating current (AC) electricity: A type of electricity created by the constant alternation of positive and negative terminals in a circuit. Voltage is often produced by electromagnetic induction, when a magnet is spun inside a coil of conductive wire. (Chapter 3)

alveolar-capillary membrane: The interface between the lung tissue and circulating blood, across which gas exchange takes place. (Chapter 12)

ampere: A unit of current; 1 ampere is equal to 1 coulomb of charge passing a point in 1 second. (Chapter 3)

amplifier: An electronic device with controls for manipulating the amplitude and morphologic characteristics of data, and also to attenuate signals with frequencies above and below user-defined filter settings. (Chapter 8)

amplitude: The vertical distance, or height, of a waveform measured from a trough to the following peak; a representation of signal voltage. (Chapter 4)

analog-to-digital (A-to-D) conversion: The conversion of analog data into binary language for digitization using an A-to-D converter. (Chapter 8)

analog-to-digital (A-to-D) converter: Instrumentation used to alter an analog waveform into binary language for digitization. (Chapter 7)

ancillary devices and equipment: A collective title for standalone devices like oximeters and capnometers when interfaced with the polygraph to supplement diagnostic or therapeutic data, and complement information recorded during a sleep study. (Chapter 4)

anemic hypoxia: Low tissue oxygenation caused by the inadequate carrying capacity of hemoglobin. (Chapter 12)

antegrade: Forward impulses of electrical activity. (Chapter 11)

apnea: The complete cessation of airflow that lasts at least 10 seconds.

apnea-hypopnea index: The number of apneas and hypopneas per hour of sleep. (Chapter 13)

arterial blood gas (ABG) analysis: The measurement of acid-base balance and oxygenation status from an arterial blood sample. This test measures arterial blood pH, partial pressure of arterial oxygen, partial pressure of carbon dioxide, and bicarbonate, and provides a calculated arterial oxygen saturation value. (Chapter 12)

arteries: major vessels that carry blood from the heart to any part of the body. (Chapter 11)

artifact isolation: The process of identifying the cause of artifact by assessing channels that share common inputs.

When only one channel is contaminated, the offending input can be isolate by changing derivations. (Chapter 10)

artifacts: Unwanted signals on the recording that can arise from the body, the environment, or the recording circuit itself. (Chapter 4)

ascending reticular activating system: A control system of the homeostatic drive. (Chapter 1)

atria: The smaller, less muscular upper chambers of the heart. (Chapter 11)

attenuate: To progressively reduce signal amplitude. (Chapter 4)

averaging or response time: A moving window within which data points collected over time are averaged for a reported value. For pulse oximetry a shortened averaging time provides more detailed data, including high and low values necessary to document the relative desaturations associated with sleep-disordered breathing. A longer averaging time results in more smoothing of the data as highs and lows are averaged out, and will reduce many false alarms like those caused by short-lived movements. A value greater than 3 seconds should never be used during polysomnography. (Chapter 12)

band width: a range of frequencies within a given period. (Chapter 4)

barrier measures: Protection between the health care professional and the source of infection. (Chapter 14)

baseline: 1. In reference to waveform characteristics, a horizontal plane that runs through the center of a wave. 2. The level of activity or other measurable characteristic of a subject in its normal state or prior to an intervention. (Chapter 4)

behavioral insomnia: insomnia arising and exacerbated by behaviors such as watching TV in bed. (Chapter 2)

beta activity: Waves with frequency greater than 14 Hz interspersed throughout the electroencephalogram with eyes opened, and alpha activity when eyes are closed. (Chapter 5)

bicarbonate (HCO_3^-): The base component responsible for acid-base balance in the blood. The renal system balances pH by producing HCO_3^- or eliminating hydrogenions. (Chapter 12)

bilevel positive airway pressure (Chapter 13)

bilevel positive airway pressure: two levels of positive pressure; one used for inspiration and another for expiration. (Chapter 13)

bioelectric signals: Data acquired using electrodes that directly represent the rising and falling of the collective electrical potential of groups of cells as obtained at the surface of the body. (Chapter 5)

biopotentials: See *bioelectric signals.*

biphasic: In reference to waveform terminology, a signal composed of two phases—one surface negative and one surface positive. (Chapter 4)

bipolar derivation: A channel derivation in which both the G1 input and the G2 input overlie an electrically active recording site. (Chapter 4)

bipolar electrode board: An electrode board with bipolar inputs. A way of interfacing input signals with the polygraph on which there are designated connections for input 1 and input 2 of each channel, from which signals are routed directly to the respective amplifier. (Chapter 4)

bipolar inputs: Connections on the electrode board that route two electrodes, or the two cables from a transducer, directly to the recording parameter's amplifier. (Chapter 4)

bipolar jack box: See *bipolar electrode board.* (Chapter 4)

bipolar montage: A montage made up of a string of bipolar derivations for each of which both the G1 input and the G2 input overlie an electrically active recording site. (Chapter 4)

bipolar recorder: The original analog recorders known as *polysomnographs,* and digital recorders that use analog amplifiers for which data are digitized between the amplifier system and the computer. (Chapter 4)

bipolar recording: The data acquired using a bipolar recorder that cannot be manipulated after the fact. (Chapter 4)

caching: The process of storing small segments of data on the hard drive. (Chapter 7)

cannula: A hollow, flexible tube used to sample gas, liquid, or pressure from the body, or to deliver a substance into the body. (Chapter 4)

capacitance: The ability of a body, or capacitor, to store a charge. (Chapter 4)

capnography: Graphical display and recording of the flow curve obtained by end-tidal carbon dioxide monitoring. (Chapter 12)

capnometer: A device used to noninvasively measure carbon dioxide values from either exhaled gas or through unbroken skin. (Chapter 4)

capnometry: End-tidal carbon dioxide monitoring. (Chapter 12)

carbon dioxide (CO_2): A waste product of cellular metabolism excreted by the body in exhaled gas. (Chapter 12)

carbon dioxide transport: The process of transporting carbon dioxide dissolved in blood plasma, red blood cells, or plasma protein to be released by the lungs. (Chapter 11)

carbon monoxide (CO): a colorless, odorless, and tasteless gas that is toxic to humans and animals when encountered in higher concentrations. It has 210 times the affinity for hemoglobin (Hb) as compared with oxygen and when bound to Hb reduces oxygen carrying capacity. (Chapter 12)

carboxyhemoglobin (COHb): The chemical combination of carbon monoxide and hemoglobin (Hb); carbon monoxide bound to Hb. (Chapter 12)

cardio-ballistic artifact: Also known as *ballisto-cardiographic artifact* and often described as *cardiac oscillations,* this represents intrathoracic pressure changes related to the changing volume of the beating heart. The slow waves are aligned with the R wave of the QRS complex, but are not related to electrical conduction. (Chapter 10)

cataplexy: A sudden loss of muscle tone triggered by strong emotion such as anger or laughing. (Chapter 2)

Centers for Medicare and Medicaid Services (CMS): Previously known as the *Health Care Financing Administration,* CMS is a federal agency within the United States Department of Health and Human Services that administers the Medicare program and works in partnership with state governments to administer

Medicaid, the State Children's Health Insurance Program, and health insurance portability standards, among other responsibilities. (Chapter 12)

central apnea: Complete cessation of airflow without respiratory effort. (Chapter 13)

central chemoreceptors: Chemical sensors in the midbrain region that detect carbon dioxide and pH changes, in the cerebrospinal fluid, directly related to blood levels. (Chapter 11)

cerebral cortex: Part of the brain responsible for the sleep-wake drive and the circadian rhythms. (Chapter 1)

channel blocking artifact: When amplifier gain or sensitivity control is set too high, or slow-wave artifact or electrode popping are extreme, channel blocking may occur. Also known as amplifier blocking, depending on software options, the positive and negative extremes of the signal may be "chopped off" for a flat appearance or the signal may intrude on adjacent channels. (Chapter 10)

chronic carbon dioxide (CO_2) retention: The condition of having a partial pressure of carbon dioxide ($PaCO_2$) level of consistently more than 45 mm Hg. In the presence of chronic CO_2 retention, the carboxic drive that normally stimulates breathing becomes blunted. As the $PaCO_2$ increases more and the drive becomes less functional, individuals with chronic CO_2 retention rely on the hypoxic drive, which stimulates inspiration when the partial pressure of arterial oxygen drops to less than approximately 60 mm Hg, to stimulate inspiration. When the hypoxic drive becomes satisfied, for example by application of too much supplemental oxygen, the body will no longer sense a need to breathe. (Chapter 12)

chronic obstructive pulmonary disease (COPD): A group of lung diseases, including emphysema, chronic bronchitis, bronchiectasis, and chronic asthma, that make it difficult to adequately exhale and result in an increased functional residual capacity. (Chapter 12)

circadian rhythm: A daily cycle of biologic activity influenced by regular variations in the environment, such as the alternation of night and day. (Chapter 1)

circulatory hypoxia (aka *stagnant hypoxia*): Tissue hypoxia resulting from inadequate cardiac output; reduced oxygen transport caused by reduced blood flow. (Chapter 12)

clinical sleep educator: A health care professional trained to provide patient education about sleep disorders. (Chapter 13)

closed circuit: A circuit in which all components are connected in one or more loops. (Chapter 3)

common mode rejection: A defining characteristic of a differential amplifier by which artifacts are minimized from amplifier output when both inputs of a derivation are contaminated by signals of identical phase and equal voltage.

common mode signal: The extraneous signal that is present when artifact is superimposed on both inputs of a recording derivation. (Chapter 4)

common referential montage: A listing of recording channels in which each channel derivation uses the same reference electrode that overlies an electrically inactive site. (Chapter 4)

common vehicle transmission: A pathway for introduction of pathogens ingested with food and water. (Chapter 14)

compliance: Measurement of specific usage determinants as related to positive airway pressure therapy. (Chapter 13)

conductor: Any material that permits the flow of electrons; the more readily a material gives up electrons determines its efficiency as a conductor. (Chapter 3)

conservation of charge: Charge can neither be lost nor created in a system; the net charge of a system remains constant. (Chapter 3)

continuous positive airway pressure: The "gold standard" treatment for obstructive sleep apnea, which acts as a pneumatic splint to maintain a patent airway. (Chapter 13)

cooximeter: A device that uses spectrophotometry to measure relative blood concentrations of oxyhemoglobin, carboxyhemoglobin, methemoglobin, and reduced hemoglobin. (Chapter 12)

cooximetry: The process of measuring additional parameters with arterial blood gas analysis when the blood sample is introduced to a blood gas analyzer that is interfaced with a cooximeter.

Coulomb's law: A scientific law that states the strength of the electrical charge is determined by the proximity of the objects to each other when interacting. (Chapter 3)

continuous positive airway pressure (CPAP)–emergent respiratory events (aka *PAP-emergent*): Central apneas as a result of the application of positive airway pressure. (Chapter 13)

critical thinking skills: The process of actively and skillfully conceptualizing, applying, inferring, analyzing, synthesizing, and evaluating information gathered from, or generated by, observation, experience, reflection, inductive and deductive reasoning, or communication, as a guide to belief and action.

cup electrodes: Small reusable electrodes, constructed from one or more precious metals, used to record electroencephalograms, which are also suitable for recording other bioelectric signals like electrooculograms, electrocardiograms, and electromyograms. (Chapter 5)

current flow: The motion of charged particles through a conductive medium. In electronics applications, current is the motion of electrons through a conductive medium moving from a lower voltage to a higher one. (Chapter 3)

cycle: Identified as any point on a wave through its corresponding point as the wave repeats (e.g., peak to peak, trough to trough, or a rise from baseline to peak followed by a drop to trough and a return back to baseline). For physiologic data, the number of cycles is determined by counting the number of peaks, whereas cycle duration is measured from trough to trough. (Chapter 4)

cyclic alternating pattern: A condition of sustained sleep and arousal instability oscillating between a greater and lesser arousal level that occurs in the presence of obstructive sleep apnea, and from which obstructive and central sleep-disordered breathing events can be differentiated. (Chapter 8)

data acquisition system: Data recorder; polysomnograph. (Chapter 5)

decay time constant: Also known as the *fall time constant,* and often simply referred to as the *time constant,* is the time it takes, in seconds, for a square wave to decay to 37% of its original amplitude. The decay time constant control setting replaces the low-frequency filter (LFF) control on some recorders. It has an inverse relationship to the LFF. (Chapter 4)

delta activity: Electroencephalogram data with frequency of 0.5-2 Hz and peak-to-peak amplitude of more than 75 μV measured over the frontal region. (Chapter 5)

depolarization: A fundamental electrical event of the heart signaling the beginning of a cardiac muscle contraction. (Chapter 11)

depolarized: When membrane potential is less negative than the resting membrane potential. (Chapter 4)

derivation: Signal derived by using recorded data from input 1 and input 2. (Chapter 4)

diagnostic polysomnogram: A sleep study recording of multiple physiologic parameters performed to aid in the diagnosis, or rule out the presence, of a sleep disorder. (Chapter 6)

diaphragm: A dome-shaped muscle group composed of the right hemidiaphragm and the left hemidiaphragm, the primary muscles of ventilation. (Chapter 11)

diaphragmatic or intercostal –electromyogram (EMG): A method of recording respiratory effort primarily used to differentiate between central and noncentral respiratory events. When electrodes are properly placed over intercostal spaces or the upper abdomen, EMG activity will be recorded anytime an effort is made to breathe. (Chapter 8)

differential amplifier: The amplifier type most commonly used for the recording of bioelectric signals because amplifier output is the difference between electrical potentials at two inputs, and artifacts are readily minimized from the recording. (Chapter 4)

diffusion: The movement of molecules across a semipermeable membrane driven by a pressure gradient; the process of oxygen and carbon dioxide exchange. (Chapter 11)

direct current (DC) amplifier: An amplifier that lacks a low-frequency filter, making it ideal for recording constant or slow-moving parameters similar to direct current electricity, after which it is named. (Chapter 4)

direct current (DC) electricity: Electrical current that is constant and flows in only one direction through a conductor. A form of electricity that does not decay and remains at full amplitude until the power source is either removed or depleted. (Chapter 3)

direct current (DC): See *direct current (DC) electricity.*

disinfection: The elimination of most disease-producing microorganisms, including bacteria, viruses, and fungi, but not spores. (Chapter 14)

duration: In sleep technology, how long something lasts in microseconds, seconds, minutes, or hours. In reference to biopotentials, how long a signal lasts as measured from trough to trough. (Chapter 4)

dynamic recording: In a dynamic recording, data are stored with settings that allow for a broad array of modifications during review. (Chapter 7)

dysrhythmia: An abnormal or irregular heart beat or rhythm. (Chapter 11)

earth ground: As required for modern electrical equipment to prevent the likelihood of shock, connects the electrical grounding wire to the earth by way of the building ground. Because the earth will always have a lower potential than a charged circuit, any electrons leaking from the circuit will be attracted to the lower potential of the earth where the current dissipates. (Chapter 6)

electrocardiogram (ECG) artifact: Usually the result of imbalanced electrode impedance within a derivation or improper mastoid reference placement, the R wave of the ECG complex is seen on channels recording biopotentials (electroencephalogram, electrooculogram, and electromyogram). (Chapter 10)

enhanced expiratory rebreathing space (EERS): Also known as *deadspace.* (Chapter 13)

electrocardiogram (ECG): The ECG is a recording of the electrical activity of the heart. For polysomnography, a single-channel bipolar derivation ECG is recorded. If chapter 8 states that it represents mechanical activity, that needs to be changed. (Chapter 8)

electrocardiography: The process of recording the electrocardiogram. (Chapter 5)

electrochemistry: The conversion of chemical energy into electrical charges. (Chapter 3)

electrode board: The input receptacle that interfaces the amplifiers and signals from the various transducers and electrodes attached to the patient. The electrode board is known by many names, including *jack box, terminal box, input board, head box,* and others. (Chapter 4)

electrode lead or wire: A small insulated wire that connects the electrode to the electrode board and through which bioelectric data travels. (Chapter 4)

electrode popping artifact: Electrode popping occurs with abrupt shifts in impedance. This can be due to a loosened electrode making intermittent contact with the skin, a fractured electrode wire, or a break anywhere in the recording circuit that occasional loses contact. (Chapter 10)

electrode: Electrodes are metal cups that readily conduct electrical activity from the scalp, along a wire, and to the input connection on an amplifier. (Chapter 4)

electroencephalogram (EEG): The recording of electrical activity of the brain. (Chapter 1)

electroencephalograph: The recording device used to record the electroencephalogram. (Chapter 4)

electromagnetic induction: The conversion of mechanical energy into electrical current by means of a conductive medium (wire) and magnet. (Chapter 3)

electromotive force (EMF): The potential difference between the terminals of an electrical energy source expressed in volts.

electromyogram (EMG): A recording of biopotentials from the skin's surface as a representation of muscle activation. (Chapter 4)

electromyography: The process of recording an electromyogram. (Chapter 5)

electronic circuit: A combination of electrical components connected by conductive mediums to perform one or more intended functions. (Chapter 3)

electrooculogram (EOG): The recording of electrical potential changes at the electrode site caused by eye movements and activity. (Chapter 1)

end-tidal carbon dioxide ($E_T CO_2$) monitoring: A method of obtaining a surrogate measure of blood carbon dioxide (CO_2) by sampling exhaled gas at the end of exhalation from which the partial pressure of CO_2 is measured. (Chapter 12)

epoch: A page of sleep study recording that appears on the computer screen; is typically a 30-second epoch for polysomnography (a paper speed of 10 mm/second). (Chapter 1)

esophageal manometry: A measure of respiratory effort derived from changes in intrathoracic pressure and the associated pressure exerted on the esophagus, as measured by placing a cannula attached to a pressure transducer, into the esophagus. The gold standard of measuring respiratory effort by which other measures are validated. (Chapter 4)

esophageal pressure: See *esophageal manometry.* (Chapter 8)

exhalation: A passive muscular event with the diaphragm relaxing resulting in expelled air. (Chapter 11)

expiratory reserve volume: Maximum volume that can be expired after a tidal breath. (Chapter 11)

exploring electrode: In reference to differential amplification, input 1 of a derivation is the exploring electrode and input 2 the reference electrode. (Chapter 4)

external respiration: The process of gas exchange between the capillary blood and the alveoli within the lungs. (Chapter 12)

eye movements: Essential data, recorded on the electrooculogram in the form of blinks, slow eye movements, rapid eye movements, and others, used to validate various sleep-wake states. (Chapter 5)

fall time constant: See *decay time constant.* (Chapter 4)

fatal familial insomnia: A rare neurologic disorder with onset in adulthood that ends in death on average 18 months after onset. It has been discovered in less than 40 families worldwide. (Chapter 2)

fomites: A form of pathogen transmission that occurs when something such as a particle of dust or liquid droplet carries an infectious agent to the host. (Chapter 14)

frequency response curve: A graphical representation of the percent amplitude attenuation applied to data at various low-frequency filter and high-frequency filter settings, as input signal frequency approaches, reaches, and surpasses the frequency cut-off, or filter settings. (Chapter 6)

frequency: The number of events observed to occur within a particular period, counted as the number of peaks when assessing physiologic data. (Chapter 4)

functional residual capacity: The amount of gas remaining in the lungs following a normal tidal breath exhalation; expiratory reserve volume + residual volume. (Chapter 11)

gain: An amplifier control used in place of the sensitivity control to increase or decrease signal amplitude. Defined as the ratio of output deflection to input signal, more simply it is a multiplication factor that represents how many times the original signal that arose from the patient was amplified for visual display. (Chapter 4)

GIGO: The acronym for *garbage in, garbage out* used to convey the concept that data must be optimized in real time if a quality recording is to be produced. (Chapter 4)

gluteraldehyde: A liquid chemical, capable of high-level disinfection with adequate exposure time, often used to process positive airway pressure (PAP) equipment used in the clinical setting. (Chapter 14)

graded potentials: Events that play an important role in nerve activity and occur when a stimulus such as heat causes part of the membrane to change potential. Unlike action potentials, graded potentials decay quickly and do not result in depolarization. (Chapter 4)

gradient: The difference between two levels, such as concentration of ions inside and outside of the cell membrane, or different gas pressures within a tube. (Chapter 4)

ground electrode (patient ground): Establishes a universal reference for all scalp potentials and the baseline at which the differential amplifier begins the potential difference calculation. Without a patent ground electrode, common mode rejection will be ineffective and artifact will readily contaminate recorded data. (Chapter 4)

ground loop: An electrical loop created when leakage current from two different electronic devices flows through the human body. (Chapter 6)

ground: A point in an electrical circuit that is assumed to have a voltage potential of zero. (Chapter 3)

head box: See *electrode board.* (Chapter 4)

health care provider orders: Instructions written by a licensed health care provider indicating the specific tests and procedures to be performed on a patient. (Chapter 9)

hemoglobin (Hb): The iron-containing oxygen-transport metalloprotein in the red blood cells of all vertebrates responsible for the majority of oxygen transport. (Chapter 12)

hemoglobinopathies: Abnormal forms of hemoglobin (Hb), such as sickle cell Hb, that result in a significant reduction in the oxygen-carrying capacity of the blood. (Chapter 12)

Hertz (Hz): The number of cycles completed in 1 second. (Chapter 3)

high-frequency artifact: An unwanted high-frequency signal recorded in addition to the signals of interest. (Chapter 6)

high frequency filter: Also known as a *low pass filter,* the amplifier control attenuates signal components with a frequency approaching, meeting, and surpassing the cut off frequency, and preserves or only nominally attenuates the signal components with a frequency below the filter setting. (Chapter 4)

histogram: A graphical summary of sleep stages and related events displayed in a compressed fashion along a common time axis. Often called a *hypnogram,* which is typically a graphical display of sleep stages only. (Chapter 1)

histotoxic hypoxia: Tissue hypoxia caused by poisoning of the cells that prevents the uptake of oxygen at the tissue level. (Chapter 12)

host: An organism invaded by a pathogen. (Chapter 14)

hypercapnia: Abnormally elevated presence of carbon dioxide in the blood; in arterial blood a arterial carbon dioxide pressure greater than 45 mm Hg. (Chapter 2)

hypercapnic: The condition of, or pertaining to, high carbon dioxide levels in the blood. (Chapter 11)

hypercarbia: See *hypercapnia.* (Chapter 12)

hypersomnia: Excessive sleepiness. (Chapter 2)

hyperventilation: Ventilation greater than that needed to meet metabolic needs as signified by a partial pressure of carbon dioxide less than 35 mm Hg. (Chapter 12)

hypnogram: See *histogram.* (Chapter 1)

hypnagogic hallucinations: Vivid, dreamlike sensations that occur at sleep onset. (Chapter 2)

hypopnea: A reduction in airflow of at least 30%, and a specific drop in the oxygen saturation level or arousal. (Chapter 1)

hypotension: Reduced systemic blood pressure. (Chapter 12)

hypoventilation: Ventilation less than that needed to meet metabolic needs as signified by a partial pressure of carbon dioxide greater than 45 mm Hg. (Chapter 2)

hypoxemia: Low amounts of oxygen in the blood. (Chapter 2)

hypoxemic: The condition of, or pertaining to, low oxygen levels in the blood. (Chapter 11)

hypoxia: Low tissue oxygenation. (Chapter 12)

hypoxic hypoxia: Tissue hypoxia that results from inadequate oxygen in inspired air. (Chapter 12)

idiopathic insomnia: Also known as *childhood onset insomnia,* idiopathic insomnia is a rare, chronic, lifelong insomnia. Onset occurs during infancy or childhood with no identifiable cause; patients are unable to initiate or maintain adequate sleep their entire lifetime. (Chapter 2)

idioventricular: Abnormal ventricular heart rhythm of unknown origin. (Chapter 14)

impedance meter: An electronic device that sends a low-voltage alternating current signal to electrodes for the assessment of impedance. (Chapter 4)

impedance: The resistance to flow of electrons in a circuit that is connected to an alternating current source of energy. (Chapter 3)

implanted electrical device: Patients may arrive for sleep testing having one of various implanted devices including, but not limited to, a pain pump, an automated internal defibrillator, a cardiac pacemaker, a diaphragmatic pacemaker, a vagal nerve stimulator, or a deep-brain stimulator. Some of these devices affect the data being acquired in the sleep laboratory, whereas others do not. (Chapter 10)

inadequate sleep hygiene: Caused by a person voluntarily avoiding sleep; is the most common type of insomnia in the general population. (Chapter 2)

inductance: When a circuit such as the patient input cable lies in close proximity, particularly when parallel, to another circuit that is carrying alternating current (AC) electricity, an AC current with opposing polarity can develop (be induced) in the other. (Chapter 4)

infrared spectroscopy: molecules containing more than one element absorb infrared light in a characteristic manner. This technology uses a gas's known absorption of infrared radiation to determine its concentration in a sample. (Chapter 12)

inhalation: Active muscular event with the diaphragm contracting downward, resulting in air intake. (Chapter 11)

input board: See *electrode board.* (Chapter 4)

inspiratory capacity: Tidal volume plus inspiratory reserve volume. (Chapter 11)

inspiratory reserve volume (IRV): Maximum volume that can be inspired following a normal inspiration. (Chapter 11)

interface: 1. To connect together (e.g., one must interface ancillary equipment with the acquisition system). 2. The general term used in reference to the patient connection for delivery of positive airway pressure, including a nasal mask, oronasal mask, direct nasal device, and oral delivery device. (Chapter 8)

interfaced: The quality of being connected together. (Chapter 5)

internal respiration: The process of gas exchange between the arterial blood and cells of the tissue. (Chapter 12)

international nomenclature: The system of organizing electrodes and associated equipment using anatomic locations where sensors are placed as labels on the input board. (Chapter 4)

jack box (head box): A device for the input and organization of numerous physiologic signals into referential, differential, and dedicated channels; also see *electrode board.* (Chapter 7)

jumper cable: A small wire device used to connect one or more electrodes or one or more inputs when the recording system does not offer the capability of accomplishing this by either manual or digital electrode selection or input switching. (Chapter 8)

K complex: A large biphasic electroencephalographic signal composed of a sharp negative deflection followed by a slower positive component with duration of 0.5 seconds or more maximally recorded over the frontal region, and prominent during stage N2 sleep. (Chapter 1)

leakage current: An unintended loss of current within a circuit. (Chapter 3)

line frequency artifact (aka *60 Hz artifact* and *electrical current noise*): Extraneous signals arising from alternating current electricity that travels into homes and businesses across power lines at 60 Hz in the United States and 50 Hz in some countries and locales. (Chapter 10)

low-frequency filter (LFF): Also known as the *high-pass filter,* the amplifier control allows signals above the cutoff frequency, or filter setting, to pass through. An LFF progressively attenuates signals with frequency approaching, reaching, and falling below the filter setting and preserves those with frequency well above it. (Chapter 4)

low-amplitude, mixed frequency (LAMF) activity: A mixture of LAMF electroencephalographic activity seen during stage wake with eyes open, N1 sleep, and REM sleep. It is also the background activity during sleep stage N2. Particularly during N1 sleep, beta activity is often interspersed throughout the pattern, and during rapid eye movement sleep sawtooth waves may appear. Alpha-range activity can be present during all associated sleep stages. (Chapter 5)

machine calibrations: Also known as *mechanical calibrations,* machine calibrations are maneuvers performed to verify the channel labels, screen order, baseline, amplifier function, filter settings, and response to amplifier control changes for each polysomnographic channel. All-channel calibrations and montage calibrations are the two types of machine calibrations. (Chapter 6)

macro shock: Occurs when the human body completes an electrical circuit and moderate to high levels of electrical current pass through it. (Chapter 6)

material safety data sheet (MSDS):   A technical bulletin prepared by the manufacturer of a chemical product and the primary source of information on the hazardous properties of the material. (Chapter 14)

medical record: A comprehensive compilation of documentation and images related to a patient's medical care. (Chapter 9)

melatonin: A hormone secreted by the pineal gland that promotes sleep. (Chapter 1)

memory capacity: 1. The amount of data a computer or hardware device is capable of storing for future use. 2. The amount of available memory required for a program to run. (Chapter 12)

micro shock: A low-level electrical current that passes through the human body. When a direct path exists to the heart, as little as 0.1 mA induces ventricular fibrillation. (Chapter 6)

microsleep: A brief episode of sleep, lasting from a fraction of a second to 30 seconds, which is terminated by an abrupt awakening. (Chapter 2)

mixed apnea: The complete cessation of airflow that is initially associated with absent effort that resumes prior to the end of the event. (Chapter 13)

modified lead II derivation: A method of recording an electroencephalogram using the right upper chest region and the left lower thorax region for electrode placement. (Chapter 11)

monophasic: In reference to waveform terminology, a signal composed of one phase that is either surface negative or surface positive, but not both. (Chapter 4)

montage calibration: A type of machine calibration performed to verify montage settings and ensure that amplifiers respond appropriately to control changes. (Chapter 6)

montage: An organized listing of the type, order, and recorder settings for each channel of data being acquired. (Chapter 7)

Moore's law: An observation about the rapid advancement of digital technology described in 1965 by Gordon Moore, later co-founder of Intel who stated in 1965 that the number of transistors incorporated in a chip will approximately double every 24 months (Chapter 7)

morphologic characteristics: The shape of a wave form. (Chapter 4)

multiple sleep latency test (MSLT):   A series of nap opportunities following a sleep study performed during the patient's habitual sleep period, to measure the degree of sleepiness. Results of the test may support the diagnosis of narcolepsy or idiopathic hypersomnia. (Chapter 1)

multiplexing: The process of combining two or more signals into a single channel that can be performed by both analog and digital processes. (Chapter 7)

muscle artifact: Unintentional 20-200 Hz signals that contaminate recorded data as the result of patient tension, body rocking, grinding of the teeth (bruxism), or pressure being applied to the offending electrode, or when muscles are activated for any reason. (Chapter 10)

narcolepsy: A sleep disorder characterized by excessive sleepiness, sleep attacks, hypnagogic hallucinations, cataplexy, and sleep paralysis (Chapter 1)

nasal cannula: A device consisting of two small tubes that fit in the nares and connect to a single larger tube used to deliver supplemental oxygen or to sample exhaled gas. (Chapter 12)

nasal pressure transducer: A device that converts pressure changes exerted on it through a small nasal cannula, into an electrical signal. The cannula transmits pressure changes inside the nares for an airflow signal on the polysomnogram. (Chapter 1)

nasopharynx: The uppermost area of the back of the throat (pharynx) beginning with the superior level of the soft palate extending into the posterior portion of the nasal cavity. (Chapter 11)

negative charge: An electrical charge arising from the presence of one or more electrons. (Chapter 3)

net charge: The sum of all electrical charges present in a system. (Chapter 3)

neuron: An excitable cell that receives and transmits information through the movement of electrical and chemical. (Chapter 5)

neurotransmitters: Any of a group of chemical agents that transmit information from one nerve to another nerve, muscle, organ, or other tissue. (Chapter 1)

noninvasive positive pressure ventilation (NPPV):   A positive airway pressure modality that augments spontaneous ventilation using pressure support and a back up rate. Effective in the treatment of alveolar hypoventilation syndromes, respiratory failure, and other disorders of ventilatory insufficiency, NPPV is administered by either an oral, nasal, or oronasal interface. (Chapter 13)

non–rapid eye movement (NREM) sleep: The sleep phase that consists of stage N1 sleep, N2 sleep, and stage N3 sleep during which rapid eye movements are atypical. (Chapter 1)

nosocomial infection: An infection acquired in a health care facility. (Chapter 14)

notch filter: An amplifier control, also known as a 60 Hz filter and line filter, that attenuates signals within a narrow frequency range surrounding 60 cycles per second, the frequency at which line current travels in the United States. (Chapter 4)

numerical nomenclature: The system of organizing electrodes and associated equipment using numbers to label the input board and electrode selector panel that have no relationship to anatomy. (Chapter 4)

Nyquist principle: For signal processing the sampling rate must be at least twice the frequency of the fastest signal of interest to minimize distortion of digitized data. (Chapter 7)

obstructive sleep apnea: Complete cessation of airflow with continued respiratory effort. (Chapter 1)

Ohm's law: Describes the relationship between voltage, current, and resistance, and is named for German physicist and mathematician George Ohm. (Chapter 3)

open circuit: A circuit in which not all components are connected by conductive mediums (wires). (Chapter 3)

opponent model of sleep: A theory describing the process by which sleep occurs, in which internal sleep pressure loads and circadian rhythm alerting signals interact during different times of the day and night. (Chapter 1)

oronasal sensor: A small device placed below the nostrils and in front of the mouth to monitor airflow. (Chapter 1)

oropharynx: The oral portion of the pharynx, which is the back of the throat from the soft palate down to the upper edge of the epiglottis. (Chapter 11)

outcomes: Clinical results of medical treatments. (Chapter 13)

outlet ground: The circuit between the electrical outlet and the common circuitry of the building breaker box that provides a path for excessive or stray current to travel. To avoid an electrical leakage current fault or a ground loop, the ground circuit must be patent between the recorder and wall outlet, wall outlet and breaker box, and from the breaker box to the earth ground. (Chapter 4)

overlap syndrome: The coexistence of obstructive sleep apnea and chronic obstructive pulmonary disease. (Chapter 2)

oximeter: A noninvasive device that estimates blood oxygen saturations. (Chapter 1)

oximetry artifacts: The most frequently encountered oximeter artifacts during sleep testing are signal loss caused by patient movement, improper attachment of the sensor, and sensor removal. These values are crucial, particularly for scoring hypopneas. The recording technologist must ensure accuracy of these data. (Chapter 10)

oxygen (O_2):   A gas needed for cellular respiration that makes up 20.95% of room air. (Chapter 12)

oxygen transport: The process of oxygen (O_2) being transported throughout the body, either attached to hemoglobin (Hb) molecules in the circulating blood or dissolved in the blood's plasma. It depends on ventilation to move gases in and out of the lungs, diffusion to move gases across the alveolar-capillary membrane, adequate Hb to carry the O_2 molecules, and circulation to move gases through the blood vessels and tissues. (Chapter 11)

oxygenation status: The assessment of how much oxygen is present in the body. (Chapter 12)

oxyhemoglobin dissociation curve: A nomogram that provides a graphical and numerical representation of the relationship between the partial pressure of arterial oxygen and saturation of peripheral oxygen under normal conditions. (Chapter 12)

oxyhemoglobin (O_2Hb) saturation: The amount of saturated hemoglobin (Hb), presumably with oxygen (O_2). A true measurement of the amount of Hb saturated with O_2 is obtained by cooximetry. When obtained by arterial blood gas analysis, the value is calculated from other measured variables. When measured by oximetry, it represents the amount of Hb saturated, but not necessarily with O_2. (Chapter 12)

oxyhemoglobin (O_2Hb):   A true measure of the percentage of hemoglobin saturated with oxygen as obtained by cooximetry. This is a direct measure of oxygen saturation. (Chapter 12)

P wave: The first wave of the electrocardiograph complex that represents atria depolarization. In polysomnography, the technologist must ensure that the P wave is upright at the start of the recording. (Chapter 5)

$P(a-et)CO_2$ gradient: The difference between the partial pressure of arterial and end-tidal carbon dioxide. (Chapter 12)

palpating: The process of examining or exploring the human body by touch. (Chapter 12)

positive airway pressure (PAP) adherence: Measurement of PAP use by objective means. (Chapter 9)

positive airway pressure (PAP)–emergent respiratory events: Central apneas as a result of the application of PAP. (Chapter 13)

paper speed: On analog recordings, paper speed established the time base from which a recording was analyzed. It is literally the speed in mm/sec that the paper is pulled under the recording pens. To record a 30-second epoch on a standard 300-mm wide chart, a paper speed of 10 mm/sec is used. For clinical electroencephalogram, a paper speed of 30 mm/sec yields a 10 second epoch on the same standard chart paper. Most digital systems offer the ability to simply choose an epoch duration, although some erroneously continue to use the convention of paper speed. (Chapter 4)

paradoxical breathing: A desynchronized breathing pattern between the thorax and abdomen that sometimes occurs with obstructive apnea. (Chapter 13)

paradoxical insomnia: Also known as *sleep state misperception, subjective insomnia,* and *pseudo-insomnia,* paradoxical insomnia is a chronic insomnia in which the patient complains that he or she is not getting adequate sleep despite objective data obtained by polysomnogram that demonstrates a normal sleep pattern. An actigraphy study may also indicate that the patient was asleep during the time the patient documents wake on accompanying sleep logs. (Chapter 2)

paradoxical sleep: Another name for rapid eye movement sleep based on its characteristics when the brain is very active but the body is atonic. (Chapter 1)

parasomnias: Abnormal behaviors during sleep. (Chapter 1)

parenteral infections: Infections acquired intravenously. (Chapter 14)

partial pressure of arterial oxygen (PaO_2):   The amount of oxygen dissolved in the blood plasma and measured by arterial blood gas analysis. (Chapter 12)

partial pressure of carbon dioxide ($PaCO_2$):   The amount of carbon dioxide dissolved in the plasma of arterial blood as measured by arterial blood gas analysis. (Chapter 12)

PASS: Acronym for use of fire extinguisher: *P*ull the pin, *A*im, *S*queeze the trigger, *S*weep side to side at the base of the fire. (Chapter 14)

pasteurization: High-level disinfection process for medical equipment using water heated to more than 166° F. (Chapter 14)

pathogen: A microorganism capable of producing disease. (Chapter 14)

patient acuity: Clinical intensity or severity of a patient's condition. (Chapter 9)

patient assessment: Comprehensive evaluation of the patient's physical, mental, and overall health status. (Chapter 9)

patient-centered care: An integrated and holistic approach to caring for patients. (Chapter 9)

peak: In reference to waveform terminology, this is the point of highest signal amplitude just before it begins to fall. Signal amplitude is measured from trough to peak and average frequency is determined by counting the number of peaks that occur within one second. (Chapter 4)

perfusion: To supply with blood; the process of delivering blood to a capillary bed in the tissue. (Chapter 12)

periodic limb movements of sleep (PLMS): A condition characterized by repetitive, very stereotypical limb movements that occur during sleep. (Chapter 2)

peripheral chemoreceptors: Chemical sensors at the level of the aortic or carotid bodies that detect decreases in the amount of oxygen in the blood. (Chapter 11)

personal protective equipment (PPE): Gowns, gloves, mask, and eye protection employed for direct contact with body substances, aerosolized and airborne pathogens, or contaminated equipment. (Chapter 14)

pH: A measure of the molar concentration of hydrogen ions in the solution; a measure of the acidity or alkalinity of the solution on a scale of 0 to 14. (Chapter 12)

photoelectricity: The conversion of photon energy into electrical charge. (Chapter 3)

photon: A light wave particle that is mass less and has a neutral charge. (Chapter 3)

photoplethysmography: A recording technology that uses light to detect the minute volume changes between the baseline component and pulsatile component of blood flow through a tissue bed to determine oxygen status. (Chapter 12)

provider orders: See *health care provider orders.* (Chapter 9)

psychophysiological insomnia: A learned insomnia usually precipitated by an event that disrupts sleep, but that continues to be problematic long after the original stressful event is completely resolved. (Chapter 2)

physiologic calibrations: A series of maneuvers performed by the patient before lights out at the beginning of each study and after "lights on" at the end of the recording to verify signal integrity and sensor function, and to obtain baseline patient data. (Chapter 6)

Pickwickian syndrome: A physiologic disorder named for a Charles Dickens character who had obesity, hypoventilation, muscular twitching, and hypersomnolence. (Chapter 1)

piezoelectric effect: The conversion of mechanical deformation of crystal lattice structures into electrical charge that is the basis for piezo crystal technology previously used to record respiratory effort. (Chapter 3)

polarity: *Polarity* is defined as having oppositely charged poles (dipoles), one positive and one negative. (Chapter 4)

polysomnogram: A recording of various physiologic parameters relating to sleep, which is also known as a *sleep study.* (Chapter 1)

polysomnography: The process of recording polysomnograms; the practice and related skillset associated with the acquisition of sleep studies. (Chapter 1)

positive airway pressure (PAP): The application of pressure above atmospheric to serve as a pneumatic splint for airway patency. (Chapter 12)

positive charge: An electrical charge arising from the presence of one or more protons. (Chapter 3)

potential difference: The amount of work done by an electrical charge moving from one point to another within a circuit. All potentials are measured from two points, hence the term *potential difference.* (Chapter 4)

power isolation: The separation of electrical currents in a circuit using an inductive transformer. (Chapter 3)

pressure support: The difference between inspiratory positive airway pressure and expiratory positive airway pressure when delivering bilevel positive airway pressure. (Chapter 13)

primary insomnia: The classification of insomnia that indicates that it is problem in and of itself and not secondary to or caused by another underlying sleep-related cause. (Chapter 2)

prions: Infectious particles of protein that cannot be destroyed and are extremely difficult to inactivate. (Chapter 14)

pulse artifact: When slow-frequency signals are in perfect alignment with the R wave of the electrocardiogram complex, they are classified as *pulse artifact.* Pulse artifact is the result of electrode placement over a pulsating blood vessel. (Chapter 10)

pulse oximeter: A noninvasive monitor for estimating the saturation of hemoglobin, presumably with oxygen. (Chapter 12)

QRS complex: The second and tallest waveform of the electrocardiogram complex that is composed of three distinct phases: the Q wave, R wave, and S wave. The QRS represents ventricular depolarization (Chapter 5)

quality health care: The degree to which health services for individuals and populations increase the likelihood of desired health outcomes and are consistent with current professional knowledge. (Chapter 9)

RACE: The acronym for the response to a fire: Rescue or Remove patients and personnel, Activate the alarm, Contain the fire, Evacuate or Extinguish the fire. (Chapter 14)

random access memory: A hardware memory storage area that initially caches collected data and allows the software to quickly read the data and apply the software filters set in the montage. (Chapter 7)

rapid eye movement (REM): A phase of sleep characterized by rapid eye movements associated with the dream state. (Chapter 1)

recording montage: The order in which the physiologic signals are displayed on the sleep data acquisition system (polygraph). (Chapter 9)

reference electrode: By convention, the electrode in the input 2 position of a derivation is the reference electrode. (Chapter 4)

referential recorder and recording: The methodology most modern digital acquisitions employ for which there is a common system reference electrode; all other electrodes are recorded as the exploring electrode against this reference. During both acquisition and review any combination of recording electrodes can be used to build any desired derivation and montage because the common reference is subtracted pout of the channel display. (Chapter 4)

referential derivation: A recording derivation in which input 1 overlies an electrically active recording area and input 2 overlies a site that is relatively inactive. (Chapter 7)

remote monitoring: Technology that provides the ability to observe PSG data in real time from remote locations. (Chapter 7)

repolarize: To return to the resting, or polarized, state; in reference to the electrocardiogram, the T wave represents repolarization of the ventricles following depolarization and contraction. Following atrial depolarization, the wave representing atrial repolarization is buried in the higher voltage QRS and cannot be visualized. (Chapter 4)

residual volume: Volume that remains in the lungs after a maximal expiration. (Chapter 11)

resistance: In reference to electronics, the ability of a material to impede the flow of electrons. (Chapter 3)

respiration: The transport of oxygen from the outside air to the cells within tissues, and the transport of carbon dioxide in the opposite direction; the process of gas exchange. (Chapter 12)

respiratory artifact: When slow-frequency artifact is aligned with the patient's breathing, it is classified as respiratory artifact. In reality these slow signals are most often caused by both respiratory movement and sweat. (Chapter 10)

respiratory belts: Sensor devices typically in a belt format placed over the chest and abdomen to collect respiratory effort data. (Chapter 1)

respiratory effort–related arousal (RERA): An arousal from sleep caused by increased work of breathing from a partial obstruction of the upper airway. (Chapter 7)

respiratory effort sensor artifact: Unwanted data is recorded on respiratory effort channels when sensors are faulty, but more often artifact emerges when belts are over-tightened, too loose, or have moved out of place. Often when respiratory airflow or effort data are discrepant, there is an issue with polarity or the gain or sensitivity control setting. (Chapter 10)

respiratory inductive plethysmography: A methodology for respiratory effort monitoring that uses an elastic belt that has a zig-zag coiled wire sewn into it through which a low-voltage sensing current flows. This creates a magnetic field that changes shape with breathing. An opposing current is induced and can be measured as a change in frequency of the applied current. The signal produced is linear and a fairly accurate representation of the change in cross-sectional area of the patient's body during breathing. (Chapter 13)

resting potential: That point at which the amount of potassium leaving a cell is very close to the amount potassium entering a cell. (Chapter 4)

restrictive lung disorder: A group of lung diseases, including kyphosis and obesity hypoventilation, that make it difficult to get air into the lungs; all lung volumes and capacities are reduced. (Chapter 12)

reticular formation: An extremely complex web of interconnecting neurons in the reticular activating system in the brain stem that promotes arousal. (Chapter 1)

retrograde: Backward impulses of electrical activity. (Chapter 11)

rise time constant: The time it takes for a square wave to reach 63% of its maximum amplitude. (Chapter 4)

salt bridge: A salt bridge is formed when a conductive material, such as sweat or an electrode cream or paste, communicates between two electrodes. Although often the result of sweat, this should not be confused with sweat artifact. (Chapter 10)

sampling rate: The number of data points stored to memory during a defined period, usually 1 second. (Chapter 4)

saturation of arterial blood with oxygen (SaO_2): A calculated value obtained by arterial blood gas analysis that approximates the oxyhemoglobin under absolutely normal conditions. (Chapter 12)

saturation of peripheral oxygen (SpO_2): The percent of saturated hemoglobin, presumably with oxygen, in the blood as measured by pulse oximetry. (Chapter 12)

sawtooth waves: Signals of 2-6 cps seen maximally in the central region during stage R sleep, often immediately before an episode of rapid eye movements. (Chapter 1)

scoring: The process of tabulating sleep study data using nationally accepted guidelines. (Chapter 9)

secondary insomnia: Classification of sleep problems that occur as the result of a primary physical, psychiatric, or substance use condition, (Chapter 2)

Seebeck effect: An effect noted by German physicist Thomas Johann Seebeck whereby temperature differences in a conducting medium or mediums are converted directly into electricity. (Chapter 3)

sensitivity: Sensitivity is the ratio of input signal to the output deflection. (Chapter 4)

sensors: Devices used to collect physiologic data, including electrodes and transducers such as those used to monitor breathing and oxygenation. (Chapter 9)

short circuit: An electrical circuit with lower resistance, or impedance, than intended. When the pathway of current flow is either continuously or intermittently disrupted, an abrupt shift in impedance occurs. (Chapter 10)

sidestream end-tidal carbon dioxide (E_TCO_2) monitoring: One method of E_TCO_2 monitoring that involves the aspiration of exhaled gas through a small tube into the sampling chamber at the point of end exhalation. (Chapter 12)

signal aliasing: Distortion of digitized data that results from an inadequate sampling rate. (Chapter 12)

signal polarity: The positive or negative condition of data that results in the respective downward or upward deflection on the polysomnograph. (Chapter 6)

signal processing: The manipulation of input data using amplifier controls, ideally to optimize the data being recorded and displayed without distorting frequencies of interest. (Chapter 10)

sinusoidal: A sinelike wave or sinusoid; waveform morphologic characteristic that is uniformly s-shaped. (Chapter 4)

sleep architecture: The fairly predictable structure and pattern of sleep as transitions are made from one sleep stage to the next throughout the sleep time. (Chapter 1)

sleep attacks: An episode of sleep in which the patient falls asleep during everyday activities, such as while eating, driving, or in conversation. (Chapter 2)

sleep efficiency: A measurement of the amount of time spent sleeping within an allowable window of time. (Chapter 9)

sleep log: A diary patients keep for a 2-week period or longer that tracks bed times, wake times, and daily activities. Used to diagnose circadian rhythm disorders and determine causes of insomnia. (Chapter 2)

sleep paralysis: A characteristic of narcolepsy in which the patient is paralyzed at awakening and cannot move immediately. (Chapter 2)

sleep spindle: A train of distinct waves with frequency 11-16 Hz (most commonly 12-14 Hz) with a duration of 0.5 seconds or longer, usually maximal in amplitude in the central derivations. Sleep spindles are a defining feature of stage N2 sleep. (Chapter 1)

sleep state misperception: See *paradoxical insomnia*, which is the recently adopted term. (Chapter 2)

sleep-disordered breathing: The all-inclusive term used to generalize about abnormal breathing events, including apneas, hypopneas, and respiratory event–related arousals. (Chapter 4)

slow eye movements (SEMs): Conjugate, reasonably regular, sinusoidal eye movements with an initial deflection usually lasting more than 500 msec. (Chapter 5)

slow-frequency artifacts: This general classification of events that are isolated to the electroencephalogram and electrooculogram channels includes respiratory artifact and sweat artifact, which often cannot be differentiated, along with pulse artifact, which is easily distinguished. Cardioballistic artifact is also slow frequency, but it is seen only on channels recording pressure and respiratory effort. (Chapter 10)

snore sensor: Either a device taped to the patient's neck to detect vibration or an electronic microphone located near the patient's head that acquires snoring sounds. (Chapter 1)

snoring: The noise produced by the airway soft tissues vibrating as the air is forced through a partially obstructed airway. (Chapter 1)

spectral analysis: An analysis of the density and power of electroencephalogram frequencies during sleep. (Chapter 7)

spectral power: Analysis of dominate waveform frequencies. (Chapter 6)

spectrophotometry: The principle that every substance has its own pattern of light absorption, and this pattern varies predictably with the amount of the substance that is present. (Chapter 12)

split-night PSG: A sleep study composed of an initial diagnostic segment followed by a therapeutic segment. (Chapter 6)

stage W: the stage of the sleep/wake cycle that represents full wakefulness.

stage N1: The first stage of sleep that represents the transition from wake to sleep.

stage N2: the secondary stage of sleep that typically incorporates up to 50% of the sleep cycle.

stage N3: The third stage of sleep that is considered deep sleep. This stage declines as we age.

stage R: the dream stage of sleep.

standard precautions: infection control precautions applied to all patients and in all situations. (Chapter 14)

standing orders: Predetermined physician orders for implementation based on protocol. (Chapter 6)

static electricity: The electrical interaction produced by two charged objects in some proximity to each other. (Chapter 3)

static recording: In a static recording, channel modifications made during acquisition are permanently written to the disk. (Chapter 7)

sterilization: A process by which all forms of microbial life, including bacteria, viruses, spores, and fungi, are destroyed. (Chapter 14)

stray capacitance: Stray capacitance is a process that results in leakage of stored electrical energy. (Chapter 6)

stray inductance: Stray inductance is a process that results in an electrical inductance of energy. (Chapter 6)

suprachiasmatic nucleus: Area of the brain that controls most of the important circadian rhythms. (Chapter 1)

sweat artifact: A slow-frequency artifact caused by perspiration loosening the electrode connection to the skin or diluting the conductive material between the electrode and the skin. Initially, baseline sway is typical on the channel, with electrode popping and channel blocking in the most extreme scenarios. (Chapter 10)

system reference artifact: For data acquisition using a referential recorder, the system reference electrode must remain patent. When this electrode becomes unstable, all channels recording bioelectric data are contaminated by artifact. For this reason, most manufacturers now offer the option for a back-up system reference, often placed at Fz, with the system reference at Cz. (Chapter 10)

system reference electrode: The common reference electrode recorded as input 2 against all recording electrodes in the background when using a referential recorder. The patency of this single electrode is crucial because it will affect the quality of all bioelectric signals if compromised. (Chapter 4)

system referencing: The process of creating derivations within the jack box or amplifier by changing input 1 and input 2 manually or electronically. (Chapter 7)

thalamus: Area of the brain that relays signals between the cerebral cortex and the reticular formation. (Chapter 1)

therapeutic intervention: The implementation of positive airway pressure therapy or another treatment such as oral appliance therapy during a sleep study. (Chapter 6)

thermoelectric effect: The conversion of thermal differences in certain conducting mediums into electrical charge. (Chapter 3)

theta: Electroencephalogram activity with a frequency of 3-7 Hz predominantly central in origin. Theta is a prominent component of low-voltage, mixed-frequency activity. (Chapter 5)

Thorax: Region of the chest formed by the sternum, the thoracic vertebrae, and the ribs. (Chapter 11)

tidal volume: Volume of gas inspired and expired with each normal breath. (Chapter 11)

time base: For digital recordings, this has largely replaced the concept of "paper speed." The time base is changed when data are compressed or stretched so either shorter or longer segments of the study can be viewed on the screen at a time (e.g., 1 second of data is stretched across the monitor versus compressing an entire hour of data to fit on the screen). (Chapter 4)

time-based capnography: Provides a numerical value of the maximum pressure of exhaled carbon dioxide for each breath, and displays either a breath-by-breath waveform or breathing trend over time. (Chapter 12)

total lung capacity: Inspiratory reserve volume + tidal volume + expiratory reserve volume + residual volume = the sum of all four lung volumes. (Chapter 11)

tracheostomy tube: An artificial airway that is surgically placed into the trachea and bypasses the upper airway. (Chapter 12)

transcutaneous carbon dioxide tension (tcPCO$_2$): The partial pressure of carbon dioxide as measured through the unbroken skin. (Chapter 12)

transcutaneous oxygen tension (tcPO^2): The partial pressure of oxygen as measured through the unbroken skin. (Chapter 12)

transducer: Any device that converts one form of energy to another. In sleep technology, a thermistor converts temperature change to an electrical signal, respiratory inductance plethysmography belts convert respiratory effort to electrical current, and the snore microphone converts sound or vibration into an electrical signal.

triphasic: The description of a waveform with three distinct phases, each of which is either surface positive or surface negative. (Chapter 4)

trough: In reference to waveform terminology, the lowest point on the wave just before it begins to rise. (Chapter 4)

T wave: the electrical representation of ventricular repolarization.

uninterruptible power supply (UPS): A battery-operated temporary power source used during electrical power failure. (Chapter 14)

vasoconstriction: A reduction in the diameter of blood vessels. (Chapter 12)

veins: Blood vessels that return blood to the heart. All veins, with the exception of the pulmonary veins, carry deoxygenated blood. (Chapter 11)

ventilation to perfusion mismatch: Abnormal distribution of ventilation to perfusion among the lung's alveolar-capillary units. (Chapter 12)

ventilation: The gross movement of gas; moving gases between the external environment and the alveoli. (Chapter 12)

ventricles: The larger, more muscular lower chambers of the heart. (Chapter 11)

vertex sharp wave: A sharp negative deflection followed by a slower positive component lasting less than 0.5 seconds in duration and prominent in the central derivations. Not required to identify any stage of sleep, they are often seen toward the end of a period of N1 sleep. (Chapter 5)

vital capacity: Tidal volume + inspiratory reserve volume + expiratory reserve volume (Chapter 11)

voltage: The potential electrical energy difference from one point to another. (Chapter 3)

wake: Sleep-wake stage identified by an electroencephalogram pattern composed of low-voltage, mixed-frequency waves with beta (>14 Hz) interspersed throughout with eyes opened, and prominent alpha activity when eyes are closed. (Chapter 5)

WYSIWYG technology: An acronym often used when discussing analog recordings that stands for *what you see is what you get,* meaning if you don't correct issues while acquiring data, they are recorded forever. (Chapter 4)

Zeitgebers: Word of German origin depicting external factors that influence and reset the human biological clock to the external environment. (Chapter 1)

ANSWERS TO END-OF-CHAPTER QUESTIONS

Chapter 1
1. A
2. D
3. B
4. A
5. A
6. C
7. A
8. C
9. A
10. B

Chapter 2
1. B
2. D
3. B
4. B
5. A
6. C
7. D
8. B
9. C
10. B

Chapter 3
1. A
2. B
3. A
4. A
5. A
6. B
7. B
8. C
9. A
10. A

Chapter 4
1. C
2. D
3. B
4. B
5. B
6. A
7. C
8. C
9. A
10. B

Chapter 5
1. B
2. A
3. A
4. D
5. B
6. A
7. D
8. C
9. A
10. A

Chapter 6
1. C
2. A
3. B
4. B
5. B
6. A
7. A
8. C
9. C
10. A

Chapter 7
1. B
2. A
3. B
4. D
5. B
6. C
7. C
8. A
9. B
10. A

Chapter 8
1. A
2. A
3. B
4. D
5. C
6. B
7. B
8. C
9. A
10. B

Chapter 9
1. D
2. A
3. B
4. A
5. C
6. B
7. B
8. C
9. D

Chapter 10
1. B
2. B
3. D
4. C
5. A
6. A
7. B
8. D
9. B
10. C

Chapter 11
1. C
2. A
3. B
4. B
5. C
6. D
7. B
8. A
9. A
10. C

Chapter 12
1. B
2. C
3. B
4. C
5. A
6. D
7. C
8. A
9. B
10. C

Chapter 13
1. A
2. A
3. A
4. C
5. C
6. A
7. C
8. A
9. B
10. B

Chapter 14
1. D
2. A
3. A
4. C
5. B
6. C
7. C
8. B

Printed and bound by CPI Group (UK) Ltd, Croydon, CR0 4YY

08/05/2025

01864688-0001